HANDBOOK OF
CARDIAC ARRHYTHMIA

HANDBOOK OF CARDIAC ARRHYTHMIA

Philip J. Podrid, M.D.
Professor of Medicine
Boston University Medical School
Director, Arrhythmia Service
Boston University Medical Hospital
Boston, Massachusetts

and

Peter R. Kowey, M.D.
Professor of Medicine
Jefferson Medical College
Thomas Jefferson University
Philadelphia, Pennsylvania
Chief, Division of Cardiovascular Diseases
The Lankenau Hospital and Medical Research Center
Wynnewood, Pennsylvania

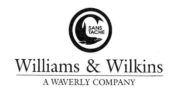

Williams & Wilkins
A WAVERLY COMPANY

BALTIMORE • PHILADELPHIA • LONDON • PARIS • BANGKOK
BUENOS AIRES • HONG KONG • MUNICH • SYDNEY • TOKYO • WROCLAW

Editor: Jonathan W. Pine, Jr.
Managing Editor: Molly L. Mullen
Production Coordinator: Linda Carlson
Copy Editor: Judith F. Minkove
Designer: Diane Buric
Illustration Planner: Ray Lowman
Composition: Mario Fernández
Printer: McNaughton and Gunn

351 West Camden Street
Baltimore, MD 21201-2436 USA

Rose Tree Corporate Center
1400 North Providence Road
Building II, Suite 5025
Media, Pennsylvania 19063-2043 USA

Accurate indications, adverse reactions, and dosage schedules for drugs are provided in this book, but it is possible that they may change. The reader is urged to review the package information data of the manufacturers of the medications mentioned.

Printed in the United States of America

First Edition,

Library of Congress Cataloging-in-Publication Data

Handbook of cardiac arrhythmia / [edited by] Philip J. Podrid and Peter R. Kowey.
   p.   cm.
  Based on the full textbook: Cardiac arrhythmia / edited by Phlip J. Podrid and Peter R. Kowey, 1995.
  Includes bibliographical references and index.
  ISBN 0-683-06909-8
  1. Arrhythmia—Handbooks, manuals, etc. I. Podrid, Philip J. II. Kowey, Peter R. III. Cardiac arrhythmia.
  [DNLM: 1. Arrhythmia—diagnosis—handbooks. 2. Arrhythmia—therapy—handbooks. 3. Antiarrhythmia agents—handbooks. 4. Arrhythmia—physiopathology—handbooks. WG 39 H2355 1996]
RC685.A65H35 1996
616.182'—dc20
DNLM/DLC
for Library of Congress
          95-45089
          CIP

The publishers have made every effort to trace the copyright holders for borrowed material. If they have inadvertently overlooked any, they will be pleased to make the necessary arrangements at the first opportunity.

96 97 98 99
1 2 3 4 5 6 7 8 9 10

This book is dedicated

to our wives,

Vivian Rubinstein Podrid

and

Dorothy Freal Kowey,

whose patience and tolerance

were critical

for the completion of this book,

and to our children,

Joshua Podrid

and

Jaime and Olivia Kowey,

our most

important legacy

PREFACE

The field of cardiac arrhythmia is rapidly changing as knowledge about mechanisms grows steadily. The enormous amount of information is reflected by the size of our full textbook, *Cardiac Arrhythmia: Mechanisms, Diagnosis, and Management*. Realizing that the amount and depth of information contained in that book is far in excess of what many physicians, students, nurses, technicians, and other paramedical personnel require for their daily practice of medicine, we have made substantial reductions in the chapters without changing the content. This handbook, therefore, serves as an abbreviated but complete review of cardiac arrhythmias, covering all aspects of arrhythmia mechanisms and management. It was our intent to deal with a very complex area of medicine in a very simple and straightforward way. We hope that we have succeeded and that all who use this manual find it useful in their daily practice of medicine.

Philip J. Podrid
Peter R. Kowey

ACKNOWLEDGMENT

Our sincerest thanks go to all of the authors who willingly contributed to the textbook upon which this handbook is based. Without their efforts, this handbook would not have been possible. We hope that by shortening their manuscripts, we did not unintentionally alter or eliminate any of the important content. A full listing of contributors follows.

We thank our editors, whose great help and guidance inspired us to complete this book. We thank our families, especially our wives Vivian Rubinstein Podrid and Dorothy Freal Kowey, who permitted us the time to accomplish this task. Most importantly, we thank our patients who, daily, inspire us to know more about the diseases that afflict them.

CONTRIBUTORS

Masood Akhtar, M.D.
Professor of Medicine, Associate Chief
Cardiovascular Disease Section
University of Wisconsin Medical
   School
Director
Arrhythmia Services
Sinai-Samaritan Medical Center
Milwaukee, Wisconsin

Jeffrey L. Anderson, M.D.
Professor of Medicine
University of Utah
Chief, Division of Cardiology
LDS Hospital
Salt Lake City, Utah

Erik Andries, M.D.
Cardiovascular Research and Teaching
Institute
Aalst O.L.V. Hospital
Aalst, BELGIUM

Uri M. Ben-Zur, M.D., F.A.C.C.
Assistant Professor of Medicine
Albert Einstein College of Medicine
Pacemaker/Arrhythmia Services
Division of Cardiology
Montefiore Medical Center
Bronx, New York

David G. Benditt, M.D.
Professor of Medicine
Department of Medicine
University of Minnesota
Minneapolis, Minnesota

Zalmen Blanck, M.D.
Assistant Professor of Medicine
University of Wisconsin Medical
   School
Milwaukee Clinical Campus
Sinai-Samaritan Medical Center
St. Luke's Medical Center
Milwaukee, Wisconsin

Pedro Brugada, M.D.
Professor of Cardiology
Cardiovascular Research and Teaching
   Institute
Aalst O.L.V. Hospital
Aalst, BELGUIM

Josep Brugada, M.D.
Director of Arrhythmia Unit
Department of Cardiology
Hospital Clinic, University of
   Barcelona
Barcelona, SPAIN

Alfred E. Buxton, M.D.
Professor of Medicine and Cardiology
Associate Chief, Cardiology Section
Temple University School of Medicine
Philadelphia, Pennsylvania

Ronald W. F. Campbell, M.D.
Professor of Cardiology
Academic Cardiology
University of New Castle-Upon-Tyne
New Castle-Upon-Tyne,
   UNITED KINGDOM

David S. Cannom, M.D.
Medical Director
Department of Cardiology
Hospital of the Good Samaritan
Clinical Professor of Medicine
Department of Medicine
UCLA School of Medicine
Los Angeles, California

Erdal Cavusoglu, M.D.
Fellow in Cardiology
Department of Cardiology
Albert Einstein College of Medicine
Bronx, New York

Jasenka Demirovic, M.D., Ph.D.
Associate Professor
Department of Epidemiology and
    Public Health
Department of Medicine
University of Miami School of Medicine
Miami, Florida

Sanjay Deshpande, M.D.
Assistant Professor of Medicine
University of Wisconsin Medical
    School
Milwaukee Clinical Campus
Sinai-Samaritan Medical Center
St. Luke's Medical Center
Milwaukee, Wisconsin

Anwer Dhala, M.D.
Sinai-Samaritan Medical Center
Milwaukee, Wisconsin

Livia Diehl, M.D.
Research Associate
Istituto di Clinica Medica
    Generale e Terapia Medica
University of Milan
Milano, ITALY

John P. DiMarco, M.D., Ph.D.
Professor of Medicine
Department of Cardiology Division
University of Virginia Health Sciences
    Center
Charlottesville, Virginia

Anne H. Dougherty, M.D.
Electrophysiology Laboratory
Division of Cardiology
Department of Internal Medicine
University of Texas Medical School
Houston, Texas

Nabil El-Sherif, M.B., B.Ch.
Cardiology Division
Department of Medicine
State University of New York Health
    Science Center
Veterans Administration Medical
    Center
Brooklyn, New York

Rodney H. Falk, M.D.
Professor of Medicine
Director of Clinical Cardiac Research
Boston University School of Medicine
Boston, Massachusetts

Richard I. Fogel, M.D.
Consulting Cardiologist
Northside Cardiology, P.C.
Indianapolis, Indiana

Peter L. Friedman, M.D.
Director, Cardiac Arrhythmia Service
    and Clinical Electrophysiology
    Laboratory
Brigham and Women's Hospital
Associate Professor of Medicine
Harvard Medical School
Boston, Massachusetts

William H. Fishman, M.D.
Professor and Associate Chairman
Department of Medicine
Albert Einstein College of
   Medicine/Montefiore Medical
   Center
Professor of Epidemiology
Albert Einstein College of Medicine
Bronx, New York

Seymour Furman, M.D.
Professor of Surgery and Medicine
Montefiore Medical Center
Albert Einstein College of Medicine
Bronx, New York

Hasan Garan, M.D.
Associate Professor of Medicine
Cardiac Unit
Massachusetts General Hospital
Boston, Massachusetts

Elsa-Grace V. Giardina, M.D.
Professor, Attending Physician
Department of Medicine
Columbia University, College of
   Physicians and Surgeons
New York, New York

Jeffrey J. Goldberger, M.D.
Assistant Professor of Medicine
Associate Director, Cardiac
   Electrophysiology
Section of Cardiology, Department of
   Medicine
Northwestern University
Chicago, Illinois

Jay N. Gross, M.D.
Assistant Professor of Medicine
Albert Einstein College of Medicine
Department of Cardiology
Montefiore Medical Center
Bronx, New York

J. Warren Harthorne, M.D.
Director, Pacemaker Laboratory
Physician
Massachusetts General Hospital
Boston, Massachusetts
Associate Professor of Medicine
Harvard Medical School
Cambridge, Massachusetts

Ram L. Jadonath, M.D.
Staff Electrophysiologist
North Shore University Hospital
Department of Cardiology
Cornell Medical College
Manhasset, New York

Mohammad R. Jazayeri, M.D.
Associate Professor of Medicine
University of Wisconsin Medical School
Milwaukee Clinical Campus
Sinai-Samaritan Medical Center
St. Luke's Medical Center
Milwaukee, Wisconsin

Jeffrey H. Johnson, M.D.
Philadelphia Heart Institute
Presbyterian Medical Center of
   Philadelphia
Philadelphia, Pennsylvania

Alan H. Kadish, M.D.
Associate Professor Internal Medicine
Director Cardiac Electrophysiology
Section of Cardiology
Northwestern University
Chicago, Illinois

Amar S. Kapoor, M.D., F.A.C.S.
Director of Interventional Cardiology
Section of Cardiology
St. Mary's Medical Center
Long Beach, California
Clinical Professor of Medicine
UCLA School of Medicine
Los Angeles, California

Harold Kennedy, M.D., M.P.H.
Professor of Medicine (Adjunct)
Distinguished Cardiologist
Department of Medicine
Section of Cardiology
Rush Heart Institute
Rush Medical College
Rush-Presbyterian-St. Luke's Medical
  Center
Chicago, Illinois

Dusan Z. Kocovic, M.D.
Associate Director of Electrophysiology
Cardiovascular Division
Hospital of University of Pennsylvania
Philadelphia, Pennsylvania

Peter R. Kowey, M.D.
Professor of Medicine
Thomas Jefferson University
Philadelphia, Pennsylvania
Chief, Division of Cardiovascular
  Diseases
Lankenau Hospital and Medical
  Research Center
Wynnewood, Pennsylvania

Karl-Heinz Kuck, M.D.
Professor of Internal Medicine
Department of Cardiology
University Hospital Eppendorf
Hamburg, GERMANY

Leslie J. Lipka, M.D., Ph.D.
Research Fellow
Department of Medicine
Columbia University, College of
  Physicians and Surgeons
New York, New York

William J. Mandel, M.D.
Director, Clinical Electrophysiology
Department of Cardiology
Cedars-Sinai Medical Center
Los Angeles, California

Francis E. Marchlinski, M.D.
Director, Arrhythmia Services
Philadelphia Heart Institute
Presbyterian Medical Center of
  Philadelphia
Philadelphia, Pennsylvania

Roger A. Marinchak, M.D.
Director, Clinical Electrophysiology
  Laboratory
Lankenau Hospital and Medical
  Research Center
Wynnewood, Pennsylvania
Associate Professor of Medicine
Department of Medicine
Thomas Jefferson University
Philadelphia, Pennsylvania

James B. Martins, M.D.
Professor of Internal Medicine
Department of Internal Medicine
University of Iowa College of Medicine
Iowa City, Iowa

Robert J. Myerburg, M.D.
Director, Division of Cardiology
Professor of Medicine and Physiology
Division of Cardiology
University of Miami School of
  Medicine
Miami, Florida

Gerald V. Naccarelli, M.D.
Professor of Medicine
Chief, Division of Cardiology
Director, Penn State Cardiovascular
  Center
The Pennsylvania State University
The Milton S. Hershey Medical
  Center
Hershey, Pennsylvania

Andrea Natale, M.D.
Assistant Professor
Department of Cardiology
Duke University
Durham, North Carolina

Philip J. Podrid, M.D.
Professor of Medicine
Boston University Medical School
Director, Arrhythmia Service
University Hospital
Boston, Massachusetts

Craig M. Pratt, M.D.
Section of Cardiology
Baylor University Medical School
Houston, Texas

Silvia G. Priori
Research Associate
Clinica Medica Generale e Terapia
Policlinico University of Milan
Milano, ITALY

Eric N. Prystowsky, M.D.
Director, Clinical Electrophysiology
   Laboratory
St. Vincent's Hospital
Indianapolis, Indiana
Consulting Professor of Medicine
Duke University Medical Center
Durham, North Carolina

James A. Reiffel, M.D.
Professor of Clinical Medicine
Department of Medicine, Division of
   Cardiology
Columbia University, College of
   Physicians and Surgeons
Attending Physician
Associate Director of the Cardiac
   Pacemaker Lab
Columbia Presbyterian Medical Center
New York, New York

Seth J. Rials, M.D., Ph.D.
Director, Basic Cardiovascular
   Research
Department of Medical Cardiology
   Foundation of Lankenau
Lankenau Hospital and Medical
   Research Center
Wynnewood, Pennsylvania

Sanjeev Saksena, M.D., F.A.C.C.
Clinical Associate, Professor of
   Medicine
University of Medicine and Dentistry
   of New Jersey
Newark, New Jersey
Director, Arrhythmia and Pacemaker
   Service
Eastern Heart Institute
Passaic, New Jersey

Melvin M. Scheinman, M.D.
Professor of Medicine
Director, Electrocardiography and
   Clinical Cardiac Electrophysiology
   Service
University of California
San Francisco, California

Michael Schluter, Ph.D.
Department of Cardiology
University Hospital Eppendorf
Hamburg, GERMANY

Peter J. Schwartz, M.D.
Istituto di Clinica Medica Generale e
   Terapia Medica
Universita' di Milano
Milano, ITALY

Lyle A. Siddoway, M.D., F.A.C.C.
Director, Cardiac Electrophysiology
  Laboratory
York Hospital
York, Pennsylvania

Bramah N. Singh, M.D., Ph.D.
Chief, Cardiology Section
Department of Cardiology
West Los Angeles Veterans
  Administration Medical Center
Professor of Medicine
UCLA Medical Center
Los Angeles, California

Bradford C. Sodowick, M.D.
Clinical Fellow
Department of Cardiovascular
  Medicine
Yale University School of Medicine
New Haven, Connecticut

Federico Soria, M.D.
Cardiology Department
Murcia General Hospital
Murcia, SPAIN

Jasbir Sra, M.D.
Assistant Professor of Medicine
University of Wisconsin Medical
  School
Milwaukee Clinical Campus
Sinai-Samaritan Medical Center
St. Luke's Medical Center
Milwaukee, Wisconsin

Gunter Steurer, M.D.
Assistant Professor of Internal
  Medicine
Department of Cardiology
University of Vienna
Vienna, AUSTRIA

Eric Taylor, Jr., M.D.
Johns Hopkins Hospital
Department of Medicine
Baltimore, Maryland

Enrico P. Veltri, M.D.
Executive Director
Department of Cardiovascular Clinical
  Research
Bristol-Myers Squibb
Princeton, New Jersey

Albert L. Waldo, M.D.
The Walter H. Pritchaw
  Professor of Cardiology and Medicine
Case Western Reserve University
Cleveland, Ohio

Bulent Zaim, M.D.
Department of Cardiology
Jewish Hospital of St. Louis
Washington University School of
  Medicine
St. Louis, Missouri

Sina Zaim, M.D.
Assistant Professor of Medicine
Department of Medicine
Hahnemann University Hospital
Philadelphia, Pennsylvania

Paul M. Zoll, M.D.
Professor of Medicine
Harvard Medical School
Attending Physician
Beth Israel Hospital
Boston, Massachusetts

Andrew C. Zygmunt, Ph.D.
Research Scientist
Department of Experimental
  Cardiology
Masonic Medical Research Lab
Utica, New York

CONTENTS

SECTION IV: CONDUCTION ABNORMALITIES

SECTION V: SYNCOPE

1   Holter Monitoring

The clinical utility of the ambulatory electrocardiogram (ECG) recording lies in its ability to continuously examine a patient over an extended period of time, permitting the patient ambulatory activity and facilitating the diurnal electrocardiographic examination of a patient in a changing environmental milieu (both physical and psychological). It has the strength of recording changing dynamic cardiac electrical phenomena that often are transient and of brief duration.

Ambulatory electrocardiography also evaluates ST segment changes (for myocardial ischemia), R-R interval changes (for heart rate variability), QRS complex measurements (for specific intervals — e.g., Q-T), and the high-resolution signal-averaged electrocardiography (for electrical fragmentation—e.g., late potentials).

PATHOPHYSIOLOGY OF CARDIAC ARRHYTHMIAS AND RATIONALE FOR USING AMBULATORY ELECTROCARDIOGRAPHY

Ambulatory electrocardiography observations from patients who experienced sudden death during examination led to the recognition that most instantaneous cardiovascular sudden deaths were caused by ventricular tachyarrhythmias, which culminated in ventricular fibrillation (VF) and death.

A 24-hour ambulatory ECG can document and identify spontaneous ectopic triggers (ventricular or supraventricular), bradyarrhythmias and tachyarrhythmias, and atrioventricular and intraventricular conduction disturbances. The ambulatory ECG can also be a valuable adjunct in recognizing abnormal substrates, as identified by fractionated late potentials. Or it can be one of the most specific sources of information in appreciating noninvasively the modulating factors of ischemia (through ST segment changes), repolarization abnormalities (Q-T or TU wave changes), or autonomic changes (R-R changes of heart rate variability).

Transtelephonic Electrographic Devices

Transtelephonic electrocardiographic devices exist as several forms of recorders and transmitters capable of direct transmission of an ECG as an audio signal by telephone (Table 1.1).

Patients can apply the device to the precordial area, obtain a recording of electrocardiographic data into solid-state memory, and later (when telephonic transmission is available) transmit the electrocardiographic data for interpretation.

Current evidence indicates that intermittent loop electrocardiographic recorders are the examination of choice in patients with recurrent or unexplained syncope who have undergone previous clinical and ambulatory electrocardiography without occurrence of symptoms or disclosure of an etiologic ECG abnormality.

1

Table 1.1
Technical and Clinical Differences of Ambulatory ECG and Transtelephonic Loop Recorder

	Ambulatory ECG	Transtelephonic Loop
Technical		
ECG data	24 or 48 hr of 2- or 3-channel ECG	4–5 min of 1-channel ECG
	Continuous ECG data	Intermittent and patient-activated ECG data
Resources needed	Holter recorder	Transtelephonic loop recorder
	Holter playback analysis system	Telephone communication with audio modem
	Operator interaction	Base station printout recorder (24-hr availability)
		Operator interaction
Cost	24-hr examination — $150–300	30-day surveillance — $200–300
Patient participation	Minimal (diary for symptoms)	Moderate/substantial (sending and recording ECG data)
Clinical		
indications	To diagnose cardiac arrhythmias with qualitative/quantitative assessment	To diagnose infrequent or rare cardiac arrhythmias qualitatively only
As first-line diagnostic test	Often	Never
As arrhythmic follow-up	Often	Rarely or special situation (e.g., sudden death cohorts or effects on Q-T interval)
As pacemaker follow-up	Often	Often

Ambulatory Electrocardiography in Arrhythmia Diagnosis

Ambulatory electrocardiography is the most widely employed technology to evaluate patient symptoms suggestive of a cardiac arrhythmia.

Such examinations serve to exclude cardiac arrhythmias as a specific cause of a patient's complaint. For less frequently occurring symptoms, transtelephonic monitoring (with or without loop memory) may be better suited and more cost-effective in the examination of an intermittent or sporadic complaint (see previous discussion). On the other hand, if symptoms are severe and potentially life-threatening (syncope, presyncope, sustained lightheadedness, etc.), it is probably more appropriate to admit the patient to the hospital for coronary care or intermediate care in-hospital telemetry long-term electrocardiography, or to utilize continuous 24- or 48-hour ambulatory electrocardiography examination within the safety of the hospital environment.

Detected electrocardiographic abnormalities of sinus bradycardias, sinus pauses, supraventricular arrhythmias, and ventricular arrhythmias are known to occur in normal asymptomatic populations. Therefore, the occurrence of such arrhythmias does not necessarily establish a causal mechanism for a transient disturbance in consciousness.

When it comes to characterizing various aspects (quantitative or qualitative) of spontaneous cardiac arrhythmias, ambulatory electrocardiography is ideally suited. It can quantitate various ectopic morphologies, qualitatively discern different morphologies, provide "onset and offset" data of various tachy- and bradyarrhythmias, permit examination of a variety of arrhythmia characteristics (e.g., coupling interval, rate dependence, changes in Q-T interval), and give deductive information concerning site of origin or pathway of reentry. This is especially true for examining paroxysmal supraventricular tachyarrhythmias, where onset and offset facilitate diagnosis of the underlying mechanism. It has been recognized for some time that the 24-hour ambulatory electrocardiography trend provides valuable heart rate data in atrial fibrillation to guide pharmacologic (digitalis, β-blocker, or calcium antagonist) therapy for control of ventricular response or to assess the control of paroxysmal events.

Prognostic Value of Ambulatory Electrocardiography in Assessing Risk

Ambulatory electrocardiography is useful to assess risk associated with cardiac arrhythmias in specific asymptomatic and symptomatic populations. Usually this is performed with the conventional 24-hour ambulatory electrocardiography recording.

CORONARY HEART DISEASE

In asymptomatic postmyocardial infarction patients, studies unequivocally demonstrated that ambulatory electrocardiography detects ventricular arrhythmias that have independent prognostic risk based upon frequency and complexity. At the same time, there is an increased risk of an adverse outcome associated with decreased left ventricular function. More recently, ambulatory electrocardiography studies of postmyocardial infarction patients have shown that heart rate variability as measured by the standard deviation of the R-R intervals in sinus rhythm is a powerful predictor of prognosis, independent of ventricular arrhythmias or left ventricular function. Patients with decreased heart rate variability have decreased vagal tone or increased sympathetic tone and may have a higher risk of VF. Decreased heart rate variability has been identified in patients who sustained sudden death during ambulatory electrocardiography.

CARDIOMYOPATHY

Ambulatory electrocardiography in patients with hypertrophic cardiomyopathy discloses that approximately two-thirds of these patients have frequent and complex ventricular arrhythmias. In addition, the presence of ventricular tachycardia (found in approximately 25%) is a reliable predictor of the subsequent occurrence of sudden death.

In ischemic or nonischemic dilated cardiomyopathy, complex and frequent ventricular arrhythmias are detected by ambulatory electrocardiography in 80–90% of patients. Some prospective follow-up studies have shown that complex repetitive ventricular arrhythmias are an independent predictor of sudden death in representative dilated cardiomyopathy populations. This association appears to be independent of hemodynamic or neuroendocrine variables, and sudden death may occur despite a seemingly favorable clinical response to medical therapy.

APPARENTLY HEALTHY PERSONS

Ventricular arrhythmias are found in 40–75% of normal persons as assessed by 24–48 hours of continuous ambulatory electrocardiography. Even frequent and complex forms have been found in 1–4% of the general population. The incidence and frequency of ventricular ectopy increase with age. When apparently healthy persons with frequent and complex ventricular ectopy are examined by careful noninvasive cardiologic evaluation and found to have no overt evidence of myocardial ischemia, dysfunction, or fibrosis, such persons have a favorable long-term prognosis. This good prognosis is even true in the presence of asymptomatic coronary artery disease.

SYMPTOMATIC VENTRICULAR TACHYCARDIA OR VENTRICULAR FIBRILLATION

An increasing number of patients have been resuscitated from sudden cardiac death or have severe coronary artery disease that predisposes them to recurrent symptomatic ventricular tachycardia. These patients have a high recurrence rate of malignant ventricular arrhythmias, when they are untreated or are treated empirically, and a decreased long-term survival.

EVALUATION OF THERAPEUTIC INTERVENTION

Ambulatory electrocardiography has proven valuable for evaluating a variety of therapies used to treat cardiac arrhythmias. Most commonly, an assessment of antiarrhythmic drug therapy and pacemaker function are the major indications for ambulatory electrocardiography.

Antiarrhythmic Drug Therapy

When serious or potentially lethal ventricular arrhythmias are discovered on ambulatory monitoring in a patient with underlying organic heart disease, physicians may treat such arrhythmias with antiarrhythmic drugs in the hope of altering an adverse prognosis. However, several pitfalls evolved from this hypothesis. One major oversight was the failure to account for the spontaneous variability of arrhythmias that occurs within each individual.

Furthermore, 25–27% of patients with benign and potentially lethal ventricular arrhythmias have spontaneous resolution of ventricular arrhythmias during 12–17 months of antiarrhythmic therapy and, therefore, do not require therapy. This variability of ventricular arrhythmia is time dependent and greater in patients with low-density ventricular arrhythmias, coronary artery disease, or frequent ventricular tachycardia runs.

The continuous conventional 24–48-hour ambulatory electrocardiography examination is the "mainstay" of such evaluations. This approach is used in the hospital or outside of the hospital to document suppression of asymptomatic arrhythmias. Commonly, a reduction in the frequency of total ventricular ectopy (70–90%), and elimination of all repetitive forms (runs and couplets), are sought to demonstrate antiarrhythmic efficacy. In addition, transtelephonic monitoring has been used to evaluate antiarrhythmic therapy and has been extended to provide "surveillance" of specific high-risk subgroups.

Evaluation of Pacemakers

It is estimated that about 90% of pacemaker patients are followed by their private physician or pacemaker surveillance service. With the emergence of pacemaker and automatic implantable cardioverter devices (AICD) technology in recent years, the need for a dedicated cardiac pacemaker follow-up clinic has become apparent.

Ambulatory electrocardiography has proven to be a valuable adjunctive assessor of pacemaker function. Because of the limited time of examination provided by the traditional clinic visit, the use of ambulatory electrocardiography has increased the diagnosis of pacemaker malfunction by examining the patient over 24 hours or more during daily activities. Enhanced detection of pacemaker dysfunction by ambulatory electrocardiography has also proven valuable in the early postimplant period, as compared with in-hospital telemetry monitoring, and has allowed therapeutic intervention prior to discharge.

SUGGESTED READING

Bachinsky WB, Linzer M, Weld L, Estes NAM. Usefulness of clinical characteristics in predicting the outcome of electrophysiologic studies in unexplained syncope. Am J Cardiol 1992;69: 1044–1049.

Bayes de Luna A, Coumel P, Leclercq JF. Ambulatory sudden death: mechanisms of production of fatal arrhythmia on the basis of data from 157 cases. Am Heart J 1989;117:151–159.

Bigger JT, Fleiss JL, Kleiger RE, Miller JP, Rolintzky LM. The relationships among ventricular arrhythmias, left ventricular dysfunction, and mortality in the 2 years after myocardial infarction. Circulation 1984;69:250–258.

Brodsky M, Wu D, Denes P, Kanakis C, Rosen KM. Arrhythmias documented by 24-hour continuous electrocardiographic monitoring in 50 male medical students without apparent heart disease. Am J Cardiol 1977;39:390–395.

Furman S, Escher DJW. Telephone pacemaker monitoring. Ann Thorac Surg 1975;20:326.

Graboys TB, Lown B, Podrid PJ, DeSilva R. Long-term survival of patients with malignant ventricular arrhythmia treated with antiarrhythmic drugs. Am J Cardiol 1982;50:437–443.

Hohnloser SH, Raeder EA, Podrid PJ, Graboys TB, Lown B. Predictors of antiarrhythmic drug efficacy in patients with malignant ventricular tachyarrhythmias. Am Heart J 1987;114:1–7.

Kennedy HL, Wiens RD. Ambulatory (Holter) electrocardiography using real-time analysis. Am J Cardiol 1987;59:1190.

Kleiger RE, Miller JP, Bigger JT, Moss AJ, and the Multicenter Post-Infarction Research Group. Decreased heart rate variability and its association with increased mortality after acute myocardial infarction. Am J Cardiol 1987;59: 256–262.

Linzer M, Pritchett ELC, Pontinen M, et al. Incremental diagnostic yield of loop electrocardiographic recorders in unexplained syncope. Am J Cardiol 1990;66:214–219.

Lipski J, Cohen L, Espinoza J, Motro M, Dack S, Domoso E. Value of Holter monitoring in assessing cardiac arrhythmias in symptomatic patients. Am J Cardiol 1976;37:102–107.

Maron BJ, Savage DD, Wolfson JK, Epstein SE. Prognostic significance of 24-hour ambulatory electrocardiographic monitoring in patients with hypertrophic cardiomyopathy: a prospective study. Am J Cardiol 1981;48:252–257.

Mason JW, ESVEM Investigators. A comparison of electrophysiologic testing with Holter monitoring to predict antiarrhythmic drug efficacy for ventricular tachyarrhythmias. N Engl J Med 1993;329:445–451.

Meinertz T, Hoffman T, Kasper W, et al. Significance of ventricular arrhythmias in idiopathic dilated cardiomyopathy. Am J Cardiol 1984;53:902–907.

Pratt CM, Delclos G, Wierman AM, et al. The changing baseline of complex ventricular arrhythmias. A new consideration in assessing long-term antiarrhythmic drug therapy. N Engl J Med 1985;313:1444–1449.

Pratt CM, Slymen DJ, Wierman AM, et al. Asymptomatic telephone ECG transmission as an outpatient surveillance system of ventricular arrhythmias: relationship to quantitative ambulatory ECG recordings. Am Heart J 1987;113:1–7.

Ruberman W, Weinblatt E, Goldberg JD, Frank CW, Chaudhary BS, Shapiro S. Ventricular premature complexes and sudden death after myocardial infarction. Circulation 1981;64:297–305.

2 Exercise Testing

Exercise testing produces a number of physiologic changes that have a role in arrhythmia management (Table 2.1). The changes that occur may result in arrhythmia, but more importantly they can have an impact on the action of antiarrhythmic drugs and their effect on the conduction system, the myocardial tissue, and ventricular contractility.

PHYSIOLOGIC EFFECTS OF EXERCISE

With exercise there is withdrawal of vagal tone and, more importantly, activation of the sympathetic nervous system and an increase in circulating catecholamines. These changes affect the balance of cardiac autonomic inputs and have significant effects on mechanical, metabolic, and physiologic parameters of myocardial function, which may be particularly important in the presence of underlying myocardial disease (Fig. 2.1). As a result of sympathetic stimulation, there is an increase in heart rate, systolic blood pressure, and myocardial contractility or inotropy. These changes cause an increase in myocardial oxygen demand, and, in patients with heart disease who have limited or impaired myocardial oxygen delivery, this results in myocardial ischemia.

Exercise testing is an adjunctive technique and should be used along with ambulatory monitoring or electrophysiologic testing for evaluating and managing the patient with a history of supraventricular or ventricular arrhythmia, particularly in the selection of an antiarrhythmic drug. It may also have a role for aiding in the stratification of patients with heart disease, in whom the risk of sudden cardiac death is increased, particularly those with a recent myocardial infarction. Exercise testing may also be of use for those patients with transient symptoms suggesting arrhythmia, in whom other techniques fail to document an etiology. Perhaps the most important role for exercise testing is in the evaluation of both the beneficial and possible harmful effects of antiarrhythmic drugs.

Table 2.1
Uses of Exercise Testing in Arrhythmia Evaluation and Management

1. Provocation of arrhythmia
2. Evaluation of antiarrhythmic drug efficacy
3. Exposure of harmful drug effects
   a. Negative inotropy
   b. Conduction abnormalities
   c. Arrhythmia aggravation
4. Prognostication—establish risk of an arrhythmic event
5. Rate control in atrial fibrillation

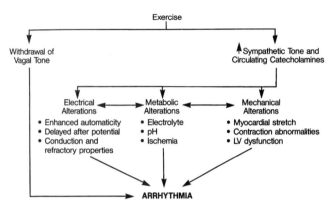

Figure 2.1. Schema of physiologic changes produced by exercise. The primary effect is activation of the sympathetic nervous system and an increase in circulating catecholamines. This results in electrical, metabolic, and mechanical changes that are important in arrhythmogenesis.

INCIDENCE OF ARRHYTHMIA DURING EXERCISE

Ventricular Arrhythmia

Ventricular arrhythmia, especially ventricular premature beats (VPBs), is commonly seen during exercise testing. The type and frequency of ventricular arrhythmia provoked by exercise are related to the presence and extent of underlying heart disease, left ventricular function, and age.

There is also an association between exercise-induced repetitive arrhythmia, particularly runs of NSVT, and the presence and extent of heart disease.

The occurrence of a serious sustained ventricular tachyarrhythmia during exercise testing is uncommon, even in those patients with underlying heart disease. When it occurs, it is most often within the first few minutes of recovery.

Supraventricular Arrhythmia

Supraventricular arrhythmia during exercise is fairly common, but the exact incidence has been difficult to establish. Most frequently observed are supraventricular premature beats, either atrial or junctional.

Although premature beats are commonly observed during exercise testing, sustained supraventricular tachyarrhythmia occurs infrequently. However, a sustained supraventricular arrhythmia is more commonly induced by exercise in patients with a history of such arrhythmia.

PROGNOSTIC SIGNIFICANCE OF VENTRICULAR ARRHYTHMIA DURING EXERCISE TESTING

There are some data showing that exercise-induced ventricular arrhythmia in patients with coronary artery disease, particularly those with a recent myocardial infarction (MI), is important prognostically. Data in other groups of patients are lacking, although a similar relationship between arrhythmia presence during exercise and mortality has also been reported in patients with chronic coronary artery disease who have not had an MI. Ventricular arrhythmia may be of prognostic significance when associated with ST segment changes indicating ischemia.

REPRODUCIBILITY OF EXERCISE-INDUCED ARRHYTHMIA

The reproducibility of exercise-induced VPBs tends to be greater in patients with underlying cardiovascular disease and a history of a sustained arrhythmia. Age may also be a factor related to reproducibility of arrhythmia during exercise.

There are no data regarding the reproducibility of exercise-induced supraventricular arrhythmia.

USE OF EXERCISE TESTING FOR MANAGEMENT OF PATIENTS WITH VENTRICULAR ARRHYTHMIA

Exercise testing has an important adjunctive role for managing patients who have already experienced a sustained ventricular tachyarrhythmia, regardless of whether noninvasive ambulatory monitoring or invasive electrophysiologic testing is used as the primary method for evaluating the patient and selecting an effective antiarrhythmic drug. However, exercise testing produces important physiologic changes that affect the myocardium and may alter or modulate the frequency and type of spontaneous VPBs (the triggers) or the properties and stability of the substrate (the reentrant circuit) (Fig. 2.2). These changes may play a role in the exposure of arrhythmia, but more importantly, exercise testing and the physiologic effects it produces (electrical, mechanical, and metabolic) have strong implications with regard to antiarrhythmic drug therapy. The changes produced by exercise testing, especially increased sympathetic tone, elevated circulating catecholamine levels, and metabolic alterations (particularly of potassium and other electrolytes, pH, and oxygen supply) may interact with, negate, or enhance antiarrhythmic drug activity. Accordingly, arrhythmia may recur or become aggravated.

Catecholamines and Antiarrhythmic Drugs

Activation of the sympathetic nervous system and an increase in circulating catecholamines are factors that may have an impact on antiarrhythmic drug action. It has been well established that, as a result of antiarrhythmic drugs, there is a decrease in membrane conductivity, prolongation of membrane refractory period and a reduction in excitability, and a decrease in membrane automaticity. In contrast, administration of catecholamines results in a shortening of the refractory period and an increase in membrane excitability, an increase in membrane conductivity, and an augmentation in automaticity, changes that are in direct opposition to those caused by antiarrhythmic drugs. Therefore, catecholamines may interfere with and negate the action of antiarrhythmic drugs by reversing their beneficial effects.

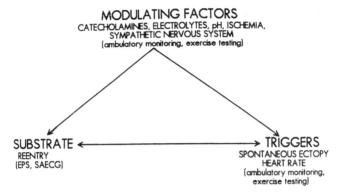

Figure 2.2. Interrelated factors important in arrhythmia occurrence. The substrate is abnormal and is capable of generating and sustaining a reentrant arrhythmia. The reentrant circuit is activated by a number of factors, especially spontaneous arrhythmia. The modulating factors or "triggers" can alter the stability of the substrate and the frequency of the trigger. Abbreviations: *SAECG*, signal averaged electrocardiogram; *EPS*, electrophysiologic study.

Exercise Testing and Exposure of Drug-Related Toxicity

In addition to its useful role for evaluating the beneficial effects of antiarrhythmic drugs on arrhythmia, exercise testing is of major importance for exposing potential toxic effects of these agents. Exercise testing, by producing an increase in heart rate, is an important technique for determining the potentially harmful effects of these agents on atrioventricular (AV) or intraventricular conduction. This may present, as a rate-related prolongation of P-R or QRS intervals and, not infrequently, a new right or left bundle branch block. In some cases this rate-dependent slowing of conduction may cause complete blockade of impulse conduction through the AV node, resulting in complete heart block. The slowing of conduction within the ventricular myocardium may, under certain circumstances, promote arrhythmia aggravation, as the slowing of impulse conduction increases the potential for reentry and arrhythmia aggravation (Fig. 2.3).

An increase in sympathetic neural activity and circulating catecholamines and the occurrence of ischemia with resultant changes of extracellular potassium levels and pH, may foster arrhythmia.

USE OF EXERCISE TESTING FOR MANAGEMENT OF SUPRAVENTRICULAR TACHYARRHYTHMIAS

Supraventricular tachyarrhythmias are infrequently provoked by exercise, and their reproducibility during exercise is poor. However, if the tachyarrhythmia is reproducibly induced, exercise testing is a useful tool for its management. Repeated exercise testing during an antiarrhythmic drug administration is an effective method for determining drug effect, and for establishing an effective program for control.

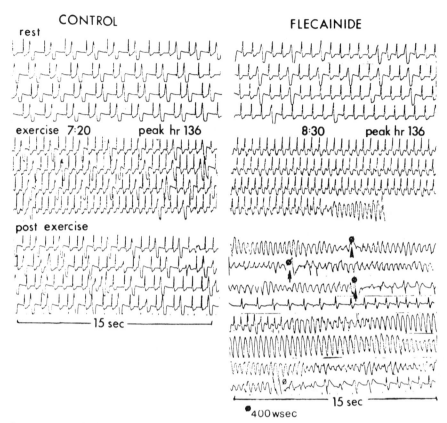

Figure 2.3. Arrhythmia aggravation exposed by exercise testing. Before therapy, there were brief episodes of nonsustained ventricular tachycardia. During therapy with flecainide, a class Ic antiarrhythmic agent, sustained ventricular tachycardia, and ventricular fibrillation, resulting in collapse, were provoked. Defibrillation was required.

Exercise testing has an important role in the management of patients with chronic atrial fibrillation (AF), to determine the ventricular rate during activity. The ventricular rate is dependent upon the state of the AV node and its electrophysiologic properties, particularly its refractoriness and ability to conduct atrial impulses to the ventricle. An important element in the management of patients with chronic AF involves slowing of the heart rate by impairing impulse conduction through the AV node.

USE OF EXERCISE TESTING FOR OTHER CONDITIONS

In addition to its important role for evaluating the beneficial or harmful effects of antiarrhythmic drugs, exercise testing has also been useful for the evaluation of other conditions associated with arrhythmia. Patients with the prolonged Q-T syndrome do not have the expected shortening of the Q-T interval during exercise, and many will develop serious arrhythmia with exercise, a result of increased sympathetic tone and further autonomic imbalance. It is possible that patients with an idiosyncratic reaction to the class Ia drugs, who develop substantial Q-T prolongation and the associated increased risk of torsade de pointes, even with low serum concentrations of drug, have a "forme fruste" of the Q-T syndrome. Exercise testing may help to identify these patients, as the Q-T will not shorten appropriately.

Exercise testing has been used to identify patients with the Wolff-Parkinson-White syndrome who are at an increased risk for sudden death. The persistence of preexcited QRS complexes during exercise testing may identify patients at risk for sudden death as determined by electrophysiologic testing (i.e., during induced AF, the shortest R-R interval is <250 msec).

SAFETY OF EXERCISE TESTING

A very important concern about the use of exercise testing in arrhythmia management, particularly in patients with advanced heart disease, is its safety. In several surveys involving thousands of patients, mortality due to the precipitation of a serious arrhythmia has been rare, with the incidence range from 0.2–0.5%.

It appears that exercise testing in patients with advanced heart disease who have a history of sustained ventricular tachyarrhythmia is a safe procedure. Although the risk of inducing a serious ventricular tachyarrhythmia during exercise testing is increased when compared with a population of patients with heart disease who have no clinical history of serious arrhythmia, the majority of events occur during antiarrhythmic drug use when exercise is performed for an evaluation of efficacy, suggesting that the arrhythmia is a result of aggravation of arrhythmia due to the antiarrhythmic drug.

SUGGESTED READING

Antman ES, Graboys TB, Lown B. Comparison of continuous intermittent electrocardiographic monitoring during exercise testing for exposure of cardiac arrhythmias. JAMA 1979;241:2802.

Califf RM, McKinnis RA, McNeer F, Harel FE, Leek L, Pryor DB. Prognostic value of ventricular arrhythmias associated with treadmill exercise testing in patients studied with cardiac catheterization for suspected ischemic heart disease. J Am Coll Cardiol 1983;2:1060.

Graboys TB, Wright RF. Provocation of supraventricular tachycardia during exercise stress testing. Cardiovasc Rev Rep 1980;1:57–58.

Jazayeri MR, Wyhe G, Avitall B, McKinna JM, Tchou P, Akhtar M. Isoproterenol reversal of antiarrhythmic effects in patients with inducible sustained ventricular tachyarrhythmias. J Am Coll Cardiol 1989;14:705.

Jelinek MV, Lown B. Exercise stress testing for exposure of cardiac arrhythmia. Prog Cardiovasc Dis 1974;16:497.

Kadish AH, Weisman HF, Veltri EP, Epstein AE, Slepian MJ, Levine JH. Paradoxic effects of exercise on the QT interval in patients with polymorphic ventricular tachycardia receiving type 1A antiarrhythmic agents. Circulation 1990;81:14.

Lown B, Podrid PJ, DeSilva RA, Graboys TB. Sudden cardiac death: management of the patient at risk. Curr Probl Cardiol 1980;4:1.

Ryan M, Lown B, Horn H. Comparison of ventricular ectopic activity during 24-hour monitoring and exercise testing in patients with coronary heart disease. N Engl J Med 1975;292:224.

Slater W, Lampert SC, Podrid PJ, Lown B. Clinical predictors of arrhythmia worsening by antiarrhythmic drugs. Am J Cardiol 1988; 61:349.

Weld FM, Chu KL, Bigger JT, Rolnitzky LM. Risk stratification with low level exercise testing two weeks after myocardial infarction. Circulation 1981;64:306.

Young D, Lampert S, Graboys TB, Lown B. Safety of maximal exercise testing in patients at high risk for ventricular arrhythmia. Circulation 1984;70:184.

3 Invasive Cardiac Electrophysiology Studies

METHODOLOGY OF CARDIAC ELECTROPHYSIOLOGY STUDIES

Basic Equipment and Personnel

A diagnostic cardiac electrophysiology study requires recording local electrograms from stimulating different cardiac sites via electrode catheters. Central components are a programmable constant current source stimulator and a multichannel data acquisition system. The stimulator must be electrically isolated and have synchronous and asynchronous pacing capability, with a cycle length range of 150–1500 msec, and with a capability of incrementing or decrementing intervals by 10 msec or less. It must also be capable of delivering a minimum of three programmable premature extrastimuli and burst pacing with an interstimulus accuracy of 1 msec. Based on experience with strength interval curves, the stimulus strength is usually set at twice the diastolic threshold (threshold should ideally be less than 1 mA), at a pulse width of 1 msec, in order to limit induction of nonspecific rhythms noted with higher currents during programmed stimulation and to maintain uniformity among different laboratories. The data acquisition system simultaneously records and stores surface electrocardiograms (ECGs), multiple intracardiac electrograms, and sometimes hemodynamic parameters recorded during the course of the electrophysiologic study. The surface ECG leads, typically I, AVF, and V1 (approximating orthogonal Frank leads X, Y, Z), are filtered according to the American Heart Association standards (0.1–100 Hz). The intracardiac signals are either bipolar, filtered below 30–40 Hz and above 400–500 Hz, or unipolar, where the recording reflects the potential difference between a single remote electrode on the catheter and an indifferent electrode placed on the body. Unipolar intracardiac recordings are typically left unfiltered because of the low frequency nature of their signal content. The signals are then amplified and displayed in real time on an oscilloscope, and simultaneous hard copies are obtained as required. The signals are recorded continuously during the study with multichannel magnetic or optical disk recorders to allow detection and analysis of unexpected transient arrhythmias.

Biplane fluoroscopy, providing right anterior and left anterior oblique views to ensure correct catheter placement is desirable, especially when intracardiac mapping and transcatheter radiofrequency (RF) ablation are performed. Induction of potentially lethal arrhythmias during the course of an electrophysiologic study depends on the type of study, and typically occurs in 20–50%. For this reason the permanent presence and maintenance of cardiopulmonary resuscitation (CPR) equipment, including a primary and a backup (second) external defibrillator in the laboratory, are mandatory.

The minimum personnel required to conduct a cardiac electrophysiology study include a clinical cardiologist with at least 1 and preferably 2 years' training in clinical cardiac electrophysiology in addition to general cardiology training, a nurse trained in acute cardiac care, and a technician familiar with the laboratory equipment, antiarrhythmic drug administration, and CPR. Because it is quite cumbersome for one cardiologist to manipulate the electrode catheter and to analyze the tracings simultaneously, the presence of a second cardiac electrophysiologist improves the efficiency of the procedure markedly. For long and labor-intensive procedures such as transcatheter RF ablation, two nurses, rather than one, may be required. An anesthesiologist should be available on demand for emergencies requiring endotracheal intubation and assisted ventilation, as well as for rare elective cases that may require general anesthesia. The services of a bioelectrical engineer or technician also need to be readily available to periodically ensure proper function and safety of the electrical equipment. It is also desirable to have the services of a cardiothoracic surgeon readily available in the event of complications, such as cardiac perforation and tamponade.

Approach to the Patient

Preparation of the patient for the electrophysiology study should begin with a clear explanation of what to expect during the sometimes protracted studies and the indications for the procedure. Informed consent specifically stating the possible risks and anticipated benefits must be obtained. Congestive heart failure, myocardial ischemia, and electrolyte abnormalities need to be treated and maintained before any invasive electrophysiology study is undertaken. For baseline studies, a period of antiarrhythmic drug washout long enough for at least 5 half-lives is required, unless there is a specific reason to perform the procedure during drug therapy. Fasting is required prior to the study as aspiration prophylaxis in case of cardioversion or intubation. Sedation is often with benzodiazepines, which have been shown to have relatively few and only mild to moderate electrophysiologic effects at the doses routinely employed.

In routine diagnostic studies the standard access is via the femoral veins. The percutaneous modified Seldinger approach is used, which allows the safe insertion of up to three sheaths for the right atrial, His bundle, and right ventricular electrode catheters. The internal jugular or subclavian vein approach facilitates entry into the coronary sinus when it is required to map left atrial and ventricular activation along the atrioventricular groove. Arterial access is not routinely required for diagnostic evaluation, but when indicated — for example, for left ventricular stimulation or mapping — may be performed retrogradely via either the femoral artery or using the transseptal catheterization technique. Lidocaine for local anesthesia should be limited to a total dose of less than 2.5 mg/kg because larger subcutaneous doses may result in therapeutic serum levels. Systemic heparinization is not routinely employed except when left heart catheterization is required or with prolonged diagnostic studies, especially when mapping and transcatheter ablation procedures require excessive instrumentation.

A comprehensive diagnostic baseline study typically requires a minimum of three electrode catheters: (a) in the right atrium at the superior vena cava and right atrial junction near the sinus node, to allow atrial pacing and to record atrial activation patterns; (*b*) across the septal tricuspid leaflet, to record His bundle potential to evaluate atrioventricular conduction; and (*c*) in the right ventricular apex, to allow ventricular stimulation and recording. If a narrow-complex tachycardia is being investigated, a fourth electrode catheter should be placed in the coronary sinus for recording of left atrial and ventricular electrograms. Follow-up antiarrhythmic drug testing may require only a single catheter placed in the right ventricular apex for programmed ventricular stimulation.

For most routine electrophysiologic studies, quadripolar electrode catheters are sufficient. This configuration allows bipolar pacing with the distal pair and simultaneous bipolar recording, with the proximal pair when used in the high right atrial and right ventricular apical position and with three contiguous or partially overlapping bipolar recording pairs when placed across the tricuspid valve for the His bundle recording. Generally bipolar pacing and recording are preferred. Bipolar and unipolar pacing thresholds are very similar, but the former has the advantage of producing smaller pacing artifacts, thus limiting distortion of recorded intracardiac signals. Bipolar electrodes are usually filtered for frequencies lower than 30–20 Hz and higher than 200–250 Hz; they provide recordings of local events with minimal far field effect, and offer good signal-to-noise ratio. The earliest onset of recorded electrical activity signifies the presence of electrical activity anywhere within the recording range of the bipole, whereas the earliest rapid deflection corresponds to the leading activation wavefront traversing midway between the recording bipole. Often bipolar waveforms are complex and manifest multiple components and more than one rapid deflection. Under these circumstances it is not possible to assign a local activation time to the electrogram with precision. Unipolar recordings, on the other hand, represent total activation, i.e., local and distant events, and therefore are generally of greater amplitude because of the far field interference and their wide filtering bandwidth. Accordingly, it is more difficult to time local events with unipolar recordings, but they provide directionality, which is not available with bipolar recordings. An activation wavefront moving toward the electrode results in a positive deflection, and one moving away produces a negative deflection. In a unipolar tracing the most rapid deflection that represents the passage of the activation wavefront under the electrode is usually bracketed between the recorded far field potentials and is labeled the intrisicoid deflection, which historically was taken to be the marker for local activation time. Laboratory studies have shown excellent correlation between bipolar and unipolar recordings and local activation times registered with intracellular recordings.

Baseline Cardiac Recordings and Analysis

Figure 3.1 shows baseline recordings obtained during a typical electrophysiologic study. The top lines are generally reserved for the (approximate) orthogonal surface electrocardiograms, which display P and QRS wave morphology and allow mean electrical axis determination. They also serve as first approximations of atrial and ventricular activation sequence and guarantee registration of the earliest

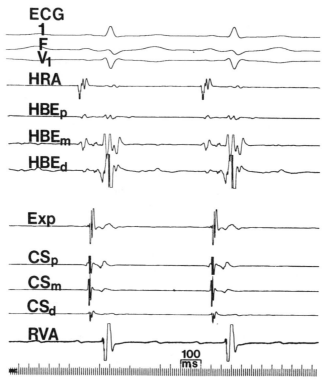

Figure 3.1. During a typical cardiac electrophysiology study, local electrograms are recorded from the high right atrium (*HRA*), His bundle (*HB*), the right ventricular apex, and from the coronary sinus (*CS*). Additional electrograms may be obtained from the right bundle branch and the left ventricle, as required by the purpose of the study. When extensive mapping is required, one or several more recording channels are dedicated to exploring (*Exp*) electrodes, which are used for multiple sequential site recording. Abbreviations: *p*, proximal; *m*, middle; *d*, distal.

surface electrical activity and frequently serve as fiducial points for proper timing of intracardiac events. Next displayed are the intracardiac electrograms, generally following the order of normal cardiac activation. The first tracing is the recording from the high right atrium close to the sinus node. Pacing at this position allows evaluation of sinoatrial node function, atrioventricular conduction, and induction of atrial arrhythmias and triggered activation-based arrhythmias in general. Recordings from this site also help determine the direction of atrial activation, i.e., high-low versus low-high and right-left versus left-right. The following tracing is the His bundle recording, which shows septal atrial, His bundle, and right high septal ventricular depolarization. The stability and reproducibility (during a given study as well as from one study to the next) of the right ventricle apex position makes it a useful site for programmed ventricular stimulation. Depending on the particular study, other required recordings may include right bundle recording, left ventricular recording, transseptal left-atrial recording, and atrial and ventricular exploring catheter tracings for mapping.

The electrophysiologic analysis begins with measuring the basic intervals that reflect the integrity of the conduction system under rest conditions. The P-A interval is measured from the onset of the earliest registered surface P wave or intracardiac atrial activation to the onset of the atrial deflection on the His bundle catheter recording from the His bundle. The proximal bipolar recording from the His bundle catheter manifests an atrial deflection from inferoposterior interatrial septum corresponding to late atrial activation. There is no general consensus on what constitutes a normal range, though normal ranges from 20 to 60 msec have been reported. Originally it was taken to represent total atrial conduction, though it is at best a rough approximation of total right atrial activation time, and more correctly a reflection of intranodal (sinoatrial to atrioventricular node) conduction. Nonetheless, prolonged P-A times do suggest abnormal atrial conduction and can be a clue to the presence of biatrial disease or disease confined to the right atrium. Rarely, diseased atrial conduction may underlie first-degree atrioventricular block (AVB). In the presence of short P-A times, one should exclude an ectopic atrial focus with more detailed atrial activation mapping.

The A-H interval is measured from the earliest rapid deflection of the atrial recording to the earliest onset of the His bundle deflection on the His bundle electrogram. This interval is taken to represent atrioventricular nodal conduction, but more correctly it is the sum of conduction through the low right atrial inputs into the atrioventricular node, the atrioventricular node proper, and the proximal His bundle. The range of this interval in normal subjects is wide, 50–120 msec, and is further influenced by the autonomic nervous system in a given individual. Short A-H intervals may be seen with increased sympathetic tone, enhanced atrioventricular node conduction, and preferential left atrial input into the atrioventricular node and in unusual forms of preexcitation. Long A-H intervals are most commonly the result of negative dromotropic drugs such as β-receptor and calcium channel blockers, enhanced vagal tone, and intrinsic disease of the atrioventricular node. Care is needed to distinguish true A-H prolongation from artifactually prolonged A-H resulting from an improperly positioned catheter mistakenly recording a right bundle branch potential as a His bundle potential. The His bundle electrogram duration reflects conduction through the short length of compact His bundle penetrating the fibrous septum. Normally it is of short duration, 15–25 msec, and composed of high-frequency deflections. Fractionation and prolongation or even splitting of the His bundle potential is seen with disturbance of His bundle conduction. The H-V interval, measured from the earliest onset of the His bundle deflection to the earliest registered surface or intracardiac ventricular activation anywhere, reflects conduction time through the distal His-Purkinje (H-P) tissue. Unlike the atrioventricular node, the H-P system is far less influenced by the autonomic nervous system, and the range in normal subjects is a narrow 35–55 msec. The most reliable method of validating the His bundle potential is His bundle pacing via the His bundle recording bipole. Demonstration of identical H-V intervals confirms that the His bundle proximal to the bifurcation of the bundle branches is indeed being recorded. A validated short H-V interval would therefore suggest ventricular preexcitation via an atrioventricular bypass tract; His bundle pacing at cycle lengths shorter than the sinus cycle length should eliminate pre-excitation, whereas atrial premature extrastimuli, which retard atrioventricular (A-V) nodal conduction, may exaggerate preexcitation. A prolonged H-V interval is consistent with diseased distal conduction in all fascicles. However, an artifac-tually prolonged H-V interval may be registered if the earliest ventricular activa-tion is missed on the surface ECG and standard intracardiac recordings, as might occur in septal infarction.

Following acquisition of baseline measurements, programmed electrical stimu-lation adapted to the specific clinical setting is carried out. The algorithms that are used for common dysrhythmias and clinical presentations are reviewed in the fol-lowing section.

SAFETY ISSUES: COMPLICATIONS OF INVASIVE CARDIAC ELECTROPHYSIOLOGY STUDIES

Complications of invasive cardiac electrophysiology studies are rare, provided that high-risk patients, such as those with critical aortic stenosis, severe hyper-trophic obstructive cardiomyopathy, or left main or severe three-vessel coronary artery disease, are excluded after cardiac catheterization and coronary angiogra-phy performed prior to electrophysiologic testing. Similarly, patients with clinical-ly unstable myocardial ischemia and uncompensated clinical congestive heart failure should be excluded or rigorously treated prior to undergoing invasive stud-ies with programmed cardiac stimulation (PCS). Serious complications of diag-nostic invasive electrophysiology studies include vascular injury, pulmonary embolism, hemorrhage requiring transfusion therapy, cardiac chamber perfora-tion resulting in pericardial tamponade, sepsis from catheterization site abscess, myocardial infarction, stroke, and death (Table 3.1). Among 359 patients under-going 1062 procedures between 1977 and 1981 at the Massachusetts General Hospital, there were no reported deaths, and a morbidity rate per procedure of 1.9%. All complications were related to the catheterization process (thromboem-bolism, infections, pneumothorax, cardiac chamber perforation) rather than to PCS. Similarly, in a series of approximately 6500 procedures performed at the Hospital of the University of Pennsylvania, there was one reported death and less than a 2% complication rate .

Recently there has been a tremendous surge in the use of intracardiac mapping and transcatheter RF ablation. Compared with the mostly diagnostic nature of these early series involving only right heart catheterization, the present studies are much longer, involve administration of higher doses of sedative and analgesic agents, require more frequent catheterization of the left heart, longer periods of radiation exposure, and more frequent change of catheters. The excessive length of some of the RF ablation procedures may raise morbidity from vascular or thromboembolic complications or from increased risk of cardiac chamber rup-ture. Other risk factors may become relevant, for example, those associated with transseptal catheterization. Furthermore, although not yet reported in the litera-

Table 3.1
Complications of Invasive Cardiac Electrophysiology Studies

Associated with percutaneous catheterization of veins and arteries
    Pain
    Adverse drug reaction
    Infection/abscess at the catheterization site, sepsis
    Excessive bleeding, hematoma formation
    Thrombophlebitis
    Pulmonary thromboembolism
    Arterial damage, aortic dissection
    Systemic thromboembolism
    Transient ischemic attack/stroke

Associated with intracardiac catheters and programmed cardiac stimulation
    Cardiac chamber or coronary sinus perforation
    Hemopericardium, cardiac tamponade
    Atrial fibrillation
    Ventricular tachycardia/ventricular fibrillation
    Myocardial infarction
    Right or left bundle branch block

Associated with transcatheter ablation
    Complete heart block
    Valvular injury/new-onset valvular insufficiency
    Coronary artery thrombosis
    Exacerbation of cardiac arrhythmias
    Myocardial necrosis
    Pericarditis

Death resulting from one of the above complications

ture as part of any large series, isolated cases of procedure-related acquired aortic and mitral insufficiency have been noted. Systemic thromboembolic events, e.g., transient ischemic attacks, must be included in the list of rare but potential complications when the procedure includes transcatheter RF ablation of a left accessory pathway or a left ventricular site of VT origin. Heart block, a possible complication of certain types of transcatheter RF ablation procedures, is also much less of a concern, if at all, for the solely diagnostic studies. Finally, the long-term safety of transcatheter RF ablation, especially when an LV site is the target of RF ablation, during the 5–10 years following the procedure, has not been established and will need careful and detailed long-term follow-up before the entire risk can be fully elucidated.

In young patients with documented supraventricular tachycardias (SVT) or VT and with no evidence of structural heart disease by noninvasive studies, including echocardiography, an invasive electrophysiology study can be undertaken with exceedingly low risk. However, if the clinical presentation is prehospital cardiac arrest or ventricular tachycardia causing hemodynamic collapse, coronary angiography and contrast right and left ventriculography should be obtained prior to invasive electrophysiologic studies with programmed cardiac stimulation, even in a young patient with no evidence of structural heart disease by noninvasive workup. There may be two notable exceptions to this "rule of thumb": Wolff-Parkinson-White (WPW) syndrome with documented AF preceding VF, and congenital prolonged Q-T syndrome, where VF has a reasonably straightforward electrophysiologic explanation. Even then, the occurrence of VF in a patient with WPW syndrome should raise the suspicion of associated ventricular disease. In patients with known organic heart disease and highly symptomatic tachyarrhythmias, cardiac catheterization and coronary angiography should precede invasive electrophysiology studies with PCS.

ROLE OF INVASIVE CARDIAC ELECTROPHYSIOLOGY STUDIES IN DIAGNOSIS AND MANAGEMENT OF BRADYARRHYTHMIAS

Symptomatic bradyarrhythmias may be broadly categorized into disorders of impulse initiation in the sinus node, e.g., sinus arrest, and disorders of cardiac conduction system, e.g., complete heart block, while realizing that both disorders may well coexist in the same patient. Correlation of symptoms of cerebral ischemia, such as dizziness, presyncope, or syncope, with episodes of severe bradycardia or markedly long pauses, is required before prescribing pacemaker therapy. This is best confirmed by continuous or episodic ambulatory electrocardiography or event-recording electrocardiography, which may document the clinical bradyarrhythmia during the symptomatic period. Permanent third-degree heart block or constant, severe, and symptomatic bradycardia do not require further documentation and are accepted indications for pacemaker therapy. More often than not, however, the problem is episodic, and ambulatory ECG monitoring techniques do not have adequate sensitivity. In these cases, findings from an EP study may complement other clinical data by unmasking suspected but previously undocumented abnormal sinus impulse formation or AV conduction (Table 3.2).

Evaluation of Sinus Node Dysfunction

The methods of assessing sinus node function are indirect. Direct recordings of sinus node potentials have been reported and appear to correlate reasonably well with indirect measurements. However, they have not yet gained wide clinical application and presently should be regarded as an investigational technique. Sinus node recovery time (SNRT), as a measure of sinus node automaticity, and the sinoatrial conduction time (SACT), as an estimate of conduction through sinoatrial tissue, are the methods employed in the electrophysiology laboratory.

SINUS NODE RECOVERY TIME

The SNRT is estimated by pacing, for at least 1 minute, from a high right atrial site close to the sinus node and measuring the interval from the last paced atrial beat to the first spontaneous sinus beat. Pacing commences at a rate slightly faster than the spontaneous sinus rate and is repeated at decreasing cycle lengths while noting the longest recovery time. Full recovery of sinus node function is necessary

Table 3.2
Different Indications for Invasive Cardiac Electrophysiology Studies

A. Established indications
    Diagnosis and management of bradyarrhythmias
        To acquire corroborative data in symptomatic patients with episodic bradyarrhythmia
        To define the level of AV block
    Diagnosis and management of tachyarrhythmias
        To define the mechanism of narrow-complex tachycardia
        To define the mechanism of wide-complex tachycardia
        To reproduce clinically documented tachycardias for intracardiac mapping prior to
          nonpharmacologic therapy (transcatheter radio-frequency ablation, map-guided
          ventricular surgery, ICD)
        To induce (? any) sustained tachyarrthmia as an endpoint to direct pharmacologic therapy
          in patients with very rare spontaneous arrhythmias
    Assessment of the integrity of the conduction system and the presence of inducible sustained VT
        in patients with syncope of suspected cardiac origin
B. Investigational indications
    Evaluation and management of patients at high risk for sudden cardiac death
        Postmyocardial infarction
        Cardiomyopathy
        History of congestive heart failure

between the pacing trains and is ensured by allowing at least 1 minute of rest between the episodes. Pacing rates up to 200 beats/minute may be employed for improved sensitivity. The P wave morphology and intraatrial activation sequence of the atrial escape beats should be consistent with sinoatrial origin; findings to the contrary suggest a shift in the atrial pacemaker or ectopic atrial escape beat and not a true postoverdrive suppression recovery beat. The normal response is a post-pacing pause, not exceeding 1400 msec, with gradual return to the baseline cycle length over the ensuing 5–6 beats. Because the absolute recovery time is a function of the spontaneous basic cycle length (BCL), adjusted parameters such as the corrected sinus recovery time (CSNRT = SNRT – BCL) or normalized recovery time (SNRT/BCL), which are less than 550 msec and 150%, respectively, in normal subjects, are probably more reliable. Note that these corrections are less accurate at lower spontaneous rates. Less commonly used is the total recovery time (TRT), the time required for the cycle length to return to the baseline value, which is usually within 5–6 beats or less than 4–5 seconds.

In sinus node dysfunction the most frequent finding is a recovery time exceeding the accepted normal value. However, marked pauses following a normal recovery time (secondary pauses) and delayed return to baseline rate (prolonged total recovery time) are also consistent with this diagnosis. It has now become apparent that more complex mechanisms underlie sinus node recovery times, and the simple assumption that prolonged sinus node recovery times reflect abnormally prolonged overdrive suppression resulting from intrinsically abnormal sinus pacemaker cell automaticity is only partially valid. More correctly, SNRT represents the sum of the conduction time needed for the last paced atrial impulse to enter the sinus node and for the succeeding sinus impulse to leave the node, in addition to the delay induced from overdrive suppression of the sinus pacemaker cell. Likewise, the number of paced impulses entering the sinus node to suppress the pacemaker cells will depend on the inward conduction characteristics of the sinoatrial tissue because with sinoatrial entrance block occurring at faster pacing rates, there will be fewer impulses per unit time to suppress the pacemaker cells. Lastly, rapid atrial pacing may alter local atrial acetylcholine concentrations, induce shifts in the pacemaker cells in the sinus node complex, and change circulating catecholamine levels, secondary to hemodynamic alterations, all of which could modify sinus node automaticity and sinoatrial conduction (see discussion that follows). These are important shortcomings that limit the clinical utility of the technique.

SINOATRIAL CONDUCTION TIME

As with sinus node recovery times, sinoatrial (S-A) conduction is assessed indirectly in the electrophysiology laboratory by analyzing the response of the sinus node to atrial extrastimuli. Most commonly used is the Strauss technique, in which a single atrial extrastimulus (A2) is initially introduced at a coupling interval just shorter than the basic cycle length and repeated every 8–10 sinus beats (A1-A1). The coupling interval is decremented by 10–20 msec until atrial refractoriness is reached, while the tester notes the timing of the return beat (A3). Thus, as diastole is decrementally scanned, the return cycle (A2-A3) intervals are measured and noted to sequentially fall into several zones of response: zone of collision, zone of reset, zone of interpolation, and zone of S-A echoes. The response, which represents collision, does not provide information on S-A conduction because of failed penetration into the sinus node region. By contrast, an atrial extrastimulus in the reset zone is able to penetrate the sinoatrial junction, enter the sinus node, and reset the sinus pacemaker cells so that the return cycle (A2-A3) exceeds (A1-A1) but is less than fully compensatory, and the following spontaneous atrial depolarization (A3) arrives earlier than expected. Thus, (A1-A2) + (A2-A3) <2 (A1-A1). Reset confirms penetration into the node, and the return interval (A2-A3) is estimated to be the sum of S-A conduction into the sinus node (SACT retrograde), the reset basic cycle length (A1-A1), and conduction of the reset impulse from the sinus node to the atrial tissue (SACT antegrade). Therefore, with the assumption that antegrade and retrograde SACTs are equal, one way SACT is measured as (A2-A3) − (A1-A1)/2. Normal SACT times generally range from 40–60 to 70–150 msec, depending on the laboratory, with the upper limits of accepted normal showing marked variation from one laboratory to the next.

There are important limitations of this technique that result from similar assumptions made when measuring SNRT. The assumption that conduction into and out of the sinus node is equal may not be valid, and recent experimental data have shown that retrograde conduction may often be slower than antegrade conduction. This finding may necessitate the use of total SACT rather than SACT/2. In the presence of marked sinus arrhythmia, the technique just described is not reliable because it might not be possible to ascertain if the alteration of the return cycle length was caused by the premature atrial depolarization or was the result of spontaneous cycle length variation.

In summary, the techniques of assessing sinus node function in the electrophysiology laboratory are flawed by assumptions that limit the validity of the techniques used and hence their clinical utility. Furthermore, although abnormal measurements correlate in general to the severity of clinical abnormality in large samples, this correlation may break down in individual cases, causing both false-negative and false-positive results. Finally, the patients in whom sinus node function or perinodal tissue conduction is most severely disturbed are symptomatic and usually have electrocardiographic evidence of bradycardia-tachycardia syndrome or spontaneous sinoatrial exit block. There is nothing to be gained by further invasive studies in these patients. If, however, sinus bradycardia is the only finding, its specificity is low enough to warrant a search for additional data before pacemaker implantation. It is then appropriate to subject these patients to an invasive study. Even then, neither SNRT nor SACT measurement can be taken as a gold standard, and they must be interpreted in the setting of other findings, including the rate response to exercise and to pharmacologic agents, such as atropine and β-adrenergic blockers, before clinical decisions are made.

Evaluation of Atrioventricular Block and Other Conduction Disturbances

Failure of conduction through the AV junction may result in symptomatic and potentially fatal bradyarrhythmias. Invasive electrophysiologic studies have little to add to diagnosis or management if spontaneous third-degree heart block, Mobitz type II second-degree heart block, or trifascicular block is documented electrocardiographically in the symptomatic patient. Invasive electrophysiologic studies may yield useful diagnostic information when symptomatic AV block is suspected, but because of its episodic nature cannot be documented by electrocardiography. Under these circumstances, His bundle recording and programmed atrial stimulation may unmask severe latent conduction system disease and, more importantly, define the level of AV conduction disturbance.

The adequacy of AV conduction is established by measuring conduction velocity and refractory periods. Conduction velocity is assessed indirectly in the electrophysiologic laboratory by measuring conduction intervals. The baseline His bundle electrogram recording provides information about AV nodal (A-H), His (H), and infra-Hissian or His-Purkinje (H-V) conduction intervals. As noted earlier, intrinsic disease of the special conduction tissue, as well as extrinsic influences, may result in abnormal prolongation of these intervals. The refractoriness of the conduction tissue is also quantitated. The relative refractory period (RRP) and effective refractory period (ERP) relate to measurements at the level of tissue input, i.e., refractoriness at the site of stimulation. The RRP is defined as the longest coupling interval of the premature extrastimulus, resulting in a fully propagated impulse but with slowed conduction. The ERP is the longest coupling interval, resulting in failure to generate a propagated impulse. The functional refractory period (FRP) of a particular cardiac tissue, on the other hand, is the minimum possible interval between two consecutively conducted beats as measured in the tissue immediately distal to it. Defined as such, it reflects tissue output because the measured intervals are remote from the site of stimulation.

ACQUIRED ATRIOVENTRICULAR BLOCK

Failure of an atrial depolarization to conduct to the ventricles, associated with the absence of a His bundle depolarization following the local atrial electrogram on the corresponding intracardiac His bundle recording, localizes the block at the AV node. Presence of a His bundle signal fragmented into separate proximal and distal components, the so-called "split His potential," or a single His potential with no ensuing ventricular depolarization, localizes the conduction disturbance at the His bundle or distal to the His bundle, respectively. If there is complete AV dissociation and the surface QRS complex is narrow, then His bundle recordings almost always demonstrate a His deflection before each ventricular depolarization. If there is bundle branch block, demonstration of a local His bundle electrogram preceding each ventricular complex, with a normal or borderline prolonged H-V interval, indicates an escape rhythm originating in the His bundle with aberrant conduction, which is more stable and reliable compared with a ventricular escape rhythm originating from a more distal His-Purkinje site. This distinction usually cannot be made electrocardiographically.

However, the combination of the electrocardiographic documentation of high-grade AV block and symptoms usually dictate therapy. Indeed, invasive electrophysiology studies have a very limited, if any, diagnostic role in patients with conduction disorders of this type. The studies may be helpful in selected situations such as 2:1 AV block, where insight into the precise site of block may influence therapy. If the block is intra- or infra-Hissian, pacemaker therapy, even in the absence of symptoms or with mild symptoms, may be indicated. If the His bundle electrogram is fragmented into a proximal and a distal component, unmasking of intra-His block by an atrial extrastimulus (proximal component present with no recorded distal component and no ventricular depolarization) is a rare but extremely specific finding that warrants pacemaker therapy. Even more rarely, His bundle recordings can diagnose pseudo-AV block, where spontaneous depolarizations that are not apparent on the surface ECG may arise from the His bundle, fail to conduct antegradely to the ventricle because of the refractoriness of the His-Purkinje conduction, and additionally prevent the proper conduction of the subsequent sinus impulse via the AV node, thus masquerading as type II AV block.

CHRONIC INTRAVENTRICULAR CONDUCTION DISTURBANCE

Patients who show true evidence of trifascicular disease on the surface ECG, i.e., right bundle branch block alternating with left bundle branch block or right bundle branch block with alternating left anterior hemiblock and left posterior hemiblock in the absence of changing antiarrhythmic drugs, do not need EP evaluation of the His-Purkinje conduction system per se, as they already have clear evidence of disease in all three fascicles.

Chronic bifascicular block is associated with mortality, even in patients who are asymptomatic. The mortality is cardiovascular in general and not from late complete heart block and reflects the usual presence of extensive organic heart disease associated with chronic bifascicular block. His bundle recordings may be of use in patients with chronic bifascicular block in predicting the risk of developing complete heart block. Finding a prolonged H-V interval in such patients signifies conduction disease in all three fascicles. An H-V interval of ≥100 msec has been found to be a useful predictor of later developing high-grade AV block over a mean follow-up period of 2 years. If there is first-degree AV block in addition to chronic bifascicular block, a His bundle recording determines whether the delay is in the AV node or in the His-Purkinje system. However, it is not clear that, based on information from an EP study, permanent pacemaker therapy in patients with even a grossly prolonged H-V interval is indicated. First, it is not certain that every asymptomatic patient with these findings, i.e., bifascicular block and prolonged H-V interval, is going to develop complete heart block. Moreover, it is unlikely that cardiovascular mortality can be substantially lowered by permanent pacing in this population. Mortality in this group of patients results mostly from other events, such as ventricular tachyarrhythmias, congestive heart failure, and recurrent ischemic events.

The AV conduction system can be stressed to reveal its functional reserve during an electrophysiology study. Rapid atrial pacing, which results in distal infra-His conduction block during 1:1 AV nodal conduction, has been shown to have prognostic importance for subsequent AV block in patients with bundle branch block, although this finding occurs with a low frequency. Administration of atropine to decrease the functional refractory period of the AV node allows more strenuous testing of the His-Purkinje system. However, absence of pacing-induced distal block has not been a dependable negative predictor of subsequent advanced AV block. Another method used to stress the AV conduction system is administration of intravenous (i.v.) procainamide, which increases conduction time in the His-Purkinje system. Infusion of up to 10 mg/kg of procainamide, while in sinus rhythm, may induce second- or third-degree distal AV block in patients with bifascicular block suspected of having intermittent advanced AV block.

Clearly, EP testing is limited in its applicability in this group of patients. In one study, only two of the 13 patients with clinically documented intermittent high-grade AV block (2 with 2:1 AV block and 11 with complete heart block) were shown to have AV conduction abnormalities when studied in the electrophysiology laboratory at a later date while in sinus rhythm, even when the techniques utilized during the electrophysiologic evaluation included baseline conduction interval determination and incremental atrial pacing before and after atropine, as well as before and after procainamide administration.

In contrast to the asymptomatic patients, those presenting with syncope or presyncopal episodes, and whose ECGs manifest bifascicular block but no other abnormality, should have an electrophysiologic study. A markedly prolonged H-V interval at rest or demonstration of intra- or infra-His block during atrial pacing or extrastimulation enhances the specificity of the electrocardiographic intraventricular conduction disturbance and may be an indication for permanent pacemaker therapy.

INVASIVE CARDIAC ELECTROPHYSIOLOGY IN THE ASSESSMENT AND MANAGEMENT OF TACHYARRHYTHMIAS

Narrow QRS Tachycardia

Narrow QRS tachycardia is almost always supraventricular in origin and in only the rarest cases, life-threatening when there is no structural heart disease. The need for invasive electrophysiologic study for a documented narrow complex tachycardia is basically reserved for its diagnostic and therapeutic role in the relief of incapacitating symptoms, and this role has increased substantially since the advent of transcatheter RF ablation. However, even if inclination is toward pharmacologic therapy for symptoms, there is always a benefit to be gained from understanding the underlying mechanism with precision for optimal treatment.

A previously published series showed that the mechanism of a regular, narrow complex tachycardia could be correctly predicted from the 12-lead ECG taken during the tachycardia in 85% of the patients. Thus, although the majority of the narrow complex tachycardias can be diagnosed correctly, provided that a 12-lead ECG can be obtained during the SVT, the incidence of correct diagnosis becomes nearly 100% after an invasive cardiac electrophysiology study. Other uses of invasive cardiac electrophysiology studies in the setting of narrow QRS tachycardia include serial electropharmacologic testing, which may be useful in finding an effective antiarrhythmic drug in patients with supraventricular tachycardia by demonstrating the effect of the drugs on the tachycardia mechanism, refractory periods, ease of electrical induction, and tachycardia rate, among other things. However, serial drug testing is being used less and less as transcatheter RF ablation techniques become more widespread. When nonpharmacologic ablative treatment is being contemplated, invasive electrophysiologic evaluation is critical to confirm the suspected mechanisms of the tachycardia and to exclude other mechanisms.

Electrophysiologic Studies in Supraventricular Tachycardia

Programmed atrial and ventricular stimulation, activation sequence mapping during supraventricular tachycardia, pacing maneuvers, such as resetting the circuit with properly timed extrastimuli during the tachycardia, and observation of the electrophysiologic consequences of pharmacologic intervention during pacing or spontaneous tachycardia will, in almost all cases, allow the diagnosis of the supraventricular tachycardia mechanism. However, before undertaking a diagnostic invasive electrophysiologic study, as much information as possible should be gathered by reviewing the 12-lead surface ECG and recordings of the clinical tachycardia when available. A-V relationship, with RP/PR ratio, demonstration of AV block, and of bundle branch block with associated cycle length alterations during tachycardia are all important observations that provide insight into possible underlying mechanism. In atrial fibrillation and typical or atypical atrial flutter, diagnostic electrophysiologic studies are generally not needed, unless the ventricular response is regular, QRS is wide, and exclusion of other diagnoses, such as VT, is needed (see discussion that follows).

An intracardiac electrophysiology study is indicated when SVT is associated with severe symptoms such as syncope or presyncopal episodes. An invasive electrophysiology study in a markedly symptomatic patient is even more strongly indicated when the resting ECG manifests the pattern of preexcitation with a δ wave or a short PR interval without a δ wave. Similarly, in patients with underlying organic heart disease who develop angina or acute heart failure during their arrhythmia, the SVT mechanism should be studied, even if its rate is relatively low.

TECHNIQUES FOR INVESTIGATING SUPRAVENTRICULAR TACHYCARDIAS

To perform a comprehensive diagnostic study for supraventricular tachycardia, electrode catheters are placed in the RA, His bundle position, RV apex, and the coronary sinus. These catheters record local electrograms from widely disparate areas of the heart: high right atrium, septal right atrium, His bundle, left atrium, left ventricle, and right ventricle, and suffice to make the diagnosis of SVT with certainty in the vast majority of cases. In more complex SVT mechanisms and in patients undergoing mapping and transcatheter ablation, additional, usually deflectable, mapping catheters are added to locate the sites of earliest activity or to record special potentials, such as accessory pathway potentials, AV nodal slow pathway potentials, right bundle potentials, and mid-diastolic potentials.

Programmed atrial stimulation is usually from the high right atrium, though in certain situations a second atrial site such as coronary sinus pacing is also employed. One and sometimes two atrial extrastimuli with progressively shorter coupling intervals are delivered following a train of eight or more drive beats at several cycle lengths until atrial refractoriness is encountered. Incremental atrial pacing in steps of 10 msec is also performed until second-degree AV block develops. During atrial pacing, AV conduction is carefully analyzed. Premature atrial extrastimuli and incremental atrial pacing may uncover disparate conduction velocities and refractory periods of the tissues responsible for the tachycardias. Ventricular preexcitation may be unmasked during atrial premature stimulation or during i.v. adenosine administration. Ventricular preexcitation in the presence of a fixed AV interval would suggest an AV accessory pathway, whereas preexcitation occurring in association with progressive increasing AV delay with a greater degree of A-H prolongation would suggest a decremental or Mahaim-type AV connection. Demonstration of antegrade dual AV nodal pathways would suggest AVNRT. Even in the absence of preexcitation and dual pathway physiology, the pattern of decremental conduction through the AV node may show marked variation from one individual to the next. Localization of the site of critical delay required for the initiation of supraventricular tachycardia identifies the mechanism and the site of the tachycardia. Critical intraatrial delay suggests sinus node reentrant tachycardia or intraatrial reentrant tachycardia (IART). Critical prolongation of the A-H interval, especially a sudden increment in A-H duration of ;≥50 msec in response to 10–20-msec shortening of the coupling interval, followed by an atrial echo beat, suggests AVNRT. AV reciprocating tachycardia may also require critical delay, but this may be intraatrial, in the AV node, in the His-Purkinje system, or in more than one tissue.

When tachycardia is induced by atrial stimulation, several important observations and maneuvers could be used to diagnose the mechanism with certainty. AVRT requires an obligatory 1:1 P-to-QRS ratio and will not sustain in the presence of AV (or VA) block. On the other hand, SNRT, IART, and atrial flutter (AFL) are likely to continue despite AV block. AV nodal reentry also manifests 1:1 AV ratio in the vast majority of cases, although, extremely rarely, atria or ventricles may be dissociated from the tachycardia circuit. Simultaneous or nearly simultaneous P and QRS activation is seen with typical AVNRT. In AVRT and in certain forms of AVNRT, the P wave follows the QRS and is usually within the first half of the R-R interval. In atypical AVNRT, and rarely in AVRT with a decrementally conducting retrograde pathway, the P follows the QRS and may be in the second half of the R-R interval.

The atrial activation sequence during the tachycardia is important. In SNRT, a high-low and right-to-left atrial activation pattern is seen, and the interatrial septum depolarizes in an anterocranial to posterocaudal direction as during a sinus beat. In IART atrial activation will usually manifest a radial spread from the focus of arrhythmogenesis, which can be located practically anywhere in the atria. However, in certain forms of AT, as well as in typical and atypical flutter, clockwise or counterclockwise rotating macroreentry circuits may be detected with the use of special catheters enabling dense mapping. In typical AVNRT the atrial activation is low-to-high septal, with the site of earliest atrial activation at the anterior interatrial septum close to the site of His bundle recording. In atypical AVNRT the atrial activation is also low to high, but with site of earliest atrial activation observed close to or within the os of the coronary sinus or at posterocaudal interatrial septum. In orthodromic AVRT the retrograde atrial activation is eccentric and originates at the site of atrial insertion of the accessory pathway. In antidromic AVRT, the retrograde atrial activation is low to high and midline because VA conduction is usually, but not always, via the H-P and AV nodal tissue. The electrophysiology study will also reveal the presence of a second accessory pathway if the proper observations are carried out. The appearance of bundle branch block during SVT with an associated increase in the tachycardia cycle length and in the ventriculoatrial interval is diagnostic of an ipsilateral retrogradely conducting accessory pathway. Introduction of synchronized atrial or ventricular extrastimuli may further confirm the reentrant mechanism and site of the tachycardia. When properly timed, such extrastimuli will enter the reentrant circuit ahead of the circulating wave of activation and advance (reset) the tachycardia. During tachycardia, if a ventricular extrastimulus synchronized with His bundle depolarization advances the following atrial electrogram and resets the SVT cycle, the presence of an extranodal AV connection is confirmed.

The assessment of VA conduction is also important in the study of supraventricular tachycardia. This is performed by ventricular extrastimulus and incremental pacing. Absence of VA conduction makes AVRT or AVNRT less likely and suggests an atrial tachycardia because the latter is independent of retrograde VA conduction. If VA conduction recovers with atropine or isoproterenol, AVNRT still remains a likely mechanism. Retrograde atrial activation during ventricular pacing may suggest the presence of an accessory pathway, if eccentric activation is noted, e.g., left atrial activation prior to interatrial septal or right atrial activation. In particular situations, administration of pharmacologic agents may be of help. Selectively blocking AV nodal conduction with adenosine may unmask latent accessory pathway conduction. Atropine or isoproterenol may be used to facilitate the induction of AVNRT or AVRT by widening of the "tachycardia zone," or the section of the cardiac cycle during which extrastimuli cause the necessary block and the critical delay to initiate reentrant activation.

Electrophysiologic Studies in Ventricular Tachycardia

In a patient with documented or suspected ventricular tachycardia (VT), the decision to proceed with an invasive cardiac electrophysiology study, as well as the stimulation protocol to be used, depends on the specific reason for which the study is requested. In addition to being a diagnostic test for precise classification of wide-complex tachycardia, the electrophysiology study may be used to investigate the etiology for syncope or severely symptomatic palpitations when VT has not been documented but suspected. In other patients, the clinician may try to use VT induction and suppression of induced VT as a guide for antiarrhythmic drug therapy. In yet others, PCS may be used to reproduce the previously documented clinical VT to assess the feasibility of nonpharmacologic therapies. For each of these different indications, the utility of cardiac electrophysiology studies is also a function of the underlying heart disease.

The standard procedure is to use bipolar pacing with a stimulation current that is twice the diastolic threshold value and a pulse width of 1 or 2 msec. Use of increased current strength for ventricular stimulation has been proposed on the basis that the associated decrease in ventricular refractory period would allow closer coupling of the extrastimuli, thereby increasing the yield of induced arrhythmias that might be accepted endpoints for the stimulation protocol; however, studies have shown a loss of specificity because of an increase in the chances of inducing previously unobserved polymorphic VT.

Different protocols exist for ventricular stimulation studies. These protocols differ in (a) electrical stimulation, (b) basic drive cycle and number of premature ventricular extrastimuli, and (c) number of sites of stimulation. Examples of adequate protocols (90% sensitivity) for VT induction, as outlined by the North American Society of Pacing and Electrophysiology (NASPE) in their 1985 report, are that which use a basic drive train of at least eight captured beats immediately followed by single, double, and if necessary, triple ventricular extrastimuli that scan electrical diastole. At least two drive trains, which differ by at least 20 beats/minute, are recommended for stimulation at the RV apex, followed by stimulation at the RV outflow tract. At least three drive trains at cycle lengths of 600, 500, and 400 msec are suggested if only the RV apex is being stimulated, although data suggest that the additional yield of a third cycle length after the first two cycle lengths is low. Left ventricular stimulation is an option, depending on the clinical circumstances, and is more commonly used if the intention is to perform activation sequence mapping for nonpharmacologic therapy. Asynchronous ventricular burst pacing for VT induction is not recommended, although a possible role may exist for synchronous burst pacing, which is less likely to induce VF.

Isoproterenol infusion during ventricular stimulation has been reported to increase the yield of VT induction and thereby the sensitivity of the technique. Isoproterenol is more commonly used for induction of "idiopathic" VT or VT of nonischemic cardiomyopathy and may be absolutely necessary for successfully inducing VT based on triggered activity. Isoproterenol is usually contraindicated if there is advanced coronary artery disease. In triggered VT and very rarely in reentrant VT, atrial pacing has also been effective in VT induction. Maintaining the extrastimulus intervals at 180 msec or greater during ventricular stimulation is a commonly accepted precaution to minimize the incidence of inducing polymorphic VT or VF, which may be endpoints of low clinical relevance, except in the patient with prehospital cardiac arrest. However, this point is controversial and has not been sufficiently investigated.

The ventricular arrhythmias induced by programmed ventricular stimulation include sustained VT (Fig. 3.2), nonsustained VT, monomorphic VT, polymorphic VT, VF, repetitive ventricular responses, and bundle branch reentry.

Variability exists in the reproducibility of VT induction by PCS and is a function of the stimulation protocol, the particular arrhythmia induced, and the underlying heart disease. Generally the short- and long-term reproducibility is high if two or three ventricular extrastimuli are used and the patient has structural heart disease secondary to coronary artery disease. One study reported 91% success in immediate reproduction of a second induced sustained VT episode after the first induction, and a 100% success of initiating a third episode after two previous inductions in patients with sustained monomorphic VT. The reproducibility of the induction technique itself was 81% after one induction and 88% after two inductions. It is important to recognize that these figures apply to induction of any sustained monomorphic VT and not necessarily to the same electrocardiographic VT morphology. Especially in the setting of advanced organic heart disease, it is common to induce several sustained monomorphic VTs with distinct surface ECG morphologies in the same patient (pleiomorphism). Although pleiomorphism of spontaneously recurrent VT is also a clinically observed phenomenon, the relationship between multiple clinical and multiple induced ECG morphologies has not been sufficiently investigated.

Finally, PCS protocols for VT must not be rigid and should be selected and modified, depending primarily on the clinical presentation (e.g., monomorphic VT vs. syncope), underlying heart disease (e.g., ischemic heart disease vs. no structural heart disease), and the indication for the study (e.g., defining an endpoint for drug therapy vs. nonpharmacologic intervention).

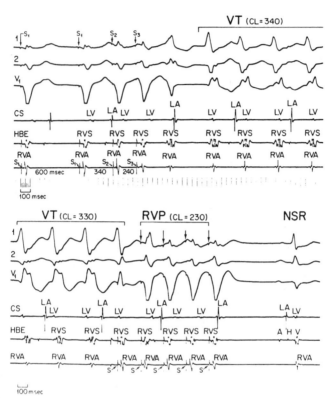

Figure 3.2. The *top panel* shows initiation of sustained monomorphic ventricular tachycardia (VT) by two programmed premature extrastimuli (S_2S_3). There is V-A dissociation during VT. In the *bottom panel*, a train of rapid ventricular pacing (RVP) results in ventricular capture with a cycle length (CL) shorter than that of VT and results in VT termination with resumption of normal sinus rhythm (NSR).

SUGGESTED READING

Akhtar M, Sheasa M, Jazayeri M, et al. Wide QRS tachycardia: reappraisal of a common clinical problem. Ann Intern Med 1988;109: 905–912.

Horowitz LN. Safety of electrophysiologic studies. Circulation 1986;73:11–28.

Horowitz L, Josephson M, Farshidi A, Spielman S, Michelson E, Greenspan A. Recurrent sustained ventricular tachycardia. III. Role of electrophysiologic study in selection of antiarrhythmic regimens. Circulation 1978;58: 986–997.

Mason J, Winkle R. Accuracy of the ventricular tachycardia induction study for predicting the long term efficacy and inefficacy of antiarrhythmic drugs. N Engl J Med 1980;303:607–613.

Prystowsky E. Electrophysiologic-electropharmacologic testing on patients with ventricular arrhythmias. PACE 1988;11:225–251.

Waldo AL, Akhtar M, Brugada P, et al. The minimally appropriate electrophysiologic study for the initial assessment of patients with documented sustained monomorphic ventricular tachycardia. J Am Coll Cardiol 1985;6:1174–1177.

Wellens H, Brugada P, Bar F. Indications for the use of intracardiac electrophysiologic studies for the diagnosis of site of origin and mechanism of tachycardias. Circulation 1987;75(suppl III):110–115.

Wilber D, Garan H, Finkelstein D, et al. Use of electrophysiologic testing in the prediction of long-term outcome. N Engl J Med 1988;318: 19–24.

Zipes D, Akhtar M, Denes P, et al. Guidelines for clinical intracardiac electrophysiology studies. A report of the American College of Cardiology/American Heart Association Task Force on Assessment of Diagnostic and Therapeutic Cardiovascular Procedures (Subcommittee to Assess Clinical Intracardiac Electrophysiologic Studies). Circulation 1989;80:1925–1939.

Zipes D, Rahimtoola S. State-of-the-Art Consensus Conference on Electrophysiologic Testing in the Diagnosis and Treatment of Patients with Cardiac Arrhythmia. Circulation 1987;75(suppl III):1–199.

4   Pharmacologic Principles of Antiarrhythmic Drugs

PHARMACODYNAMICS

Pharmacodynamics defines the mechanism of action of a drug and the relationship between the concentration of drug at the site of action and the effect produced. For antiarrhythmic drugs, pharmacologic effects are mediated primarily by actions at the myocardial cell membrane. Sites of action include various membrane ion channels and adrenergic, cholinergic, and purinergic receptors.

Antiarrhythmic drugs are frequently classified according to prominent electrophysiologic effects. The most widely used classification was originated by Vaughan Williams. This system, shown in Table 4.1, categorizes drug effects into four general classes. Class I drugs block rapid inward sodium channels. The avidity of binding of these drugs varies with different stages of the action potential. Lidocaine and mexiletine appear to bind more strongly to "inactive" channels during the plateau phase of the action potential. Drugs that prolong action potential duration (and the duration of the plateau phase) theoretically would enhance the efficacy of lidocaine or mexiletine. This phenomenon is believed to be responsible for the enhanced efficacy of the combination of mexiletine and quinidine as compared with the individual drugs alone. Classes III and IV are described by effects of drugs on other membrane ion channels. Class III drugs block outward potassium channels, thus slowing repolarization of the cell and prolonging action potential duration. Class IV drugs block slow inward calcium channels, with resultant depressant effects on tissue, in which depolarization of the cells is predominantly caused by those currents, including the sinoatrial (SA) and atrioventricular (AV) nodes. Class II drugs are defined by their inhibition of β-adrenoreceptors.

The Vaughan Williams classes correlate reasonably well with specific membrane effects of the drugs. However, this classification system has a number of shortcomings. First, it does not take into account the presence of multiple effects produced by a single drug. For example, quinidine has effects of both class I and class III drugs, sotalol has effects from both classes II and III, and amiodarone has properties of all four drug classes. Second, drugs within a given class can produce quite disparate "secondary" effects. For example, some class I drugs block more than one type of ion channel, and the kinetics of the interaction of these drugs with the sodium channel can vary widely. The subdivision of class I drugs into three subclasses (classes Ia, Ib, and Ic), based on electrocardiographic effects of the drugs, corrects for much of this variability (Table 4.1). Finally, this classification does not take into account active metabolites, which may have disparate effects from their "parent" drugs. For example, procainamide blocks inward sodium channels and outward potassium channels, making it a class Ia drug. In contrast, its major metabolite, N-acetylprocainamide (NAPA, acecainide), blocks

Table 4.1
Classification of Antiarrhythmic Drugs

Class	ECG Effect	Membrane Effect	Examples	Arrhythmias Treated
Ia	↑ QRS, ↑ Q-T	Na^+ channel block, intermediate kinetics K^+ channel block	Quinidine Procainamide Disopyramide	SVT AF VT
Ib	↓ Q-T	Na^+ channel block, rapid kinetics	Lidocaine Tocainide Mexiletine	VT
Ic	↑↑ QRS	Na^+ channel block, slow kinetics	Fleicainide Propafenone ?Moricizine	SVT AF VT
II	↓ HR, ↑ P-R	β-Receptor inhibition	Propranolol and others	SVT AF*
III	↑ Q-T	K^+ channel block	NAPA Sotalol Amiodarone	SVT AF VT
IV	↓ HR, ↑ P-R	Ca^{++} channel block	Verapamil Diltiazem	SVT AF*
Digitalis	↑ P-R, ↓ Q-T	Na^+, K^+-ATPase inhibition	Digoxin Digoxin	SVT AF*
Adenosine	↓ HR, ↑ PR	Purinergic receptor agonist	Adenosine	SVT

^{a}↑, increase; ↓, decrease; HR, heart rate; SVT, supraventricular tachycardia; AF, atrial fibrillation/flutter; AF*, atrial fibrillation/flutter (control of ventricular response); VT, ventricular tachycardia and other ventricular arrhythmias.

outward potassium channels but has no effect on inward sodium currents, making NAPA a class III drug. The type of pharmacologic effect produced during procainamide therapy depends to an extent on the relative concentrations of procainamide and NAPA, which are in turn dependent on such factors as renal function and genetically determined drug metabolism pathways.

Despite its shortcomings, the Vaughan Williams classification scheme does provide a useful shorthand for describing antiarrhythmic drug effects. Drugs within a given class have similar antiarrhythmic efficacy for specific types of arrhythmias. The classes also predict some types of drug toxicity. For example, a drug slowing conduction (class I, III, or IV) would be ill-advised in patients with extensive underlying conduction disease, and a drug-prolonging Q-T interval (class Ia or III) could present an excessive proarrhythmia risk in a patient with preexisting Q-T prolongation.

Adenosine and digitalis produce antiarrhythmic effects that are not described in the Vaughan Williams classification scheme. Adenosine stimulates a specific receptor, A1, which is coupled by inhibitory G proteins to adenyl cyclase and to the time-dependent outward potassium channel. Cardiac effects of adenosine include S-A and AV node depression. Adenosine effect is blocked by the methyl-xanthines caffeine and theophylline.

Digitalis mediates its effects through both direct and indirect routes. Digitalis-induced blockade of Na^+, K^+-ATPase causes an increase in intracellular sodium concentration and, indirectly, an increase in intracellular calcium concentration. (Increased intracellular sodium concentration leads to reduced exchange of extracellular sodium for intracellular calcium.) In addition, digitalis also appears to directly increase inward calcium currents and to shorten action potential duration. These effects lead to enhanced myocardial contractility and reduced AV node conduction.

Indirect effects of digitalis are mediated through the autonomic nervous system. At therapeutic concentrations, digitalis increases efferent vagal tone and reduces efferent sympathetic activity. This results in reduced sinus rate, increased atrial rate during atrial fibrillation (AF) and flutter (due to shortened atrial refractory period), and reduced AV conduction. The combination of an increase in atrial rate and a reduction in AV node conduction slows down the ventricular rate during AF and flutter. Also, treatment of supraventricular tachycardia with digitalis is based on the AV node-slowing effects of the drug. At toxic digitalis concentrations, sympathetic activity is enhanced, phase IV automaticity is increased, and delayed afterdepolarizations are produced, with a resultant increase in ventricular arrhythmia.

Antiarrhythmic drug effects can be altered in a variety of circumstances, including hypoxia, ischemia, acidosis, electrolyte disorder, and conditions of high sympathetic tone. The common thread of many of these effects is a change in resting membrane potential. The resting membrane potential of atrial and ventricular myocytes and Purkinje fibers is dependent in large part on the relative concentrations of potassium inside and outside the cell. In the presence of increased extracellular potassium concentrations, as are seen in the presence of ischemia, acidosis, or hyperkalemia, the cell membrane becomes partially depolarized. This causes a change in configuration of some fast sodium channels from an excitable state to an inexcitable state. As a result, the magnitude of the inward sodium current during cell excitation is reduced. This leads to reduced conduction velocity in surrounding tissues. Because antiarrhythmic drugs will block some remaining excitable sodium channels, conduction will be slowed by these drugs to a greater extent than usual in these circumstances and conduction block may be more likely. In the presence of hypokalemia, duration of the action potential is prolonged, and proarrhythmia related to long Q-T intervals may be seen in patients receiving class Ia antiarrhythmic drugs.

In the presence of catecholamines, there is an increase in intracellular calcium. In some circumstances, this can lead to delayed afterdepolarizations and resultant proarrhythmia. This situation is similar to the proarrhythmia seen during digitalis intoxication. Also, increased intracellular calcium levels cause enhanced depolarization of calcium-dependent tissues such as sinus and AV nodes, with resultant increase in heart rate and conduction. Thus, catecholamines can reduce the effectiveness of calcium channel blockers and β-adrenergic blockers.

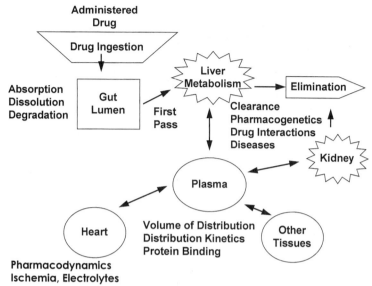

Figure 4.1. Pharmacokinetic factors to be considered from drug ingestion to pharmacologic effect to elimination.

PHARMACOKINETICS

Pharmacokinetics describes the relationship between drug dose and plasma concentration over time. Because drug effect is usually related to plasma concentration, pharmacokinetic data can be extrapolated to predict the time course of drug effect. Pharmacokinetic analysis of a drug encompasses all elements of its absorption into the body, distribution to various body tissues, metabolism, and elimination (Fig. 4.1). Pharmacokinetic parameters for antiarrhythmic drugs are listed in Table 4.2.

Absorption

Absorption is defined as the passage of unchanged drug from the gut lumen to the systemic circulation. The efficiency of absorption is defined by the term bioavailability, which is defined as the portion of administered drug that reaches the systemic circulation unchanged. By definition, a drug given intravenously is 100% bioavailable. However, for an orally administered drug to be bioavailable, it must be released into the gut lumen, passed through the gut wall into the portal circulation, and circulated through the liver unchanged.

The release of drug into the gut lumen can be profoundly influenced by the formulation of the drug. Most drugs are formulated as tablets, which must break down in the stomach or intestine for drug to be released. The methods of making these tablets can have important effects on drug release. For example, in a classic report by Lindenbaum et al. in 1971, the bioavailability of different formulations

Table 4.2
Pharmacokinetics of Antiarrhythmic Drugs[a]

	Major Route of Elimination	Elimination Half-life	Protein Binding	Active Metabolites
Quinidine	Hepatic (50–90%) Renal (10–30%)	7–18 hr	85–95%	3-OH-Quinidine
Procainamide	Hepatic (40–70%) Renal (30–60%)	2.5–4.7 hr	15%	N-Acetyl procainamide
Disopyramide	Renal (36–77%) Hepatic (11–37%)	7–9 hr	Dose-dependent 20–60%	Mono-N-dealkyl disopyramide
Lidocaine	Hepatic (90%)	1.5–4 hr	70%	MEGX, GX[b]
Mexiletine	Hepatic (90%)	8–12 hr	70%	
Tocainide	Renal (50–60%) Hepatic (40–50%)	12–15 hr	10%	
Flecainide	Hepatic (70%) Renal (25%)	11 hr	40–60%	
Encainide	Hepatic (90%)	2–9 hr[a]	70%	ODE, MODE
Propafenone	Hepatic (99%)	2–32 hr[a]	90%	5-OH-Propafenone
Moricizine	Hepatic (90%)	6–13 hr	76–96%	Probable
Bretylium	Renal (90%)	4–16 hr	<10%	
Sotalol	Renal (90%)	10–20 hr	0%	
Amiodarone	Hepatic (99%)	3–15 wk	99.9%	Desethyl amiodarone
Verapamil	Hepatic (70%)	4 hr	90%	Norverapamil
Diltiazem	Hepatic (90%)	3–5 hr	78%	Desacetyl and demethyldiltiazem
Adenosine	Vascular, endothlium, erythrocytes	<10 sec		
Digoxin	Renal (60%)	30–50 hr	25%	

[a]Inherited variability in metabolism.
[b]MGEX, monoethylglycyllxylidide; GX, glycylxylidide; ODE, O-desmethylencainide; MODE, methoxy-O-desmethyl-encainide.

of digoxin was found to vary from 40–90%. Much of this variability was related to differences of dissolution of different manufacturers' preparations. Because of that experience with digoxin, more rigid standards were developed for "equivalency" of generic drugs. However, there is still potential for significant differences between formulations. Therefore, when using a drug with a narrow therapeutic margin, it is advisable to avoid changing preparations after a satisfactory dosage has been determined.

The problems of drug release from sustained-release preparations are more complex. First, there is no clear standard for generic equivalency of these preparations. Because of this, if it is necessary to change from one sustained-release preparation to another, it is wise to confirm adequate drug levels and antiarrhythmic response after the change. Second, in evaluating these sustained-release formulations, one must assess not only the extent of drug release but also the time course of release. A formulation with very slow release may not be completely released during the transit through the bowel, particularly in situations associated with rapid gastrointestinal transit time. For example, bioavailability of one sustained-release procainamide preparation was found to be markedly reduced in patients with a colostomy. If adequate drug effect or plasma concentration cannot be achieved with sustained-release preparations, use of a standard-release preparation may be more effective.

The switch from a standard preparation to a slow-release preparation of an antiarrhythmic agent can be problematic, as there are no clear guidelines for dosage equivalence of standard and sustained-release preparations of quinidine, procainamide, and propranolol. For these drugs, it is best to treat the sustained-release preparation as a totally new drug and to perform dose titration and assess response accordingly. For disopyramide and verapamil, the usual recommendation is that the drugs be kept at the same total daily dosage, with first dose of the sustained-release preparation given 6–12 hours after the last dose of standard formulation. During any formulation change, it is important to verify that the response is maintained and that there is no significant change in plasma concentrations of drug after the change.

Drug Distribution

After absorption, the drug is distributed to the various tissues of the body. The pattern of drug distribution immediately after administration of an intravenous (i.v.) bolus is largely dependent on the perfusion of different tissues. Initially a drug goes into plasma and highly perfused tissues such as heart, liver, brain, and kidney. These tissues can be conceptualized as comprising a central compartment, which is the initial volume into which a drug distributes. The drug may redistribute from the central compartment, to other tissues, or to sites of metabolism and elimination (Fig. 4.2). Drug redistribution to less perfused tissues such as muscle, skin, and adipose tissue occurs later, after drug administration. These less perfused tissues make up peripheral compartments. For some drugs, there is very slow distribution to some tissues, which comprise the deep compartment. The relative concentrations of drug in these various compartments ultimately reach an equilibrium, termed steady state.

The pharmacokinetic compartments are mathematical entities and do not correspond closely with specific physiologic entities. They are useful in predicting the time course of plasma concentrations after administration of a drug, but do not necessarily allow prediction of drug concentration in specific organs.

The plasma concentration achieved after administration of a given dose of drug is dependent on the volume into which it is diluted. The volume of distribution is a theoretical volume that describes the relationship between dose and plasma con-

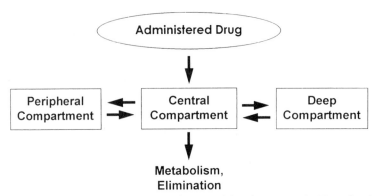

Figure 4.2. Pharmacokinetic compartments. Administered drug first enters a highly perfused central compartment and is then redistributed to peripheral compartments and more slowly equilibrating deep compartments.

centration and is usually expressed as a function of body weight (e.g., liter/kg). The magnitude of the volume of distribution is dependent on (*a*) the perfusion of various tissues (that can change in congestive heart failure or shock, as described below); (*b*) the concentration of plasma and tissue proteins that bind to the specific drug; and (*c*) the physicochemical properties of the drug and the resultant ability of the drug to be bound by tissue and plasma proteins or to be concentrated in lipid. The first two of these can show intraindividual or interindividual variability and hence should be considered in predicting circumstances in which the dose of a drug must be altered.

After administration of an i.v. bolus of drug, the volume of distribution is relatively small, reflecting the volume of the readily accessible central compartment (Vc). The volume of this central compartment is changed in some pathologic situations. For example, in congestive heart failure (CHF), Vc of lidocaine is reduced by about 40%, presumably because of the reduction of perfusion of many organs (including liver, kidney, and splanchnic bed). Therefore, bolus doses of lidocaine must be reduced in patients with CHF to avoid toxicity.

The volume of distribution is larger at steady state. Steady state is the time when there is equilibrium between the various tissues of the body. At that time, there is no net redistribution of drug, and the amount of drug administered is equal to the amount eliminated. The steady-state volume of distribution, Vss, reflects entry of drug into less perfused tissues. Steady-state volume of distribution is useful in predicting the plasma concentration that will be achieved during chronic administration of a given drug dosage. Like Vc, Vss can also be changed in various pathologic circumstances. For example, Vss of digoxin is reduced by quinidine because of dislodgment of digoxin from tissue-binding sites. This is an important contributor to quinidine-related digoxin intoxication.

Volume of distribution is determined by a number of factors, including the ability of the drug to infiltrate various tissues, the extent to which the drug is bound to proteins in plasma and tissues, and the lipophilicity of the drug. Most antiarrhythmic agents are weak bases and are bound to varying extents in plasma by α-1-acid glyprotein. Digoxin and weakly acidic drugs are bound in plasma, primarily to albumin. The drug must be free in plasma (not bound to plasma proteins) to reach its site of action and to produce a pharmacologic effect.

The extent to which drugs are bound to plasma and tissue proteins can change in different clinical situations, with resultant changes in volume of distribution and in the amount of unbound drug available to produce a pharmacologic effect. The most common causes of protein-binding changes are changes in the concentration of the binding proteins, changes in the concentration of the drug, interactions with other drugs competing for binding by the same proteins, and change in pH.

Changes in plasma concentration of drug-binding proteins can have clinical consequences. As mentioned previously, most antiarrhythmic agents are weak bases that are bound to the acute phase-reactant α-1-acid glycoprotein. The concentration of this protein increases during acute illness. For example, the concentration of α-1-acid glycoprotein increases after an acute myocardial infarction, causing an increase in protein binding of such antiarrhythmics as quinidine and propranolol. Because most drug assays measure total drug and do not differentiate bound from unbound drug, the increase in the bound portion of drug (and reduction in active unbound fraction) would be apparent only in the observation that a higher total concentration of drug is required to produce the same pharmacologic effect. This phenomenon would be expected with any drug highly bound to α-1-acid glycoprotein, and has been demonstrated with both quinidine and lidocaine.

Drug interactions can alter the extent of binding of drug to plasma and tissue-binding sites. This scenario was just described with regard to the quinidine-digoxin interaction. It is also seen in the interaction between phenylbutazone and warfarin, in which phenylbutazone displaces warfarin from plasma albumin-binding sites and thus potentiates warfarin effect.

The concentration of drug can alter protein binding for some drugs. For some drugs the available plasma protein-binding sites are limited and are nearly completely filled at usual pharmacologic concentrations of the drug. As the concentration of the drug increases, it fills the remaining binding sites remains unbound, or binds to weaker binding proteins. This leads to a disproportionate rise in unbound drug concentration as the total concentration increases. Among cardiovascular drugs, this phenomenon is most commonly seen with disopyramide and phenytoin. Disopyramide is extensively bound to plasma proteins at low concentrations; but when the concentration of drug is increased, the fraction of drug that is protein bound is reduced because of saturation of binding sites. As a result, as dosage of drug is increased, the concentration of active unbound drug increases out of proportion to the total concentration. This can be demonstrated at usual dosages during a single dosing interval. A formulation of drug that leads to a more steady total disopyramide concentration produces less fluctuation in unbound disopyramide concentration, and could lead to reduction in concentration-related drug toxicity.

Changes in plasma and tissue pH can theoretically alter protein binding by changing the ionized state of antiarrhythmic drugs. This has not been clinically described, presumably because of the narrow range of normal physiologic pH maintained by the body. In conditions of marked acidosis, changes in protein binding and volume of distribution of a drug could occur. In view of other physiologic alterations during marked acidosis, however, the clinical results of such changes are difficult to predict.

Drug Metabolism and Elimination

Drug elimination can occur via a number of routes. The most common are direct elimination by the kidneys and hepatic metabolism of drug, followed by biliary or renal elimination.

CLEARANCE

Clearance (Cl) describes the rate of removal of drug from plasma, and is defined as the volume of plasma cleared of drug per unit time. Discrete rates of clearance can be defined for different organs, e.g., renal clearance and hepatic clearance. The sum of these individual clearances is called total body clearance or systemic clearance. Total systemic clearance is most commonly defined by one of the following equations:

For i.v. infusions, Cpss equals Steady-state plasma concentration:

$$\text{Clearance} = \frac{\text{Dosing rate}}{\text{Cpss}}$$

For oral dosing, AUC equals the area under the plasma concentration versus time curve for a single dosing interval:

$$\text{Clearance} = \frac{\text{Dose}}{\text{AUC}}$$

Clearance is the most reliable indicator of the rate of metabolism and elimination of drug. Assessment of drug elimination by other variables, such as half-life, is less satisfactory because half-life can be altered both by changes in clearance and by changes in volume of distribution, as described in the following paragraphs.

First-pass or presystemic clearance, as described earlier, is the metabolism of a drug during passage through the liver before reaching the systemic circulation. A number of drugs undergo extensive first-pass clearance. For example, lidocaine is nearly completely metabolized, making its oral use clinically ineffective. Propafenone, metoprolol, propranolol, and verapamil also show extensive first-pass clearance. For these drugs, the oral dosage required for therapeutic effect is much higher than the i.v. dosage, because the intravenously administered drug dose bypasses the portal circulation and hence has no first-pass clearance. For most drugs the portion of drug passing unmetabolized through the portal circulation is relatively constant, leaving a linear relationship between oral dose and plasma concentration. However, as discussed earlier with regard to absorption, propafenone exhibits "saturable kinetics," with saturation of the liver-metabolizing capacity for the drug and resultant nonlinear rise in plasma concentration after an increased oral dosage. For example, following a 3-fold dosage increase from 300 to 900 mg/day, the plasma concentration of propafenone increases nearly 9-fold. The clinical implications of this rapid rise in plasma concentration are complex, however, because of a drop in production of the active metabolite 5-hydroxypropafenone when the debrisoquine system is saturated.

DRUG METABOLISM

Most antiarrhythmic agents are nonpolar and lipid soluble, traits that facilitate reabsorption of drug from the renal tubules and from the gastrointestinal tract. Metabolism of drug produces more polar metabolites that are more readily eliminated than the parent drug. Drug metabolism can be divided into phase I reactions, which change the drug into more polar metabolites via oxidation-reduction reactions, and phase II reactions, which conjugate the drug or its phase I metabolites to an endogenous ligand such as glucuronide, sulfate, or acetate. Most phase I drug metabolism occurs in the liver, with oxidative metabolism usually occurring via the cytochrome P-450 enzyme systems. However, metabolism of some rapidly cleared drugs occurs in the lungs, plasma, vascular endothelium, or blood cells. Adenosine, for example, is rapidly taken up by erythrocytes and vascular endothelium and metabolized.

Although most drug metabolites are pharmacologically inactive, several antiarrhythmic drugs do have active metabolites that may contribute to their pharmacologic effects. Findings suggesting the presence of an active metabolite include a disparity between the concentration of a drug and its pharmacologic effect, discrepancy between a short drug half-life and a long duration of pharmacologic effect, and demonstration of a population of patients who have a different response to the drug than the rest of the population. Table 4.2 lists known active metabolites of antiarrhythmic drugs, as well as other general pharmacologic data pertinent to antiarrhythmic drug dosing.

PHARMACOGENETICS

Genetically determined differences in drug metabolism have been demonstrated for several antiarrhythmic drugs. The most important sources of inherited variability in metabolism ("polymorphic metabolism") for antiarrhythmic drugs are N-acetyltransferase and the cytochrome P-450 "debrisoquine pathway."

N-Acetyltransferase is responsible for the acetylation of procainamide to form the metabolite NAPA (acecainide). The same enzyme system is responsible for interindividual variability in hydralazine, dapsone, and isoniazid metabolism. Patients may be divided into "fast" or "slow" acetylator phenotypes, based on the extent of acetylation of these compounds. Fast acetylators have about twice as much enzyme as slow acetylators. Approximately 45% of white and black populations carry the slow acetylator trait, whereas it is found in only 10–20% of Asians.

The polymorphism of procainamide metabolism has two clinical implications. First, rapid acetylators may develop high enough plasma concentrations of NAPA to produce pharmacologic effects. This may contribute to the antiarrhythmic effect of procainamide. NAPA, however, differs electrophysiologically from its parent, procainamide, in that it produces significant Q-T prolongation (outward potassium channel blockade), although having no effect on inward sodium channels. NAPA is renally eliminated and can accumulate to toxic levels in patients with renal failure. Thus, in fast acetylators the presence of NAPA, with its potential electrophysiologic and toxic effects, must be kept in mind. A second result of polymorphic metabolism is seen in the development of procainamide-induced lupus syndrome. Slow acetylators develop positive antinuclear antibody and procainamide-induced lupus syndrome earlier in therapy than do fast acetylators. Slow acetylators, with limited acetylation capacity, shunt more procainamide to alternative oxidative metabolism pathways. Apparently, free radicals formed during oxidative metabolism can bind to nuclear histones, inducing the production of antinuclear antibodies.

Polymorphic metabolism has also been demonstrated in varying degrees for propafenone, encainide, flecainide, and metoprolol. The enzyme system responsible for this is an oxidative P-450 enzyme called the "debrisoquine pathway," named for the drug for which this enzyme system was first identified. Population studies have shown this enzyme system to be expressed in a bimodal pattern, with subjects termed "extensive" or "poor" metabolizers. The poor metabolizer phenotype is expressed in approximately 9% of the population. In poor metabolizers the parent drug plasma concentration is increased, clearance is reduced, and elimination half-life is prolonged. The debrisoquine pathway is involved in metabolism of several cardiovascular drugs including encainide, propafenone, and metoprolol.

The debrisoquine pathway produces active metabolites of encainide and propafenone, and the relationship between drug concentration and effect is altered in poor metabolizers. For example, the major metabolite of encainide, O-desmethylencainide (ODE), produces greater conduction slowing than does encainide. In poor metabolizers, the concentration of encainide is much higher, yet the degree of QRS prolongation is reduced and antiarrhythmic efficacy appears to be reduced.

The major active metabolite of propafenone is 5-hydroxypropafenone. This metabolite appears to have similar electrophysiologic effects to the parent drug but with slightly less potency. In poor metabolizers, the propafenone concentration required for a therapeutic response is higher, but there is no significant difference in dosage or response rates in those patients. There does, however, appear to be a higher incidence of central nervous system side effects of propafenone in poor metabolizers, suggesting that propafenone produces greater neurotoxicity than does its metabolite. The β-adrenoceptor blocking effect of propafenone is greater in poor metabolizers than in extensive metabolizers, consistent with in vitro findings that propafenone is a more potent β-blocker than its major metabolite.

Specific drug interactions have been observed for the debrisoquine pathway. Quinidine, even in single doses as low as 80 mg, is a potent inhibitor of the debrisoquine pathway. Patients taking quinidine show drug clearance patterns typical of poor metabolizers. Propafenone reduces metabolism of other debrisoquine pathway substrates. Clearance of warfarin, which is partially metabolized by the debrisoquine pathway, can be reduced by propafenone, potentially leading to excessively prolonged prothrombin time and bleeding complications.

Familiarity with drugs metabolized by the debrisoquine pathway can lead to predictions of potential drug interactions. Drugs metabolized at least in part by this pathway include (*a*) the tricyclic antidepressant desipramine; (*b*) the β-blockers propranolol, metoprolol, and timolol; (*c*) the antiarrhythmics propafenone and flecainide; (*d*) dextromethorphan; and (*e*) warfarin. Reduced clearance and elevated plasma concentrations could be seen with these drugs in poor metabolizers and in patients receiving other drugs metabolized by the pathway (e.g., propafenone) or inhibitors of the pathway (e.g., quinidine). These interactions would be expected to be most pronounced for desipramine, metoprolol, timolol, propafenone, and dextromethorphan, drugs for which the major route of clearance involves the debrisoquine pathway. For drugs with only minor clearance by the debrisoquine pathway, such as propranolol, warfarin, and flecainide, these drug interactions would not be expected to be clinically significant, except when other major routes of clearance are impaired.

HALF-LIFE

The half-life (T1/2) of a drug is defined as the time required for plasma concentration to drop by 50%. This value can be determined from analysis of concentration versus time curves after a dose of drug, or can be derived from clearance and volume of distribution using the equation:

$$T\tfrac{1}{2} = ln\ 2 \times (volume\ of\ distribution/clearance)$$
$$= 0.693 \times (volume\ of\ distribution/clearance)$$

Using half-life to describe the rate of change in plasma concentration over time acknowledges the fact that for most drugs, including antiarrhythmic agents, the rate of removal of drug from plasma by distribution or elimination is dependent on the plasma concentration of drug. The drop in plasma concentration occurs as an exponential function, and can be transformed to a linear function by plotting log of concentration against time. In the first half-life, plasma concentration drops by 50%; in the second half-life, half of the remainder is lost (75% drop from the initial plasma concentration), and so forth. The rate of rise in plasma concentration after initiation of therapy is also dependent on elimination half-life, as shown in Figure 4.3.

For drugs characterized by more than one pharmacologic compartment, more than one half-life may be defined. In the most common instance, the drop in plasma concentration after administration of an i.v. bolus of a drug can be divided into

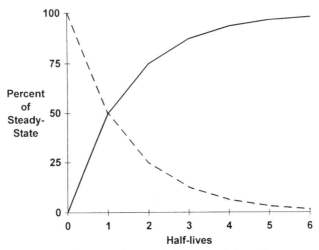

Figure 4.3. Time required for accumulation and elimination of drug. After initiation of drug therapy (solid line), 50% of steady-state drug concentrations are achieved in 1 half-life and 90% in 3.3 half-lives. Similarly, after drug is stopped (broken line), concentration drops by 90% after 3.3 half-lives.

a rapid "distribution" period, when drug is distributed from the central to the peripheral compartment, and an "elimination" period, when drug is cleared from the central compartment by metabolism or elimination. For example, when lidocaine is given as a single i.v. bolus, the plasma concentration initially drops rapidly, reflecting the relatively short time required for redistribution of drug from the central compartment to the peripheral compartment. The time required for plasma concentration to drop by 50% during this phase is called the "distribution half-life," which for lidocaine is approximately 7 minutes. After equilibration with the peripheral compartment has occurred, the rate of decline of plasma concentration is slower and is described by the "elimination half-life," which for lidocaine is approximately 100 minutes. If a single bolus of lidocaine is given at a dosage required to produce an instantaneous plasma concentration twice the minimum effective concentration, the plasma concentration would drop to ineffective levels after approximately 7 minutes. In contrast, after discontinuation of a chronic infusion producing the same plasma concentration at steady state, plasma concentration would not fall to ineffective levels for 100 minutes. Because of this relatively slow decline in plasma concentration after stopping a steady-state infusion, the common practice of "weaning" lidocaine by slowly dropping the infusion rate may not be necessary.

When a drug is administered orally, it is absorbed slowly, usually at a rate slower than the distribution rate of the drug, and the distribution phase is masked by the slow absorption of the drug. Because of this, only elimination half-life is of importance in planning oral dosage regimens for most antiarrhythmics.

Amiodarone is an exception to the rule that distribution kinetics are unimportant for orally administered drugs. Amiodarone, whose distribution kinetics are much slower than its absorption kinetics, requires a prolonged "loading" period to rapidly achieve (in a few days) and maintain pharmacologic effect. The additional drug-given during the loading period, replaces drug distributed from the central compartment to peripheral compartments over the first several weeks of therapy. After steady state has been achieved, usually 3 months or more, there is no net distribution out of the central compartment, and maintenance dosing to replace metabolized or eliminated drug will maintain steady plasma concentrations.

LOADING DOSE, MAINTENANCE DOSING

The time required to achieve steady-state plasma concentration during chronic therapy can be estimated based on the elimination half-life, as shown in Figure 4.3. After approximately 3.3 half-lives, 90% of the steady-state plasma concentration is achieved. Thus, for a drug with a half-life of 8 hours, a 24-hour period of treatment is sufficient to effectively reach "chronic" drug levels.

If the time to steady state is longer than is clinically acceptable for achievement of a therapeutic effect, a "loading dose" may be given to bring plasma concentrations into the desired concentration range more rapidly. This approach is commonly used with lidocaine. If lidocaine is given at a fixed infusion rate without loading boluses, more than 6 hours will be required to reach steady-state plasma concentration. This is obviously too long a delay for treatment of life-threatening arrhythmias. To achieve arrhythmia control more rapidly, a loading dose is given to reach and maintain steady-state plasma concentrations within minutes. Conceptually, these loading bolus regimens are designed to give extra lidocaine to fill the central compartment and to replace the drug that is leaving plasma through distribution to peripheral compartments. At steady state, when there is no net movement of drug from central to peripheral compartments, the "extra" lidocaine is no longer needed. Drug is then administered as a "maintenance infusion," i.e., drug is given at the same rate at which it is eliminated.

Loading dosage regimens are also used for amiodarone, as discussed earlier, and for procainamide, quinidine, and bretylium. For procainamide, a loading dose of 10–15 mg/kg is given over 30–60 minutes, either as a number of small boluses separated by 5–10 minutes, or as an infusion. Rapid rates of administration of procainamide can cause adverse effects, and the patient must therefore be monitored closely and the infusion stopped or reduced if hypotension or excessive QRS prolongation is noted. When given orally, a loading dose of 1500 mg has been reported to be effective. For quinidine, a loading dose of 10 mg/kg is given as an infusion over 30–60 minutes. The infusion rate must often be reduced because of hypotension, presumably resulting from the α-blocking effects of quinidine. When used orally, the loading dose used is 600 mg. For bretylium, the initial bolus dose causes an immediate increase in heart rate, blood pressure, and cardiac excitability because of release of catecholamines from sympathetic nerve endings. Subsequently, the ganglionic blocking effects (postural hypotension) and antiarrhythmic effects are seen.

As illustrated previously, loading regimens are often limited by drug side effects. When a drug is given rapidly and allowed to reach relatively high plasma concentrations, as usually happens during loading, there is an increased incidence of adverse effects. For this reason, antiarrhythmic drug-loading regimens should be used only when the necessity of earlier antiarrhythmic drug effect outweighs the potential toxicity of the rapid loading regimen.

DESIGN OF DRUG DOSING SCHEDULES

Knowledge of elimination half-life can be helpful in designing dosing regimens for antiarrhythmic drugs. The main considerations in determining how frequently the drug should be administered are the elimination half-life of the drug and the acceptable range between minimum and maximum plasma concentrations. If the maximum concentration can safely be four times as great as the minimum effective concentration, the dosing interval can be as long as 2 half-lives. Similarly, for an 8-fold spread between minimum and maximum concentrations, a dosing interval up to 3 half-lives may be used.

One precaution in using half-life to design a dosing regimen is that the half-life of the active element must be considered. For drugs with a prominent active metabolite with a half-life longer than that of the parent drug, dosing schedules based only on the parent drug elimination half-life can lead to overdosing of the active metabolite. For example, encainide is a drug with a half-life of approximately 1.8 hours. Its major active metabolite, ODE, is more potent than encainide itself and has an elimination half-life of approximately 10 hours. In its early clinical use, before ODE was recognized, encainide was dosed at 3–4-hour intervals, and changes in dosage were made at intervals of less than a day. This led to adverse effects in a number of subjects because of unexpected accumulation of ODE.

Changes in Drug Disposition Because of Disease States

Drug disposition is altered in a number of disease states. Those most commonly encountered in patients receiving antiarrhythmic drug therapy are CHF, renal failure, and liver disease (cirrhosis). Pharmacologic changes related to concomitant illness and coadministered drugs are discussed here and outlined in Tables 4.3–4.5.

CONGESTIVE HEART FAILURE

In the presence of CHF, liver blood flow is reduced, leading to reduction in clearance of drugs with high extraction ratios. Lidocaine clearance is reduced by approximately 40%, leading to a need for a lower maintenance infusion rate. Also, as discussed earlier, the central volume of distribution of lidocaine is reduced in CHF, necessitating reduction in initial loading dose. Other antiarrhythmic agents have not been shown to have significantly altered kinetics in the presence of CHF.

Antiarrhythmic agents with negative inotropic effects should be avoided, if possible, in patients with overt CHF. Antiarrhythmics with the greatest negative inotropic potential are disopyramide, flecainide, and β-blockers.

Table 4.3
Precautions for Antiarrhythmic Drug Use in Common Disease States

	Renal Failure	Liver Disease	Congestive Heart Failure
Quinidine	Lower therapeutic range	Reduce dosage	
Procainamide	NAPA dominant Reduce dosage		Reduce dosage
Disopyramide	Reduce dosage		Avoid, negative inotropic effect
Lidocaine		Reduce dosage	Reduce dosage
Mexiletine		Reduce dosage	
Tocainide	Reduce dosage		
Flecainide	Reduce dosage		Avoid, negative inotropic effect
Propafenone Moricizine Sotalol	Reduce dosage		Caution, negative inotropic effect
Amiodarone Verapamil			Caution, negative inotropic effect
Digoxin	Reduce dosage		

RENAL FAILURE

Drug and metabolite accumulation can occur in patients with renal failure. This has been best documented with procainamide and its metabolite, NAPA. Because of potential toxicity due to accumulation of these drugs, procainamide should be avoided in patients with renal failure. Other renally excreted drugs, and drugs with renally excreted metabolites, should also be used with caution in patients with renal failure.

LIVER DISEASE

Hepatic metabolism is not materially altered by liver disease, except in the presence of severe hepatic dysfunction, as seen in patients with cirrhosis. Lidocaine clearance is reduced in cirrhotics, with no change in volume of distribution. A reduction in maintenance infusion rate is therefore required, with no change in initial loading dose. Dosages of other hepatically metabolized drugs may also require reduction.

PHARMACOKINETICS IN THE ELDERLY

Most alterations in medication therapy for the elderly are based on pharmacokinetic considerations. The most important of these is reduced renal function in

Table 4.4
Antiarrhythmic Drug Interactions with Common Cardiovascular Drugs

	Digoxin	β-Blockers	Ca++ Blockers
Quinidine	↑ Digoxin level		
Procainamide			
Disopyramide		Additive negative inotropic effect	Additive negative inotropic effect
Lidocaine		↑ Lidocaine level	
Mexiletine			
Tocainide			
Flecainide	↑ Digoxin level	Additive negative inotropic effect	Additive negative inotropic effect
Propafenone	↑ Digoxin level	↑ β-Blocking effect	Additive negative inotropic effect
Moricizine			Inhibits diltiazem metabolism
Sotalol			
Amiodarone	↑ Digoxin level	↑ β-Blocking effect	Potential bradycardia
Verapamil	↑ Digoxin level	Additive bradycardia and negative inotropic effect	

Table 4.5
Antirrhythmic Drug Interactions with Common Noncardiovascular Medications

	Warfarin	Cimetidine	Phenytoin
Quindine		↑ Quinidine level	↓ Quinidine level
Procainamide		↑ Procainamide level	
Disopyramide			↓ Disopyramide level
Lidocaine		↑ Lidocaine level	
Mexiletine			↓ Mexiteline level
Tocainide			
Flecainide		↑ Flecainide level	
Propafenone	↑ Prothrombin time	↑ Propafenone level	
Moricizine			
Sotalol			
Amiodarone	↑ Prothrombin time		

the elderly. Even in patients with normal serum creatinine, glomerular filtration rate is significantly reduced in older patients, as shown by the commonly used formula for estimating creatinine clearance:

$$CCr = [(140 - age) \times weight\ (kg)]/[72 \times serum\ creatinine\ (mg/dL)].$$

Because of this, initial dosage of renally eliminated drugs should be reduced in elderly patients. Age-related changes in hepatic function and serum proteins could potentially alter drug selection and dosing, but currently available data do not allow specific recommendations for antiarrhythmic agents. A prudent approach in the elderly patient is to begin with a lower antiarrhythmic drug dosage than usual, and to titrate upward slowly, as needed.

Drug Interactions

The most common mechanisms of drug interactions are (a) inhibition or enhancement of drug metabolism, (b) displacement of drug from plasma or tissue binding sites, (c) competition for receptor sites, and (d) additive pharmacologic effects. Common drug interactions are outlined in Tables 4.4 and 4.5. Cimetidine inhibits hepatic metabolism of a number of drugs, including quinidine, procainamide, lidocaine, flecainide, propafenone, and propranolol. This drug interaction is the result of direct inhibition of hepatic metabolic P-450 enzyme systems. Phenytoin, phenobarbital, and rifampin induce (enhance) hepatic oxidative metabolism, with a resultant drop in plasma concentrations and shortening of elimination half-life for such drugs as quinidine, disopyramide, and mexiletine. Quinidine and propafenone both inhibit oxidative metabolism through the debrisoquine pathway, as discussed previously. Digoxin clearance is reduced by quinidine, flecainide, propafenone, amiodarone, and verapamil. The mechanism of this interaction is best understood for quinidine, which dislodges digoxin from tissue-binding sites leading to potentially toxic digoxin levels. β-Blockers reduce liver blood flow, with resultant reduction in clearance of high-extraction drugs such as lidocaine.

Although the interactions mentioned above are all pharmacokinetic, pharmacodynamic drug interactions can also be clinically important. For example, β-blockers and calcium channel blockers reduce heart rate, AV nodal conduction, and contractility. These effects may be additive to the effects of antiarrhythmics.

SUGGESTED READING

Benet LZ, Williams RL. Design and optimization of dosage regimens; pharmacokinetic data. In: Gilman AG, Rall TW, Nies AS, Taylor P, eds. The pharmacologic basis of therapeutics. New York: Pergamon Press, 1990.

Drayer DE, Lowenthal DT, Woosley RL, Wies AS, Schwartz A, Reidenberg MM. Cumulation of N-acetylprocainamide, an active metabolite of procainamide, in patients with impaired renal function. Clin Pharmacol Ther 1977;22:63–69.

Reidenberg MM, Drayer DE, Levy M, Warner H. Polymorphic acetylation of procainamide in man. Clin Pharmacol Ther 1975;17:722–730.

Riddell JG, McAllister CB, Wilkinson GR, Wood AJJ, Roden DM. Constant plasma drug concentrations—a new technique with application to lidocaine. Ann Intern Med 1984;100:25–28.

Siddoway LA, Roden DM, Woosley RL. Clinical pharmacology of old and new antiarrhythmic drugs. In: Josephson, ME, ed. Sudden cardiac death. Cardiovascular clinics. Philadelphia: FA Davis, 1985:199–248.

Thomson PD, Melmon KL, Richardson JA, et al. Lidocaine pharmacokinetics in advanced heart failure, liver disease, and renal failure in humans. Ann Intern Med 1973;78:499–508.

Woosley RL, Roden DM, Duff HJ, Carey EL, Wood AJJ, Wilkinson GR. Co-inheritance of deficient oxidative metabolism of encainide and debrisoquine. Clin Res 1981;29:501A.

5   Class I Antiarrhythmic Drugs

CLASS IA ANTIARRHYTHMIC AGENTS: QUINIDINE, PROCAINAMIDE, AND DISOPYRAMIDE

QUINIDINE

CLINICAL ELECTROPHYSIOLOGIC AND ELECTROCARDIOGRAPHIC EFFECTS

In patients with the sick sinus syndrome, quinidine may depress the sinus node (Table 5.1). Quinidine has a direct suppressant effect on the sinoatrial node (S-A node) as well as an indirectly mediated vagolytic or sympathomimetic effect.

The direct actions of quinidine prolong AV nodal (A-H interval) and His-Purkinje (H-V interval) conduction times. In addition, via a direct effect, quinidine decreases heart rate and increases the atrial effective refractory period ERP). In the innervated human heart, quinidine may shorten the A-H interval, while in the denervated heart, it has the opposite effect. Quinidine decreases the A-H interval in patients because of a vagolytic influence and an enhancement of sympathetic tone via the baroreceptor reflex.

In humans, therapeutic concentrations of quinidine produce changes on the surface electrocardiogram (ECG) (Table 5.1), including a slight increase in heart rate, probably secondary to its anticholinergic actions on the sinus node, as well as an increase in reflex sympathetic activity. In patients with cardiac conduction system disease, the drug may produce a slight prolongation of the P-R interval. In most patients, the QRS complex widens, usually by less than 40 msec, as the quinidine concentration increases. Lengthening of the Q-T interval by as much as 25% is the most prominent effect of therapeutic concentrations on the ECG.

CLINICAL PHARMACOLOGY

Several preparations of quinidine are used clinically, including quinidine sulfate, quinidine gluconate, and polygalacuronate preparations (Table 5.2). Bioavailability of the oral sulfate and gluconate preparations is approximately 80 and 70%, respectively. Quinidine sulfate is absorbed rapidly; peak plasma concentrations are attained in approximately 90 minutes. Quinidine gluconate is absorbed more slowly after an oral dose; peak concentrations are achieved in approximately 4 hours. Thus, gluconate preparations can be administered every 8–12 hours. Quinidine is also available for intramuscular injection and produces a higher and earlier peak plasma concentration. However, the intramuscular drug causes pain and necrosis at the site of injection, and absorption is only 87%. Quinidine can also be administered intravenously if administered slowly, but hypotension may be problematic.

Table 5.1
Electrocardiographic and Electrophysiologic Effects of Class Ia Antiarrhythmic Agents

	Quinidine	Procainamide	Disopyramide
Sinus rate	↓0↑	0	↓0↑
P-R interval	↓0↑	0↑	0
Q-R-S interval	↑	↑	0↑
Q-T interval	↑	↑	↑
A-H interval	↓0↑	0↑	0↑
HV interval	↑	↑	↑
A ERP	↑	↑	↑
AVN ERP	0↑	0↑	0↑
H-P ERP	↑	0↑	↑
V ERP	↑	↑	↑
AP ERP	↑	↑	↑

↓0↑, changes may be variable.
A, atrial; ERP, effective refractory period; AVN ERP, AV nodal; H-P ERP, His-Purkinje; V ERP, ventricular; AP ERP, accessory pathway.

Table 5.2
Pharmacokinetics of Class Ia Antiarrhythmic Agents

Variable	Quinidine	Procainamide	Disopyramide
Bioavailability	70–80%	75–95%	70–90%
Peak concentration (hr)	1–3	1–2	0.5–2
Therapeutic concentration range (μg/mL)	2–6	4–10	2–5
Half-life elimination (hr)	6–7	3–6	4–10
Volume of distribution (L/kg)	2–3	1.5–2.5	0.5–1.5
Total body clearance (mL/min)	200–300	300–700	100–200
% Metabolized	60–80	30–50	25–35
Active metabolite	(3S)-3-Hydroxyquinidine 2'-oxyquinidinone	N-Acetylprocainamide	Mono-N-dealkylate d disopyramide
Protein binding	Albumin (80%)	Albumin (20%)	Albumin (30%) α-1-Acid Glycoprotein
Peritoneal dialysis	(–)	(–)	(–)
Hemodialysis	(±)	(+)	(±)

Quinidine's metabolism occurs mainly via the liver. Most metabolites are hydroxylated at one site; either on the quinoline ring or on the quinuclidine ring. A small amount of dihydroxy compounds are also produced. The metabolism of quinidine varies among patients; some of the drug's metabolites are cardioactive. In addition, laboratory assays may variably include some drug metabolites in their measurements. Thus, the assayed quinidine concentrations may be misleading in clinical situations, such as renal failure, where active and inactive metabolites accumulate. Quinidine is filtered at the glomerulus and secreted by the proximal renal tubule. Metabolites and approximately 20% of the parent drug are renally excreted. The half-time of elimination is approximately 7 hours, but elimination is reduced in congestive heart failure (CHF), hepatic dysfunction, or renal disease. Because quinidine is a weak base, reabsorption is reduced and excretion is increased with acidic urine.

DRUG DOSING

The standard oral maintenance dose of the sulfate is 200–400 mg four times daily; it reaches steady-state within 24 hours (Table 5.3). A 30% greater dose of the gluconate or 38% greater dose of the polygalacturonate is necessary; dosing may be decreased to every 8 hours with the slow-release preparations. The ECG is monitored for excessive Q-T prolongation and if the Q-Tc prolongs more than 25%, the dose is reduced or discontinued, although no study has conclusively determined the Q-Tc length beyond which repolarization is dangerously prolonged. If quinidine is tolerated, therapy continues. The therapeutic serum quinidine concentration is 2–6 µg/mL. The gluconate can be administered intravenously at a rate of 0.5 mg/kg/minute to a maximum of 10 mg/kg with careful monitoring. Any fall in blood pressure should be treated with intravenous (i.v.) saline and the infusion decreased.

HEMODYNAMIC EFFECTS

Quinidine lowers the blood pressure and produces hypotension, particularly when administered intravenously. Hypotension is secondary to the α-blocking effect of the drug. Hemodynamic studies of patients administered quinidine indicate that it produces peripheral vasodilation without a decrease in cardiac output or myocardial performance. Studies in recipients of human cardiac transplants reveal that quinidine reduces cardiac output by venodilation and not via a negative inotropic action.

INDICATIONS

Quinidine is useful in the treatment of both supraventricular and ventricular arrhythmias. Quinidine is also effective in the prevention and treatment of atrial premature contractions (APC) and junctional premature contractions (JPC). However, in light of its potential for proarrhythmia, quinidine's use for APC or JPC should be limited to symptomatic patients where a β-blocker or digitalis therapy has been ineffective or contraindicated.

Table 5.3
Dose and Method of Administration of Class Ia Antiarrhythmic Agents

Method of Administration	Quinidine Sulfate	Procainamide	Disopyramide
Oral			
Conventional			
Total daily dose (mg)	800–1600	2000–6000	400–800
Dosing interval (hr)	6–8	4–6	6–8
Steady state (days)	1.–1.5	1–2	1–1.5
Sustained release			
Total daily dose (mg)	1200–1800	2000–6000	400–800
Dosing interval (hr)	8–12	6–8	12
Steady state (days)	1–1.5	1–2	1–1.5
Intramuscular	Not widely used	Not widely used	Not approved USA
Intermittent intravenous injection			
Loading dose	6–10 mg/kg at 0.3 to 0.5 mg/kg/min	6–15 mg/kg at 0.2 to 0.4 mg/kg/min	1–2 mg/kg for 15 min[a] 1–2 mg/kg for 45 min
Unit dose	60–100	100	80
Dosing interval (min)	5	5	5
Maximum total dose (mg)	___[b]	1000	___[b]
Constant rate i.v. infusion			
Rate (mg/min)	1–2	2–6	___[b]
μg/kg/min	10–30	15–80	___[b]
Time to 90% steady state (hr)	20	12	___[b]

[a]Investigational
[b]___, not applicable.

Quinidine is used to chemically cardiovert atrial fibrillation (AF) or flutter to normal sinus rhythm by prolonging the atrial ERP and decreasing conduction velocity of the atrium, resulting in slowing of the circus movement rate. Quinidine has also been hypothesized to reduce atrial inhomogeneity. These effects result from the direct effect of the drug, as well as from its vagolytic effects. Quinidine is efficacious in maintaining normal sinus rhythm in patients with AF or atrial flutter. A metaanalysis of six randomized trials examining its efficacy in the maintenance of sinus rhythm found that in quinidine-treated patients, 69, 58, and 50% maintained sinus rhythm 3, 6, and 12 months after cardioversion compared with 45, 33, and 25% of the control patients. Mortality in quinidine-treated patients, however, was three times greater. Examination of deaths reveal many of noncardiac or unknown etiology; a greater number of patients with ischemic heart disease were randomized to quinidine, although this was not statistically significant.

Quinidine effectively suppresses ventricular premature complexes (VPCs) in more than 60–70% of patients and is used to treat VPCs if they produce discomfort or hemodynamic compromise. Low-dose quinidine-mexiletine combination therapy has been shown to be more effective and better tolerated than quinidine monotherapy to suppress VPCs and nonsustained ventricular tachycardia (VT).

Table 5.4
Relative Frequency of Adverse Effects with Class Ia Antiarrhythmic Agents

Adverse Effects	Quinidine	Procainamide	Disopyramide
Cardiovascular			
Sinus arrest	+	+	+
AV block	±	±	±
Prolonged Q-T	++	+	+
Torsade de pointes	+++	++	++
Proarrhythmia	+++	++	+
Hypotension	++	+	+
Heart failure	+	+	++
Gastrointestinal			
Diarrhea	+++	+	(−)
Constipation	(−)	+	++
Nausea, abdominal			
pain	++	++	+
Hepatotoxicity	+	+	+
Central nervous system			
Cinchonism	++	(−)	(−)
Psychosis	++	++	+
Depression	+	++	+[a]
Blurred vision	+	+	++[a]
Hematologic			
Thrombocytopenia	+++	+	+
Agranulocytosis	+	+++	+
Hemolytic anemia	+	+	+
Hypoprothrombinemia	+	(−)	(−)
Genitourinary			
Urinary retention	(+)	(±)	++[a]
Other			
Dry mouth	(−)	(−)	++[a]
Hypoglycemia	(−)	(−)	++
Fever	+	+	+
SLE-like syndrome	+	++	(−)

[a]Secondary to anticholinergic properties.

SIDE EFFECTS

Adverse effects preclude long-term quinidine therapy in up to 30% of patients (Table 5.4). The most frequent adverse effects of oral treatment are gastrointestinal and include nausea, diarrhea, and abdominal bloating and discomfort. Gastrointestinal (GI) effects may be less severe with the gluconate preparation. Central nervous system (CNS) toxicity, referred to as cinchonism, includes tinnitus, hearing loss, confusion, delirium, disturbances in vision, and psychosis. Immune-mediated reactions, such as rash, fever, hemolytic anemia, leukopenia, hepatotoxicity, and anaphylaxis, have also been reported. Thrombocytopenia is produced by antibodies to quinidine-platelet complexes, which cause platelets to agglutinate and lyse. In addition, a lupus-like syndrome, similar to that induced by procainamide, may occur.

Quinidine cardiac toxicity manifests itself by slowed cardiac conduction (QRS widening), slowed repolarization (Q-T prolongation), and sinus or AV nodal conduction block. Ways to diminish toxicity include administration of sodium lactate and increasing pH, which favors binding of free quinidine to serum albumin. At the level of the sodium channel, alkalosis promotes the neutral form of the drug and hyperpolarizes the cell by reducing external potassium, enhancing recovery of the sodium channel from block.

Quinidine exhibits proarrhythmic effects, as reported by many investigators. Although there are many forms of arrhythmia aggravation, of particular concern is "quinidine syncope" due to self-terminating polymorphic VT, known as torsade de pointes. Although the reported incidence is variable, Roden et al. reported it to be 1.5%. Significant Q-T prolongation is seen with torsade de pointes. Torsade de pointes may occur because of triggered activity produced by early afterdepolarizations and may be precipitated by bradycardia, hypokalemia, diuretics, or digitalis. Syncope is not related to plasma quinidine concentration nor to duration of treatment.

DRUG INTERACTIONS

Several drug interactions occur after quinidine administration that may confound treatment. Phenytoin, phenobarbital, and rifampin induce hepatic enzymes that increase quinidine clearance and decrease the plasma drug concentration. Amiodarone and cimetidine decrease the clearance of quinidine and increase the plasma concentration. The digoxin-quinidine interaction is well described. Quinidine increases the steady-state plasma concentration of digoxin, and the digoxin dose should be decreased prior to starting quinidine. The serum concentration of both agents should be followed and the size of doses decreased where necessary. Nifedipine decreases serum concentration of quinidine, and verapamil increases the quinidine half-life and, therefore, the serum concentration. When quinidine is administered with coumarin anticoagulants, a reduction in clotting factor concentrations occurs, and prothrombin time should be monitored and the coumarin dose adjusted. Quinidine competitively inhibits the debrisoquin-metabolizing isozyme, P450, which metabolizes many commonly used medications; care must be exercised in administering quinidine to patients using these agents.

PROCAINAMIDE

CLINICAL ELECTROPHYSIOLOGIC AND ECG EFFECTS

Effects on sinus rate in patients studied in the clinical electrophysiology laboratory are variable, although a slight increase in heart rate (7%) has been reported, as well as a significant decrease in sinus cycle length, uncorrected sinus recovery time, and sinoatrial conduction time. Sinus node dysfunction may be aggravated by procainamide.

Procainamide is associated with increased atrial refractoriness (Table 5.1). At therapeutic concentrations, it causes slight prolongation of AV conduction and variable effects on ERPs and functional refractory periods (FRPs) of the AV node; a vagolytic effect may account for such variability. Even at low doses, it significantly increases the H-V and His-Purkinje FRP and relative refractory periods (Table 5.1). In patients with preexisting intraventricular conduction defects, procainamide causes modest, approximately 18%, prolongation of the H-V interval.

Interindividual variability in the surface ECG is observed (Table 5.1) and, like the others in its class, prolongation of the P-R, QRS, and Q-Tc intervals can be expected after procainamide, although it has no significant effect on the R-R interval. Procainamide widens the QRS slightly at usual doses but can markedly increase the QRS at faster rates or at high plasma concentrations. Progressive prolongation of the QRS as the plasma concentration increases is useful to assess the myocardial effect. Likewise, widening of the QRS interval greater than 25% is recommended as an endpoint to dosing. As the plasma drug concentration increases, the coupling interval of VPC is prolonged, suggesting progressive prolongation of His-Purkinje conduction. Because both procainamide and its metabolite, N-acetylprocainamide, prolong the ERP, prolongation of the Q-Tc interval is often noted. Procainamide also prolongs the total electrical systole of ventricular premature depolarizations such that the QRS and Q-Tc intervals of the VPC are also prolonged.

CLINICAL PHARMACOLOGY

The bioavailability of procainamide is large and ranges from 75–95% (Table 5.2). Peak plasma concentration is reached within 1–2 hours. A small amount is protein bound, i.e., 10–20%; however, binding to the acute phase reactant, α^{-1}-acid glycoprotein, is not as important as for quinidine or disopyramide. Procainamide is a weak base, and it follows urine pH-dependent excretion in dogs but not in humans. The apparent volume of distribution is very large, ranging from 1.5–2.5 liters/kg body weight (Table 5.2) and can be significantly reduced under conditions such as CHF or cardiogenic shock. At steady state, the myocardium to plasma procainamide concentration ratio is 3:1.

Approximately 30–50% of procainamide is metabolized by the liver, and at least three metabolites have been recognized and two identified. Although 7–24% of the major cardioactive metabolite, N-acetylprocainamide, is recovered in the urine, another metabolite, desethyl-N-acetylprocainamide is less well characterized. The $t^{1/2}$ elimination half-life of procainamide ranges from 3–6 hours; however, patients with diminished renal function or severe renal disease have a markedly prolonged elimination half-life and reduced clearance, and smaller doses or less frequent dosing intervals are necessary. Total body clearance ranges from 300–700 mL/minute. N-acetylprocainamide kinetics studied in normal subjects and in cardiac patients reveal that its half-life varies between 4 and 15 hours, and total body clearance is about 200–300 mL/min, 2.5 times less than the parent compound. Renal clearance of N-acetylprocainamide is important in patients with cardiac disease, the elderly, and functionally anephric patients, for whom elimination may be more than 40 hours. The effective N-acetylprocainamide concentration is 9–12 mg/L.

DRUG DOSING

Procainamide is a very versatile agent that may be given orally, intravenously, or (rarely) intramuscularly (Table 5.3). Oral administration is most widely used, and 500–1500 mg every 4–6 hours is a satisfactory schedule. Cardiac patients may have a significantly longer half-life of elimination than do normal patients, because of decreased renal function and/or low output states. Thus, dosing should be individualized. Moreover, because N-acetylprocainamide has antiarrhythmic effects, even longer dosing intervals may be possible. Sustained release formulations, based on delayed GI absorption, improve patient compliance and avoid peak and nadir plasma concentrations. Daily doses, ranging from 3–7.5 g, are given in divided doses 3 to 4 times a day.

The therapeutic antiarrhythmic plasma concentration range of procainamide for VPC suppression following myocardial infarction (MI) is 4–12 mg/liter (Table 5.2). The average plasma concentration required for suppression of chronic VPCs is higher (range, 2–17 mg/liter) and the concentration that prevents sustained ventricular tachyarrhythmias is even higher (range, 5–32 mg/liter). An effective procainamide plasma concentration after sustained-release formulations ranges from 7–10 mg/liter, and for N-acetylprocainamide from 9–12 mg/liter. Intramuscular administration is possible but not widely used, probably because it offers little advantage. Indeed, peak plasma concentrations and the time needed to reach the peak approximate those of oral therapy.

In acute situations, where the drug must be administered rapidly, intermittent i.v. procainamide can be given at 100-mg doses for 5 minutes through an indwelling i.v. catheter to a maximum of 1–1.5 g. Blood pressure is measured every 5 minutes following a dose, and continuous electrocardiographic monitoring to determine the QRS and Q-Tc intervals should be performed. An alternate method of procainamide administration is to administer the drug via a rapid constant-rate infusion, e.g., to administer the same dose at a constant-rate infusion (10–20 mg/minute). Once acute arrhythmia is controlled, an i.v. infusion may be started.

HEMODYNAMIC EFFECTS

Procainamide does not significantly modify arterial blood pressure, as determined in models of anesthetized or conscious dogs. In anesthetized dogs, procainamide causes an initial fall in blood pressure that is related to the speed of administration, while a vasodilatory effect, resulting from inhibition of ganglionic transmission, has also been demonstrated. Rapid and large i.v. injections cause systemic hypotension, a decrease in pulmonary vascular resistance, a fall in pulmonary artery pressure, local vasodilation, and a decline in cardiac output.

INDICATIONS

Procainamide's efficacy in terminating VT or preventing induction of VT, using programmed electrical stimulation, ranges from 15–50%. Incremental procainamide increases tachycardia cycle length, increases the effective ventricular refractory periods, and potentiates rate-dependent prolongation of the QRS duration (Table 5.1). It increases the VT cycle length; however, this is not predictive of efficacy, and some arrhythmias are more easily induced or difficult to terminate after procainamide. Procainamide's effectiveness may be enhanced in combination with the class Ib drugs, phenytoin, lidocaine, and mexiletine, or with β-blockers, agents that possess different electrophysiologic properties.

Patients with stable VPCs, VPCs post-MI, and with lethal and potentially lethal ventricular arrhythmias have been treated. Reduction of ventricular arrhythmias in 90% of patients with VPCs and 80% with nonsustained VT has been documented in the acute setting. Sixty-five percent of 218 patients with chronic ventricular arrhythmias had an antiarrhythmic effect, and others have reported similar results with chronic ventricular arrhythmias. Sustained-release procainamide has been effective against chronic stable and potentially lethal VPCs, and 76% of patients have at least a 75% reduction in VPC frequency and complex forms when treated with 3.0–7.5 g/day.

Procainamide suppresses premature atrial depolarizations, paroxysmal atrial tachycardia, AF, and flutter. During its development, reports indicated that it was more effective against ventricular than supraventricular arrhythmias; however, it has proven to be as effective as quinidine against supraventricular arrhythmias. Procainamide converts AF to sinus rhythm in patients with normal left atrial size and reduces premature atrial depolarizations, atrial tachycardia, and atrial echo beats. It prolongs atrial flutter cycle length, atrial refractoriness, and atrial conduction, and during atrial pacing, procainamide may convert atrial flutter to normal sinus rhythm. Because the atrial rate in fibrillation and flutter decreases, procainamide probably slows the maximum repetition rate for a cell until it is not possible for a circulating wave front of excitation to find a mass of excitable cells. Procainamide effectively terminates paroxysmal AF, especially when given intravenously for arrhythmia associated with coronary artery bypass surgery.

Procainamide effectively suppresses antegrade and retrograde conduction over an AV bypass tract in some patients with Wolff-Parkinson-White (WPW) syndrome, who are susceptible to AF. This is a reflection of prolongation of the refractory period, as well as a slowing of conduction velocity in atrial, ventricular, and accessory pathway tissue.

SIDE EFFECTS

GI symptoms (anorexia, nausea, vomiting), CNS symptoms (headache, insomnia, dizziness, psychosis, hallucination, and depression), fever, rash (morbilliform urticaria), myalgias, digital vasculitis, and Raynaud's phenomenon have been reported. A potentially life-threatening event is pancytopenia or agranulocytosis in a patient receiving procainamide. This requires drug withdrawal and, if necessary, treatment with appropriate antibiotics. This may be an allergic or hypersensitivity reaction or immunologically mediated. It occurs days to weeks after starting procainamide, and recovery of the white cell blood count is variable after stopping the drug. Radionuclide studies of customary doses indicate procainamide decreases left ventricular function slightly, but toxic concentrations diminish myocardial performance, and large i.v. doses cause significant hypotension.

A worrisome adverse effect associated with procainamide is the systemic lupus erythematosus (SLE) syndrome that occurs in 15–25% of patients taking the drug for more than 1 year (Table 5.4). The syndrome is associated with arthralgias and arthritis and a serositis involving lungs, pleura, and pericardium. Approximately 15–20% of patients receiving procainamide develop antinuclear antibodies (ANAs) but not the SLE-like syndrome, suggesting that ANAs are not pathognomonic for the clinical expression of SLE. To determine if the potential for developing the SLE-like syndrome is predictable, several investigators tested the rate of acetylation from the fraction of N-acetylprocainamide in urine or plasma samples versus the acetylation phenotype determined with isoniazid, dapsone, or sulfamethazine. Slow acetylators develop positive ANA as well as the SLE-like syndrome more rapidly and at a lower dose than fast acetylators. However, acetylation phenotype does not reliably predict all adverse events, and fast acetylation phenotype does not offer protection from other adverse effects.

The effects of quinidine on the Q-T interval are significantly greater (P <.001) than procainamide and are unrelated to differences in cycle length, QRS duration, serum potassium level, concomitant drug administration, or relative serum drug levels of quinidine or procainamide. Quinidine prolongs the Q-T interval to a greater extent than procainamide explaining why quinidine is more frequently associated with torsade de pointes than procainamide. Other forms of proarrhythmia and nonfatal cardiac arrest have been observed in 3–12% of patients taking procainamide and do not appear as common as with the type Ic drugs, encainide or flecainide.

DRUG INTERACTIONS

In contrast to quinidine, procainamide does not interact with digoxin; however, treatment with amiodarone results in increased procainamide concentrations. Procainamide, cimetidine, and ranitidine are secreted by an active transport mechanism in the proximal tubule, and cimetidine and ranitidine may decrease systemic clearance of procainamide, in part by inhibiting its active secretion by the kidneys. Inhibition of renal clearance and prolongation of the half-life of elimination of procainamide and its metabolites cause higher procainamide concentrations, and the procainamide dose may need to be reduced. There is conflicting evidence regarding the effects of procainamide in combination with β-blockers. Some studies indicate that β-blockers have no significant effect on the kinetics of procainamide or N-acetylprocainamide, while others suggest that the half-life of elimination is increased and clearance decreased. Ethanol causes a significant reduction of the half-life and increases total clearance of procainamide without affecting either volume of distribution or renal clearance, which could account for an unpredictably low plasma drug concentration in patients whose alcohol intake is increased. Ethanol also increases the percentage of N-acetylprocainamide measured in blood and urine.

DISOPYRAMIDE

CLINICAL ELECTROPHYSIOLOGIC AND ECG EFFECTS

The electrophysiologic effects in humans are dependent on the dual action of disopyramide (Table 5.1). These effects studied in humans indicate that spontaneous sinus cycle length does not change but may decrease secondary to disopyramide's anticholinergic effects, and in the presence of atropine, cycle length increases. When given intravenously, sinus node recovery time is shortened, atrial functional and effective refractory periods are prolonged, and the AV nodal refractory period shortens slightly. However, pretreatment with atropine causes a prolonged sinus node recovery time and cycle length and prolongs the A-H interval and FRP of the AV node. Although patients with normal sinus function have normal sinus node recovery time and S-A conduction time, these may be depressed in patients with sinus node dysfunction. The variable effects of disopyramide on sinus node function appear to be influenced by its class Ia-electrophysiologic effects plus anticholinergic effects.

After disopyramide in humans, the A-H interval usually remains unchanged, while the H-V interval prolongs. Although it can cause high-grade AV block in patients with bifascicular disease, for the most part disopyramide is well tolerated. Atrial and ventricular refractory periods are increased; AV nodal ERP and FRP are unchanged, although AV nodal ERP may be slightly decreased and AV nodal FRP may be increased.

The electrocardiographic effects of disopyramide in normal and cardiac subjects are similar to quinidine and procainamide; however, the magnitude of ECG changes are not as great as after either quinidine or procainamide (Table 5.1). Disopyramide may increase sinus rate via its substantial anticholinergic effects. Its effect on the P-R interval is variable, with some reports indicating an increase while others note a decrease. The QRS increases from 2.7—39% (average, 15%) at therapeutic concentrations, and the Q-T and Q-Tc intervals are prolonged.

CLINICAL PHARMACOLOGY

Disopyramide is a racemic mixture of two *d*- and *l*-isomers. Absorption is rapid and complete, with a 70–90% absorption rate. In healthy subjects, peak plasma levels are attained in 2 hours (Table 5.2). Approximately 15% undergoes "first-pass" elimination via the liver. The mean plasma half-life of disopyramide is 6.7 hours, with a range of 4–10 hours, and the therapeutic plasma concentration range is 2–50 µ/mL. Disopyramide is excreted primarily in the urine; about 65–75% is excreted as the parent drug and the rest as the potentially active mono-*N*-dealky-lated metabolite (20%), mono-*N*-dealkylated disopyramide, and other minor metabolites (10%). Significant accumulation occurs at doses greater than 3 mg/kg, and in some, the plasma concentration of the major metabolite exceeds the parent compound. Metabolism is increased by agents that enhance hepatic enzymes (rifampin, phenytoin, and barbiturates), and plasma concentration is reduced in their presence. Because elimination is primarily via renal excretion, the dose must be decreased in patients with renal impairment and in the elderly.

DRUG DOSING

The usual adult dose of conventional disopyramide is 400–800 mg/day orally, given in divided doses of 100–150 mg every 6 hours or, for sustained release disopyramide, 300 mg every 12 hours (Table 5.3). In cases of refractory arrhythmias, maintenance doses of 1200 mg/day have been given. Occasionally, for rapid control of an arrhythmia, an oral loading dose of 300 mg of conventional disopyramide is recommended, followed by a maintenance regimen of 400–800 mg/day, i.e., 150 mg every 6 hours. Higher maintenance doses following the initial loading dose have been used, particularly if there are no adverse effects; however, careful electrocardiographic and blood pressure monitoring or hospitalization are necessary to avoid drug overdose.

HEMODYNAMIC EFFECTS

Animal studies have documented the substantial negative inotropic effect of disopyramide. As little as 1 mg/kg of body weight given intravenously causes a marked reduction in myocardial contractility in dogs. At higher doses (5–10 mg/kg), the decrease in contractile force is 50–100% greater than with quinidine. Compared with quinidine, stroke volume, left ventricular stroke work, and fractional shortening are reduced, and end-diastolic segment length is increased in dogs receiving intravenous disopyramide. At relatively low doses of 1–2 mg/kg, cardiac output is decreased about 18%, and at larger doses, 5–10 mg/kg, cardiac output decreases even more, by 22–49%. In patients with ventricular dysfunction, disopyramide may reduce cardiac output by 8–25% and increase peripheral vascular resistance. The drug may also cause cardiogenic shock.

INDICATIONS

A number of clinical studies have shown that disopyramide is effective in suppressing VPCs in about 65% of patients and is as effective as quinidine in suppressing VPCs by 75%. This finding was demonstrated in an 8-week double-blind study in which disopyramide, 400–800 mg/day, was compared to quinidine, 1300 mg/day. Lower doses in combination with mexiletine are more effective and better tolerated than monotherapy with either disopyramide or mexiletine. A combination of disopyramide (mean dose = 524 mg/day) and mexiletine (652 mg/day) in smaller doses is well tolerated, avoids dose-related side effects, and is more effective than either drug used alone or in higher doses.

Disopyramide has been shown to be effective in suppressing sustained VT. Studies using programmed electrical stimulation fail to induce VT in 4–34% at plasma levels in midrange, i.e., 3–5 µg/mL. In uncontrolled studies it is effective in preventing the recurrence of spontaneous VT by diminishing recurrence rate or eliminating further episodes. Disopyramide is as effective as other class Ia agents in its ability to suppress sustained VT assessed by programmed electrical stimulation. There is no concordancy or discordancy in effect between disopyramide and others in its class, and, thus, lack of efficacy with quinidine or procainamide should not preclude a trial of disopyramide.

Disopyramide is as effective as quinidine in suppressing atrial premature complexes, and a double-blind study of patients successfully cardioverted showed disopyramide to be as effective as quinidine in preventing recurrence of AF and more effective than placebo. The negative inotropic effect and the potential to worsen heart failure limit its use, particularly in patients with a history of heart failure and AF. Disopyramide, however, is a reasonable choice for younger patients without heart failure. The effect of disopyramide on atrial flutter is similar to quinidine in that a reduction in atrial flutter rate and a vagolytic effect on AV conduction may lead to 1:1 conduction and consequent rapid ventricular response. Thus, when used for atrial flutter, treatment with each of the class Ia agents should be preceded with an agent to slow AV nodal conduction, such as digoxin, a β-blocker, or calcium channel antagonist.

Disopyramide has been moderately useful in managing supraventricular tachycardia, and doses ranging from 200–600 mg/day prevent episodes of supraventricular tachycardia. It has been used to treat persistent supraventricular tachycardia; however, other agents, in particular calcium channel antagonists and β-blockers, have been used with greater success.

In the WPW syndrome, disopyramide prolongs both antegrade and retrograde refractory periods of the accessory pathway and depresses conduction in the accessory pathway. Thus, it has potential usefulness in treating arrhythmias that involve a reentrant pathway. Disopyramide terminates AF in 82% of patients with AF and the WPW syndrome, in the absence of atrial enlargement, using i.v. administration over 10 minutes. R-R intervals during AF are significantly prolonged after the drug (by <80%), and AF was more tolerable, even if conversion to sinus rhythm does not occur.

The usefulness of disopyramide for vasovagal syncope has recently been noted. Its autonomic and hemodynamic properties may (a) antagonize vagally mediated bradycardia (anticholinergic) and (b) attenuate or substantially reduce hypercontractility with its associated chamber obliteration via its negative inotropic properties. In addition, its vasoconstrictor properties may support or maintain systemic pressure, decreasing the need for increased peripheral catecholamines, which are partly responsible for the increased contractility.

Negative inotropic effects of disopyramide have been used to treat a small number of symptomatic adults and children with idiopathic hypertrophic subaortic stenosis. Intravenous disopyramide infusion resulted in abolition of the resting outflow gradient, increase in exercise capacity, and decrease in symptoms.

SIDE EFFECTS

The safety profile of disopyramide has been well established, and its most commonly observed side effects are anticholinergic, including dry mouth (32%), urinary hesitancy (14%), and constipation (11%). Because of its anticholinergic actions, disopyramide should not be used in patients with glaucoma, myasthenia gravis, or urinary retention. Some of the anticholinergic effects may be diminished by concomitant use of physostigmine, pyridostigmine, or bethanechol. These agents may selectively reverse the troublesome anticholinergic effects without affecting its electrophysiologic or antiarrhythmic properties. Compared with others in its class (Table 5.4), there is a low incidence of CNS adverse effects, and the SLE-like syndrome and agranulocytosis seen with procainamide are very rarely found. The most severe side effects result from its negative inotropic effects, which are more marked than others in its class. The proarrhythmic potential for disopyramide (6%) is less than quinidine (15%) or procainamide (9%).

Acute CHF may occur as early as 48 hours following the administration of disopyramide. An important predictor of heart failure is a past history of CHF. Worsened heart failure occurs in 55% of patients with such a history compared with an incidence of 5% in those without. Heart failure is usually promptly reversed on discontinuation of disopyramide but in some may require treatment with diuretics, inotropic agents, or afterload-reducing agents.

Like others in its class, disopyramide has been reported to aggravate ventricular arrhythmias and cause Q-T interval prolongation and "torsade de pointes." Disopyramide syncope associated with Q-T prolongation has been described. As with quinidine and procainamide, proarrhythmia is frequently associated with hypokalemia, hypomagnesemia, and bradyarrhythmias. In a series of patients with torsade induced by class Ia drugs, lidocaine was found to be inconsistently effective, while atrial or ventricular pacing was effective and tolerated. Intravenous magnesium sulfate was useful in patients with Q-T prolongation when given as an initial bolus of 2 g with repeated doses as needed. The mechanism of action of this benefit may be secondary to suppression of afterdepolarizations.

DRUG INTERACTIONS

Disopyramide's interactions with other drugs are considerably less than quinidine's. It may potentiate the effect of coumadin, but this does not appear to be a significant interaction. Nevertheless, prothrombin time should be checked in patients taking disopyramide, particularly when the dose is stopped or changed. In contrast to quinidine, disopyramide does not interact with digoxin. There is no effect of either propranolol or diazepam on disopyramide kinetics; however, drugs

with negative inotropic effects including β-blockers and/or calcium channel antagonists may have pharmacodynamic interactions and should be used cautiously in
view of disopyramide's myocardial depressant effects. Because there is a significant
kinetic interaction with drugs that induce hepatic enzymes (phenytoin, barbiturates, or rifampin), the concentration of the metabolite relative to the parent compound may be increased and the incidence of adverse anticholinergic effects may
also be increased. Drugs such as scopolamine or atropine will enhance the anticholinergic effect of disopyramide, aggravating dry mouth and urinary retention.

CLASS IB ANTIARRHYTHMIC AGENTS: LIDOCAINE AND MEXILETINE

LIDOCAINE

CLINICAL ELECTROPHYSIOLOGIC AND ECG EFFECTS

Lidocaine was in widespread clinical use before the advent of clinical electrophysiology and has not been as systematically investigated using electrophysiologic
procedures have as many newer antiarrhythmic agents. In patients with normal
sinus and AV nodal function, no consistent effect on spontaneous heart rate or P-
R interval is seen, and QRS complexes are unchanged. In patients with sinus node
disease, lidocaine is well tolerated. In one study, sinus node dysfunction was not
aggravated in nine patients with preexisting disease, and in 17 patients with AV or
H-V interval disorders, no clinically untoward effects were produced by a 100-mg
i.v. bolus of lidocaine. In five of the total of 26 patients treated, however, an intraventricular conduction disorder was produced. By contrast, in randomized clinical
studies, asystole and sinus bradycardia have been reported. Most incidents appear
to have passed quickly, but in one study, resuscitation was necessary for some
patients. Thus, lidocaine can rarely and unexpectedly disturb sinus node and perhaps AV nodal function. Atrial, AV nodal, and ventricular effective refractory periods are usually unchanged.

CLINICAL PHARMACOLOGY

Lidocaine undergoes extensive first-pass hepatic metabolism and must be
administered either intravenously or intramuscularly. It is metabolized to glycine
xylidide and monoethylglycine xylidide. These have weak antiarrhythmic properties, and both may contribute to toxicity. Lidocaine has a relatively short elimination half-life of 3 hours, necessitating constant infusion or multiple intramuscular
administrations to maintain therapeutic plasma concentrations. For these reasons,
lidocaine is appropriate only for the acute treatment or short-term prophylaxis of
ventricular arrhythmias.

DRUG DOSING

Lidocaine is generally administered as an i.v. bolus of 1.0–1.5 mg/kg (often translated in emergency situations as 100 mg for an average adult) delivered over 3 minutes, followed by an infusion of 4 mg/minute for 1 hour, 3 mg/minute for 1 hour, and then 2 mg/minute thereafter. The half-life of a single bolus is approximately 15 minutes, because of rapid hepatic metabolism as well as dissipation to adipose tissue, where the drug is avidly bound. Because an infusion will require 2–3 hours before steady-state therapeutic levels are achieved, repeated boluses of the drug may be necessary to maintain efficacy during this time. This is also the case if an increased dose and infusion rate are necessary. The maintenance infusion level should be decreased in patients with liver disease and for those in heart failure. During prolonged i.v. therapy (>24 hours), there is a risk of toxic accumulation, and in this situation the dose should be guided by plasma concentration estimates. When lidocaine is being used for acute termination of an arrhythmia, a second bolus of 50–100 mg over 5 minutes can be given, if the initial administration is unsuccessful and if clinical circumstances are consistent with continuing a drug approach. The second bolus should not be given within 5 minutes of the first for fear of producing neurotoxic effects.

Lidocaine accumulates in adipose tissue during a constant infusion, creating high levels in the body. When the infusion is discontinued, the drug is released into the blood from these stores over the next 2–3 hours. Hence there is no reason to "taper" lidocaine.

HEMODYNAMIC EFFECTS

In clinical practice, lidocaine is hemodynamically well tolerated. There are only rare reports of hemodynamic collapse caused by lidocaine, but detailed studies have revealed a dose-dependent depressive effect on left ventricular performance. Lidocaine increases preload (left ventricular end diastolic pressure [LVEDP] rises) and contractility is impaired (fractional shortening and ejection fraction fall). At "therapeutic" concentrations, the effect is minimal, but when high doses of lidocaine are given, cardiac output and blood pressure may be significantly depressed. The elderly and patients with preexisting functional abnormality are most vulnerable. Nonetheless, lidocaine is remarkably well tolerated, even by patients with overt heart failure; its relatively short half-life provides an important safeguard, inasmuch as any deleterious effect can be contained by prompt cessation of therapy.

INDICATIONS

Early studies indicated that lidocaine might be used for prophylaxis against primary ventricular fibrillation (VF in the absence of shock or failure) complicating acute MI. In the 1960s and 1970s, primary VF complicated about 10% of hospitalized MI patients and was held responsible for the substantial out-of-hospital mortality of the condition.

Only three studies have provided statistically secure positive evidence that prophylactic lidocaine prevents VF. In one study, VF was not the assessed endpoint; the patients were not monitored. Sudden death was analyzed and found to be significantly less frequent in those who received active lidocaine. This result, however, was obtained in a randomized study in which 156 patients received lidocaine and 113 received placebo. This imbalance has been attributed to the unblinding of therapy by some of the participating general practitioners, and it has cast doubt on the reliability of the result. In another study, i.v. lidocaine was proven effective, but this investigation provided little information about the safety of lidocaine, particularly in those patients who later were proven not to have had an MI. A prethrombolytic trial was conducted by paramedics and concentrated on the first hour after lidocaine administration. The authors predetermined that analysis of VF would be made in the first 15 minutes (when intramuscular lidocaine was unlikely to have been absorbed sufficiently to achieve therapeutic plasma concentrations) and in the subsequent 15–60 minutes. VF was significantly reduced in this latter period (0.4%, placebo; 0.07%, lidocaine), but in that same time period, asystolic events were significantly increased in lidocaine-treated patients. This study provides the best proof that lidocaine can prevent primary VF which complicates acute MI, but it reveals a risk of provoking potentially serious asystolic events.

SIDE EFFECTS

The unwanted cardiac effects of lidocaine have already been described. They comprise sinus slowing, asystole, hypotension, and shock. These problems are not common but are particularly associated with overdosing or with overly rapid administration of the drug. Moreover, the elderly and those with significant preexisting disease are at greatest risk. Remarkably little is known of lidocaine's capacity to provoke tachyarrhythmias. Its specificity of action and relatively short elimination half-life probably provide a great degree of safety. Although lidocaine's proarrhythmic potential has not been systematically evaluated, many years of use in the unstable phase of MI should have provided ample opportunity for any significant risk to have been identified.

Lidocaine commonly produces unwanted noncardiac effects. They are principally related to CNS toxicity and usually are trivial. One of these, tremor, is useful as a bedside sign of toxicity. High plasma concentrations of lidocaine can provoke seizures; this is of particular concern when lidocaine infusions are continued more than 24 hours, inasmuch as subtle accumulation may occur. Paradoxically, in a study specifically addressing the toxicity of prophylactic lidocaine, the first 12 hours of drug use represented the greatest risk period. Unwanted effects were greater in those who had not suffered an MI, raising concern about the use of the drug in an undefined chest pain population. Undesired effects were loosely correlated with plasma concentrations.

MEXILETINE

CLINICAL ELECTROPHYSIOLOGIC AND ECG EFFECTS

Mexiletine reduces conduction velocity in the ventricular myocardium, with an insignificant prolongation of the H-V interval. Sinus and AV node function and atrial refractoriness are usually unaffected, but as with lidocaine, mexiletine increases the functional refractory period of the AV node. In overdoses, mexiletine may cause asystole, sinus arrest, and AV block. In normal therapeutic doses, mexiletine produces no consistent ECG effects.

CLINICAL PHARMACOLOGY

Mexiletine, although available for parenteral use, is rarely used in this way. Lidocaine offers easier administration and a greater margin of safety through its shorter elimination half-life; the principal attraction of mexiletine is that it is active when taken orally. Mexiletine's important pharmacokinetic properties are detailed in Table 5.5. It is well absorbed from the GI tract and suffers no significant first-pass hepatic metabolism. After oral ingestion, peak plasma concentrations are achieved in about 90 minutes in normal subjects, but in patients with acute myocardial infarction, there is a delay of up to 5 hours between administration and peak plasma levels.

DRUG DOSING

Mexiletine has a large volume of distribution, and some have recommended that oral loading doses be given in an attempt to hasten the time taken to achieve stable plasma concentrations. Although this approach has some merit, in practice, little time is gained. Moreover, substantial oral loading doses may be poorly tolerated and prejudice patients against continuing therapy. The standard maintenance dose of mexiletine is 200–400 mg three times a day using conventional capsules or 360 mg twice daily of the slow-release form.

Mexiletine is metabolized in the liver; 15–20% is excreted unchanged in the urine. Renal excretion is dependent upon the pH level and on the presence of urinary alkalosis. The renal excretion of the drug is impaired, and blood levels increase. The magnitude of the effect is rarely large enough to be of clinical relevance. No active metabolites are known. Mexiletine's elimination half-life in MI patients is between 12–15 hours, but, importantly, this is prolonged in those with hepatic disease. The half-life is shorter in normal individuals (8–10 hours), and in those with "lone" arrhythmias (10–14 hours). The half-life is shorter in smokers

Table 5.5
Pharmacokinetic Properties of Mexiletine and Tocainide

	Mexiletine	Tocainide
Oral absorption	>90%	>95%
Elimination t½	10–15 hr	9–40 hr
Mean	12 hr	14 hr
Volume of distrubution	6–9 L/kg	1–3 L/kg
Protein binding	60–70%	4–20%
Elimination	80% metabolized	65% metabolized
Plasma concentration range	1–2 µg/mL	4–10 µg/mL
Daily dose	200–400 mg t.i.d.	400–800 mg t.i.d.

than in nonsmokers, but the clinical significance of this observation is uncertain. Mexiletine's half-life is little affected by heart failure, although a reduction in hepatic and renal blood flow can reduce clearance and increase the half-life. Renal function abnormalities do not affect clearance, at least until creatinine clearance values reach about 10 mL/minute.

HEMODYNAMIC EFFECTS

Studies involving i.v. mexiletine administration have shown minor and clinically unimportant decreases in blood pressure and cardiac output. In a comparison with lidocaine and propranolol, mexiletine produced a similarly minimal hemodynamic effect as its sister compound, lidocaine. When given to patients with impaired left ventricular performance, oral mexiletine does not alter either right or left ventricular ejection fractions. In clinical studies, mexiletine, particularly oral mexiletine, has been well tolerated hemodynamically, with only rare reports of hypotension, although the drug does cause a mild reduction in peripheral vascular resistance. More recent studies have confirmed the fairly modest depressant properties of mexiletine. The incidence of CHF exacerbation is low (2–3%) and is seen primarily in patients with a history of heart failure.

INDICATIONS

Mexiletine is indicated for the acute and chronic management of symptomatic ventricular arrhythmias, including VT. In uncontrolled studies, efficacy rates of 60–80% have been observed in patients with chronic stable ventricular arrhythmias. In the few controlled trials, "success" rates of 55–73% were reported. When tested in an electrophysiologic study against inducible monomorphic VT, it achieved an efficacy rate of 40%, but when used for similar but previously drug-resistant VTs, electrophysiologically established efficacy ranged from only 6–35%. Other assessment techniques, principally Holter monitoring, achieved a higher success rate. Mexiletine's relative lack of left ventricular depression has led to its use in patients with impaired cardiac function, for whom the drug appears to be reasonably effective and well tolerated. Nonetheless, such patients may be very sensitive to any negative inotropism, and mexiletine should be used very cautiously and only for clear indications.

Recently, there has been interest in the role of mexiletine as a component of combination antiarrhythmic therapy, and impressive anecdotal results have been reported. For the present, despite some theoretical attraction and the specific advantages of mexiletine, no antiarrhythmic drug combination has been subjected to sufficient research for general recommendation.

SIDE EFFECTS

Like other antiarrhythmic drugs, mexiletine may create new arrhythmias (Table 5.5). The proarrhythmia rate reported varies from 0–29%, which might suggest that in some circumstances proarrhythmia is a serious risk. Clinical usage indicates

Table 5.6
Side Effects of Mexiletine and Tocainide

Central nervous system
  Dose-related
    Dizziness
    Lightheadness
    Tremor
    Slurred speech
    Nystagmus
    Paresthesias

  Not dose-related
    Hallucinations
    Personality change
    Emotional instability
    Memory impairment
    Insomnia
    Seizures

Gastrointestinal
  Abdominal discomfort
  Nausea
  Vomiting
  Anorexia
  Diarrhea
  Liver function test abnormalities

Cardiovascular
  Arrhythmia aggravation
  Congestive heart failure
  Hypotension
  Bradycardia and asystole (mexiletine)

Hematologic
  Thrombocytopenia (mexiletine)
  Agranulocytosis (tocainide)

Other
  Positive ANA
  Fever
  Rash
  Pulmonary fibrosis (tocainide)

that the proarrhythmia risk is low, perhaps less than 5%. Polymorphic tachycardia can occur, but it is relatively uncommon. Some researchers have suggested a positive role for mexiletine in the management of long Q-T-associated torsade de pointes, but, despite some theoretical attractions, this cannot be recommended with confidence at present. Registry evidence does not confirm this concept, although possibly there is a responsive Q-T subgroup that is as yet unidentifiable. Mexiletine may aggravate or provoke heart failure; this is not common except in those with preexisting cardiac decompensation. Bradycardia, hypotension, and AV nodal blockade are rarely observed.

The majority of mexiletine's unwanted effects are noncardiac. Nausea and vomiting and CNS effects, including ataxia, tremor, dizziness, speech disorders, and rarely seizures significantly limit the use of mexiletine. Although these CNS effects are usually dose-related, others, including memory and personality changes, insomnia, and hallucinations, are not. The CNS side effects are identical to those caused by lidocaine.

Serious noncardiac unwanted effects are rare but include thrombocytopenia, hepatitis, and ANA positivity. Other reports have documented that in some patients a positive ANA has become negative upon changing antiarrhythmic therapy to mexiletine.

CLASS IC ANTIARRHYTHMIC AGENTS: PROPAFENONE, FLECAINIDE, AND MORICIZINE

PROPAFENONE

CLINICAL ELECTROPHYSIOLOGIC AND ECG EFFECTS

The clinical electrophysiology of propafenone has been studied extensively in both human volunteers and patients with various degrees of cardiac disease. Propafenone significantly increases the P-R interval (by 12–22%) and the QRS duration (by 6–17%) in a dose-related fashion (Table 5.7). It prolongs the Q-T interval minimally, and because most of the Q-T prolongation is due to QRS widening, a more appropriate measurement of repolarization time is the J-T interval, which is not altered. Given the wide variability in metabolism and resultant blood levels, only estimates can be given for the average changes in electrocardiographic intervals caused by propafenone. AV nodal conduction is significantly increased. Thus, care is necessary when propafenone is used in patients with suspected sick sinus syndrome or heart block. Sinus cycle length is usually unchanged by oral administration of propafenone. However, the drug does have β-receptor and calcium channel blocking effects; thus, it can cause sinus node depression and dysfunction, especially in patients with underlying sinus node dysfunction. Both atrial and ventricular refractoriness are increased during propafenone therapy. A potentially important observation is that antegrade and retrograde accessory pathway conduction are significantly increased in patients with the WPW syndrome.

Propafenone has structural similarities to β-adrenergic antagonists. The oral administration of propafenone results in an increased density of β-adrenergic receptors on human lymphocytes, and propafenone administration results in typical clinical β-blocking effects, although the drug is estimated to be only 1/40th as potent as propranolol. Thus, propafenone should be used cautiously in asthmatics or patients with sick sinus syndrome.

The degree to which propafenone produces β-blocking effects in individual patients is partially related to the dose administered as well as the degree to which the drug is metabolized (normal or slow metabolizer) and the resulting plasma

Table 5.7
Electrophysiologic and Electrocardiographic Effects of Class Ic Antiarrhythmic Agents

	Propafenone	Flecainide	Moricizine
Sinus rate	Decreased	NSC[a]	Decreased
A-H interval	Increased	NSC	Increased
H-V interval	Increased	Increased	Increased
Atrial ERP	Increased	NSC	NSC
AV node ERP	Increased	NSC	NSC or increased
Ventricular ERP	Increased	Increased	NSC or increased
Accessory pathway ERP	Increased (antegrade and retrograde)	Increased (antegrade and retrograde)	Increased (antegrade and retrograde)
P-R interval	Increased	Increased	Increased
QRS interval	Increased	Increased	Increased
JTc	NSC	NSC	NSC or increased

[a]NSC, no significant change; ERP, effective refractory period.

propafenone level. In general, the degree of heart rate slowing in patients taking therapeutic doses of propafenone is modest compared with that of a nonselective β-blocker.

CLINICAL PHARMACOLOGY

The metabolism of propafenone is complex, resulting in a large variability of plasma levels (Table 5.8). Propafenone is well absorbed from the GI tract and reaches peak plasma concentrations in 2–3 hours. Food and antacids reduce the rate of absorption and delay the time to peak concentrations but do not alter the level achieved. The drug is strongly protein bound. In the majority of patients (40%), propafenone metabolism is rapid via the liver cytochrome P-450 system with an elimination half-life of 3–12 hours. A specific cytochrome P-450 enzyme responsible for propafenone metabolism has been identified. The primary metabolites are 5-hydroxypropafenone and N-depropylpropafenone, both of which possess modest antiarrhythmic activity. In approximately 7–10% of patients, the metabolism of propafenone is slower, and propafenone metabolites are not formed or minimally detected, because of the absence of this single hepatic cytochrome P-450 enzyme. In patients lacking this enzyme, the elimination half-life is dramatically prolonged (10–32 hours). Thus, there are significant resultant differences in the plasma concentration of propafenone, with the slow metabolizers achieving concentrations up to two times the extensive metabolizers.

Elimination of the drug is primarily by hepatic metabolic and fecal excretion, with <1% of the original dose excreted unchanged. The drug exhibits nonlinear pharmacokinetics. As the dose increases, hepatic metabolic sites become saturated, metabolism decreases, and blood levels and half-life increase. The mean steady-state plasma elimination half-life ($t_{1/2}$) is significantly longer for poor metabolizers (17.2 hours) than in the more than 90% of patients who metabolize the drug rapidly,

Table 5.8
Clinical Pharmacology of Selected Class Ic Antiarrhythmic Agents

	Propafenone	Fleicainide	Moricizine
Dose	Oral, 150–300 mg t.i.d.	Oral 50–15· mg t.i.d.	Oral 200–400 mg. t.i.d.
Absorption	Rapid, complete	Rapid, complete	Rapid, complete
Bioavailability	Dose-related 13–55%; (first-pass hepatic clearance)	95%	30–40% (first-pass hepatic metabolism)
Peak levels	2–5 hr	3–4 hours	1–3 hours
Protein binding	90–95%	40%	95%
Volume of distribution	3.0 liter/kg (200–300 liters)	10 liters/kg	11.6 liters/kg (200–300 liters)
Half-life	6 hr (3–12 hr) in extensive metabolizers; 17 hr (10–32 hr) in poor metabolizers	20 hr (11–30)	2–4 hr (10–13 hr in patients with heart disease)
Therapeutic blood levels	Variable	0.2–1.0 µg/mL	Variable
Metabolism	Hepatic (99%) (rapid in extensive metabolizers, 90% of patients)	Hepatic (70%)	Hepatic (>99%)
Metabolites	5-Hydroxypropafenone N-Depropylpropafenone	meta-O-Dealkylated flecainide meta-O-Dealkylated lactam flecaininde Probably inactive	Inactive (approximately 8)

in which the $t_{1/2}$ averages 6 hours. As would be expected, the half-life of propafenone is increased in patients with significant liver disease. Caution should also be used when administering propafenone to patients with severe renal disease, including patients on hemodialysis, because of renal elimination of the active propafenone metabolites in the urine. Propafenone is not significantly cleared by hemodialysis. The majority of clinical trials that have investigated the relationships between plasma concentration, dose, and the antiarrhythmic effects of propafenone have concluded there is no clinically useful correlation.

INDICATIONS

Propafenone is presently indicated only for use in life-threatening ventricular arrhythmias. The relevant clinical trials of propafenone relate to its ability to suppress inducible sustained VT during electrophysiologic studies (EPS). The reported studies of propafenone-related suppression of inducible VT provide wide estimates of efficacy rates from 8–36% (Table 5.9). The differences in individual studies are explained by the small sample sizes and the fact that the patient populations as well as efficacy definitions vary. A reasonable expectation is that the acute response rate to the suppression of inducible VT by propafenone is probably 15–25%. Even less can be said about estimating the long-term efficacy of propafenone in this population. Only small and uncontrolled clinical trial observations are available, comprised of varying protocols, doses, and definitions of efficacy.

Table 5.9
Results of Therapy with Class Ic Antiarrhythmic Agents

	Propafenone	Flecainide	Moricizine
Efficacy[a]			
VPBs	70–80	80	50–70
NSVT	50–70	80–85	50–60
VT (EPS)	15–25	10–20	10–15
AF	40–60	70	?
SVT	70	80	?
Toxicity[b]			
Proarrhythmia	5–9	4–19	3–12
CHF	5	5–15	2–12
Noncardiac	14–20	20–30	20–25
Discontinuing for toxicity	5–10	5–10	6–10

[a]Percent of patients with arrhythmia suppression
[b]Percent of patients having side effect.

There has been a published experience from 27 studies involving 394 patients on propafenone who underwent EPS; the studies were small, uncontrolled trials (average 14 patients per report). Of the 394 patients, 25% had no arrhythmia induced on propafenone. Subjective assessment of long-term efficacy (mean 14 months) was reported as 67%, a number that should be interpreted cautiously.

Propafenone suppressed VPCs by 70–80% in more than 70% of patients tested (Table 5.9). Elimination of couplets and runs of nonsustained ventricular tachycardia (NSVT) occur in 50–70%, an observation consistent with the effectiveness of most antiarrhythmic drugs tested. It is important to note that, based on the results of these clinical trials, a dose-response relationship can be identified that shows a proportional increase in the reduction of VPCs, couplets, and runs of VT using propafenone doses of 450–900 mg. At the 900 mg/day dose, 68% of patients achieved a mean VPC reduction of 80%.

The efficacy of propafenone for AF has also been studied in many trials (Table 5.9). In a study of 100 patients randomly selected to receive propafenone or sotalol, patients with chronic AF were followed for 1 year. The rate of patients remaining in sinus rhythm at 3, 6, and 12 months on propafenone was 46, 41, and 30%, respectively, whereas similar proportions of sotalol-treated patients remained in sinus rhythm at the same time intervals (49, 46, and 37%, respectively; P not significant). Thus, both of these agents were only modestly effective in maintaining sinus rhythm. The long-term efficacy of propafenone has also been investigated. In 60 patients presenting with either paroxysmal AF (PAF) or chronic AF, 40% of patients remained free of symptomatic arrhythmia recurrences at 6 months. However, the patients who remained in chronic AF benefitted from the β-adrenoreceptor-blocking effects of propafenone, which produced a decrease in the ventricular response rate. These modest efficacy results demonstrate limited expectations with propafenone in this population. In a trial of 33 patients with either paroxysmal AF (N = 17) or paroxysmal supraventricular tachycardia (N =

16), propafenone administration resulted in a prolonged time to first symptomatic arrhythmia recurrence (P <.004). Recurrence rates on propafenone were reduced 80%, compared with recurrence rates on placebo, but complete long-term freedom from arrhythmia recurrence is an unrealistic expectation.

Propafenone prolongs the antegrade and retrograde refractory periods in patients presenting with supraventricular arrhythmias and WPW syndrome. Propafenone was more effective than procainamide in slowing the ventricular response due to AF in these patients with WPW syndrome, although there was a trend to a better conversion rate with procainamide. The majority of these patients are now treated by catheter ablation, but propafenone is an attractive alternative in the long-term management of paroxysmal AF associated with the WPW syndrome.

SIDE EFFECTS

In patients with life-threatening ventricular arrhythmias, proarrhythmia associated with propafenone has been reported to occur in 4–19% of patients. A overview of 684 patients with a variety of ventricular arrhythmias, Hernandez and co-workers estimated the serious proarrhythmia rate at 3.6%. In the ESVEM trial, 24% of patients receiving propafenone had some adverse cardiovascular event that was similar to that caused by the other drugs: imipramine (43%); mexiletine (27%); pirmenol (23%); procainamide (24%); quinidine (24%); and sotalol (26%). However, ventricular tachyarrhythmias during drug titration occurred more often in patients who received propafenone than in patients who received any of the other six antiarrhythmic drugs. Importantly, nearly half of these effects occurred within 2 days of the initiation of propafenone therapy and were not related to either rapid dose escalation or drug accumulation in slow metabolizers.

Propafenone can cause new cardiac conduction abnormalities including AV block and bundle branch block. These are infrequent and resolve with drug withdrawal or dose reduction. Overall conduction abnormalities are observed in up to 8.4% of patients receiving propafenone. First-degree heart block occurs most frequently (2.5%), while second- or third-degree heart block is uncommon (0.6 and 0.2%, respectively). Propafenone can also result in a worsening of CHF because of a combination of its electrophysiologic class Ic effects combined with its β-adrenergic receptor and perhaps calcium blocking effects. The frequency with which this occurs appears to be both dose dependent and related to the degree of underlying structural heart disease.

Approximately 14–20% of patients taking propafenone experience noncardiac complaints. Mild CNS symptoms are common and include dizziness, headache, and blurred vision. Because of the drug's β-blocking effects, exacerbation of asthma occurs but is uncommon. GI symptoms occur occasionally and include nausea, anorexia, vomiting, constipation, and altered (metallic) taste, probably resulting from secretion of the drug in saliva.

DRUG INTERACTIONS

Propafenone has β-blocker activity; thus, concomitant use of β-blockers may result in an enhanced sympatholytic effect. Propafenone blood levels may become elevated because of competitive liver metabolism. Prothrombin time may increase when warfarin is coadministered. Cyclosporin levels may increase as a result of propafenone, and digoxin levels increase by 37–63%, although clinical relevance is not certain. Concomitant quinidine and cimetidine administration will increase propafenone levels, a result of metabolic interaction in the liver.

FLECAINIDE

CLINICAL ELECTROPHYSIOLOGIC AND ELECTROCARDIOGRAPHIC EFFECTS

Flecainide slows cardiac conduction in all tissue, producing dose-related increases in P-R and QRS intervals (Table 5.7). Although there is a small but significant rate-corrected increase in the Q-T interval, this is primarily due to the marked QRS prolongation; the J-T interval, which more accurately represents the time for repolarization, is unchanged. During EPS, A-H and H-V intervals are prolonged, reflecting slowing of conduction. Average increase in the P-R interval is 25% (40 msec), with first-degree heart block commonly seen. The increase in QRS duration may be as high as 25%.

CLINICAL PHARMACOLOGY

Flecainide is available in the United States for oral use only, and the recommended dose is 100–200 mg orally twice a day (Table 5.8). Flecainide is well absorbed after oral administration, and peak plasma levels are achieved by 3 hours. Foods and antacids do not affect absorption. Approximately 75% of the drug is metabolized in the liver. There are two major metabolites that are conjugated and undergo renal excretion. They have only modest electrophysiologic activity but are of little clinical importance. The remaining 25% of the drug is excreted unchanged by the kidney. The plasma half-life averages 20 hours, with steady-state levels reached in 3–5 days. Elimination half-life averages 14 hours, and the oral administration of flecainide is usually twice a day. The drug is not extensively bound by plasma proteins (i.e., 40%). In patients with CHF, the plasma half-life is increased because of a reduction in renal and hepatic blood flow. The elimination half-life is also prolonged in patients with CHF and with end-stage renal disease and may be as long as 27 hours.

INDICATIONS

A review of the literature emphasizes that, although flecainide is approved for use in patients with life-threatening ventricular arrhythmias, its efficacy is poor and the likelihood of serious toxicity is high. Thus, at this time in clinical practice, it is very infrequently considered for these patients. Previous small uncontrolled clinical trials estimate the likelihood of preventing inducibility of sustained VT to be very low, probably in the range of 10–15% (Table 5.9).

A number of placebo-controlled, short-term clinical trials documented that flecainide is very potent in suppressing VPCs, couplets, and runs of NSVT (Table 5.9). Despite such impressive potency and superiority over class Ia and Ib drugs, the clinical benefit of asymptomatic arrhythmia suppression was not investigated until the Cardiac Arrhythmia Suppression Trial (CAST), which evaluated one group, i.e., those with a recent myocardial infarction. As described in numerous reports, the trial was terminated prematurely after a mean time of 10 months of follow-up because of an excess mortality in patients treated with encainide and flecainide. The CAST provided unequivocal data to contraindicate the use of flecainide in patients surviving MI with asymptomatic ventricular arrhythmia. The problem is the degree to which CAST results can be extrapolated to the use of flecainide in other patient populations (e.g., VPCs in other forms of heart disease, atrial arrhythmias).

Of practical interest is the use of oral flecainide in the treatment of both paroxysmal and chronic AF. In a pivotal clinical trial, 64 patients with paroxysmal AF were treated with flecainide if they had two or more documented attacks of paroxysmal AF within the 4-week baseline run-in period. Flecainide (200–400 mg/day every 12 hours) was administered in a 4-month double-blind, randomized, crossover comparison trial with placebo. Symptomatic attacks were documented by transtelephonic ECG monitoring. In the placebo group, the first episode of recurrent AF occurred after a median of 3 days of placebo administration, as opposed to 14.5 days on flecainide (P < .001). The time interval between attacks was also lengthened from 6.2 days in placebo-treated patients to 27 days in flecainide-treated patients (P <.001). Whereas 31% of flecainide-treated patients had no recurrence of AF during the 4-month study, only 9% of placebo-treated patients were free of recurrent attacks of AF (P = .013). Although the results of this study were highly statistically significant, they also point out the limited expectations of drug therapy for paroxysmal AF in that at least one recurrent episode of AF on flecainide will occur within 4 months in two-thirds of patients. Thus, such therapy should be initiated with the understanding that it will decrease the frequency of episodes but will probably not totally eliminate them, especially over a long-term period.

In a trial of 34 patients with paroxysmal supraventricular tachycardia (SVT), flecainide was associated with a 79% freedom from symptomatic paroxysmal SVT (29/34) events, while 15% (8/34) of patients on placebo had no arrhythmia recurrences (P <.001).

SIDE EFFECTS

In a metaanalysis of all controlled trials in which flecainide was used as prophylactic therapy after an acute MI, the risk of cardiac death during flecainide therapy was increased, with an odds ratio of 1.82 (95% confidence interval (CI) = 0.94–3.53; P = .07). In a review of 1835 patients with supraventricular arrhythmias treated with flecainide, the overall incidence of cardiac side effects and toxicity was 8%. Exacerbation of supraventricular arrhythmias occurred in 1.6% of patients, and there was a 1.9% incidence of ventricular proarrhythmia. Therefore, the overall proarrhythmia rate was 3.5%. Like propafenone, flecainide may convert AF to atrial flutter, with a more rapid ventricular response. In a review of 80 studies reported in abstracts involving 1371 patients, adverse cardiac events included worsening arrhythmias in 28 patients (2.1%), conduction disturbances in 15 patients, and worsening CHF in five patients. The incidence of ventricular proarrhythmia is substantially greater and the reported incidence is as high as 19% in patients with heart disease. Flecainide has significant negative inotropic activity, and left ventricular (LV) ejection fraction may be reduced by 10–18%. The incidence of worsening of the CHF in patients with impaired LV function is reported to be as high as 15%.

The most common noncardiac side effects are those of the CNS, including dizziness, lightheadedness, headache, fatigue, and tremors. A variety of other CNS complaints are uncommonly seen. However, visual disturbances, which include blurred vision, difficulty focusing, and spots before the eyes, have been reported to occur in up to 15% of patients. GI side effects such as nausea, vomiting, diarrhea, dyspepsia, and anorexia are uncommon and usually not severe.

DRUG INTERACTIONS

A number of drug interactions are important during flecainide therapy. Both cimetidine and amiodarone may increase flecainide levels and effect. This is also true of concomitant use of propranolol. Other negative inotropic drugs such as disopyramide, β-blockers, and verapamil should be used with caution with flecainide because negative inotropic effects are additive. The concomitant use of flecainide and digoxin may result in increased digoxin levels.

MORICIZINE

CLINICAL ELECTROPHYSIOLOGIC AND ECG EFFECTS

The clinical electrophysiologic effects of moricizine show significant dose-related changes in all intervals on the ECG (Table 5.7). There is a dose-related increase in P-R and QRS duration. The Q-T and Q-Tc intervals are modestly prolonged. His bundle recording studies document A-H and H-V interval prolongation. Moricizine does not dramatically affect atrial conduction or atrial refractory periods. Moricizine also does not change the refractory periods of the ventricle, AV node, or His-Purkinje system. In addition, antegrade and retrograde conduction of accessory pathways is slowed.

CLINICAL PHARMACOLOGY

Moricizine is available only for oral administration, and the recommended dose is 200–400 mg three times a day (Table 5.8). Absorption from the GI tract is almost complete, and levels peak 1.5–3 hours after administration. It has a bioavailability of approximately 30–40%, which results from a first-pass effect. Hepatic metabolism is primarily responsible for the elimination of moricizine, resulting in a large number of metabolites whose antiarrhythmic properties have not been characterized. There is substantial protein binding, approximately 95% in the plasma as well as in the peripheral tissue. Moricizine can be administered three times a day, although in some patients it is effective when used twice per day. The mean elimination half-life after a single oral dose of moricizine is 1.5–3.5 hours in normal subjects, which is significantly increased in cardiac patients to over 13 hours, especially in those with CHF. Drug elimination occurs primarily through the GI tract with less than 1% of the drug excreted unchanged in the urine. The extent of drug accumulation in patients with either severe hepatic or severe renal disease has not been adequately identified; thus, when it is administered to such patients, caution is justified. Database analysis of concomitant administration of digoxin, warfarin, propranolol, and cimetidine revealed no significant interactions. In contrast, moricizine may induce hepatic enzymes enhancing the metabolism of theophylline, and therefore theophylline levels may be reduced and must be monitored.

INDICATIONS

The clinical experience with moricizine in the treatment of life-threatening arrhythmias is limited. A total of 117 patients (mean age 60 years) with life-threatening ventricular arrhythmia underwent programmed electrical stimulation studies before and after moricizine administration. A total of 75 of these 117 patients had inducible sustained VT during the control EPS; of these 75, 19 (25%) were not inducible on moricizine. A wide variety of doses were used (500–1275 mg/day), with a mean daily dose of 936 mg. Therapy had been administered for an average of 6 days before the EPS. Suppression of inducible sustained VT with moricizine appeared comparable to other class Ia agents (10–15%) (Table 5.9).

Recent single-center trials of moricizine have been quite pessimistic. In a study of patients with coronary artery disease (mean LVEF, 32%), EPS was performed before and after the administration of moricizine. Of the 20 patients who had inducible sustained VT, moricizine was ineffective in preventing inducibility in any of these patients. In addition, possible proarrhythmic responses occurred in four patients. In a separate uncontrolled clinical trial, 26 patients with sustained VT were treated with 400–1000 mg of moricizine daily, and efficacy of moricizine was assessed by programmed electrical stimulation. Although only three of the 26 (12%) patients became noninducible during moricizine therapy, seven patients were observed to develop serious ventricular proarrhythmia during moricizine loading. These included three patients who developed sustained VT. In addition, one had a cardiac arrest and one patient died of intractable VF.

A number of early placebo-controlled trials demonstrated that moricizine is moderately effective in suppressing VPCs, couplets, and runs of NSVT (Table 5.9). In these trials, which involved patients with heart disease, many of whom had sustained VT or VF, ambulatory monitoring was used to assess drug effect. Up to 80% of patients had suppression of spontaneous arrhythmia, although the drug was less effective in patients who had serious arrhythmia and only 40% of such patients responded. In the Cardiac Arrythmia Pilot Study (CAPS), moricizine was more effective (66%) than imipramine (52%) and placebo (37%) but less effective than flecainide (83%) or encainide (79%) in achieving VPC suppression. Moricizine was selected as one of the drugs for use in CAST I and II. After encainide and flecainide were dropped from CAST, the study continued with only moricizine in CAST II, which compared the use of moricizine versus placebo in a group of patients with LVEF <40% who survived an MI. Although the difference in mortality between the two groups was not significantly different, the likelihood of demonstrating any potential patient benefit by prolonging the trial was low and it was halted.

SIDE EFFECTS

The early proarrhythmic toxicity of moricizine (incidence, 2.1%) identified in CAST II has been discussed. A review of 908 patients treated with moricizine for ventricular arrhythmias in the pharmaceutical database yields an overall proarrhythmia rate of 3.2%. Of the 29 proarrhythmic events, 26 occurred within 7 days of drug initiation. Proarrhythmia did not result in death. In patients with life-threatening ventricular arrhythmia, the proarrhythmic incidence may be higher. A recent trial summarizes the experience with moricizine in 144 patients representing a mixed population of patients with life-threatening ventricular arrhythmias and other symptomatic arrhythmias. The incidence of moricizine-associated proarrhythmia was 15%. The most severe ventricular proarrhythmic events included VF in six patients, including three who expired; incessant VT in seven patients; and new sustained VT in four patients. A profile of a patient considered more likely to have a proarrhythmic event on moricizine therapy might show a history of a sustained VT, lower LVEF, the presence of CHF, and a history of previous drug-induced proarrhythmia.

In a study of 908 patients in the United States pharmaceutical database, the estimate of the overall frequency of aggravation of CHF was 12.8%, although attributable to moricizine in only 3%. The mean LVEF of patients with exacerbation of CHF was 26%. The data obtained in CAST II provide an accurate representation of the incidence of CHF in a postinfarct population characterized by baseline LV dysfunction (mean LVEF, 32%). During long-term follow-up (mean 18 months), the incidence of new or worsening CHF was 13.2% in placebo, versus 17.6% in moricizine-treated patients, a difference of 4.4%. In a separate report of patients with life-threatening ventricular arrhythmias, moricizine was used in 125 patients. Of these, 2.4% of patients experienced moricizine-induced CHF. However, the incidence was 4.8% in those with a prior history of heart failure, while CHF was not observed in patients without a history of failure.

From review of all available patients in the pharmaceutical database and those in the CAST II trial, the overall drug discontinuation rate is <10%. It is also apparent that a majority of the common complaints during moricizine therapy are relatively mild and dose-related. In the lower dose range (600 mg/day), side effects are primarily minor GI complaints, including nausea, vomiting, abdominal discomfort, and diarrhea occurring in approximately 10–11% of patients. The other most common symptoms are neurologic and include dizziness, tremor, ataxia, and lightheadedness, which occur in up to 15% of patients. These complaints usually subside with continued dosing or down-titration. Phenothiazine-like side effects (dry mouth and urinary retention) do occur, but are uncommon and are usually dose related.

SUGGESTED READING

Anderson JA, Gilbert EM, Alpert BL, et al. Prevention of syptomatic recurrences of paroxysmal atrial fibrillation in patients initially tolerating antiarrhythmic therapy: a multicenter, double-blind, crossover study of flecainide and placebo with transtelephonic monitoring. Circulation 1989;80:1557–1570.

Campbell RWF. Mexiletine. N Engl J Med 1987;316:29–34.

Clyne CA, Estes NAM, Wang PJ. Drug therapy: moricizine. N Engl J Med 1992;327:255–260.

Funck-Brentano C, Kroemer HK, Lee JT, Roden DM. Drug therapy: propafenone. N Engl J Med 1990;322:518–525.

Giardina EGV, Fenster PE, Bigger JT, Mayersohn D, Marcus FI. Efficacy, plasma concentrations and adverse effects of a new sustained release procainamide preparation. Am J Cardiol 1980;46:855–861.

Greenspan AM, Horowitz LN, Spielman SR, Josephson ME. Large dose procainamide therapy for ventricular tachycardia. Am J Cardiol 1980;46:453–462.

Hernandez M, Reder RF, Marinchak RA, Rials SJ, Kowey PR. Propafenone for malignant ventricular arrhythmia: an analysis of the literature. Am Heart J 1991;121:1178–1184.

Lerman BB, Waxman H, Buxton AE, et al. Disopyramide: evaluation of electrophysiologic effects and clinical efficacy in patients with sustained ventricular tachycardia or ventricular fibrillation. Am J Cardiol 1983;51:759–763.

Mason JW, Hondeghem LM. Part IV. The electrophysiology, pharmacology, and clinical efficacy of classic cardiac antiarrhythmic agents: quinidine. Ann N Y Acad Sci 1984;432:162–176.

Morady F, Scheinman M, Desai J. Disopyramide. Ann Intern Med 1982;96:337–343.

Podrid PJ. Moricizine (Ethmozine HCl) — a new antiarrhythmic drug: is it unique? Am J Cardiol 1991;68:1521–1525.

Rademaker AW, Kellen J, Tam YK, Wyse DG. Character of adverse effects of prophylactic lidocaine in the coronary care unit. Clin Pharmacol Ther 1986;40:71–80.

Roden DM, Woosley RL. Drug therapy: flecainide. N Engl J Med 1986;315:36–41.

Roden DM, Woosley RL, Primm RK. Incidence and clinical features of the quinidine-associated long QT syndrome: implications for patient care. Am Heart J 1986;111:1088–1093.

Stein J, Podrid PJ, Lamapert S, Hirsowitz G, Lown B. Long-term mexiletine for ventricular arrhythmia. Am Heart J 1984;107:1091–1098.

6   β-Blockers

β-blockers have therapeutic efficacy in patients with systemic hypertension, angina pectoris, and cardiac arrhythmias. Some β-blockers have also been shown to reduce the risk of mortality and sudden death in survivors of acute myocardial infarction (MI).

PHARMACOLOGY OF β-BLOCKING DRUGS

The β-blocking drugs are competitive inhibitors of catecholamines at β-adrenoreceptor sites. They act to reduce the effect of the catecholamine agonist on a sensitive tissue. In the presence of the drug, the dose-response curve of the agonist is shifted to the right, i.e., a higher concentration is required to provoke the response.

The chemical structures of most β-blockers have several features in common with the agonist isoproterenol. Most β-blockers exist as pairs of optical isomers and are marketed as racemic mixtures. Almost all of the β-blocking activity is found in the negative (–) levorotatory stereoisomer, which can be up to 100 times more active than the positive (+) dextrorotatory isomer.

β-Blockers are also classified as selective or nonselective (Table 6.1), based on their abilities to antagonize the actions of sympathomimetic amines in some tissues at lower doses than other tissues. Drugs have been developed with a degree of selectivity for two β-adrenoceptor subgroups: β_1-receptors, such as those in the heart, and β_2-receptors, such as those in the peripheral circulation and bronchi. It has been known for some time that selective β_1-blockers such as acebutolol, atenolol, esmolol, and metoprolol inhibit cardiac β_1-receptors but have less influence on bronchial and vascular β_2-adrenoceptors. There is no evidence that nonselective and selective β-adrenergic blockers differ in their antiarrhythmic potency.

Table 6.1
Pharmacodynamic Properties of β-Adrenoceptor Blocking Drugs Used In Arrhythmias

	β_1 Blockade Potency Ratio (Propranolol = 1.0)	Relative β_1_ Selectivity	Intrinsic Sympathomimetic Activity	Quinidine-Like Membrane Stabilizing Activity	Type III Antiarrhythmic Action
Acebutolol	0.3	+	+	+	0
Atenolol	1.0	++	0	0	0
Esmolol	0.02	++	0	0	
Metoprolol	1.0	++	0	0	0
Propranolol	1.0	0	0	++	0
Sotalol	0.3	0	0	++	0
Timolol	6.0	0	0	0	0
Isomer					
D-Propranolol	0	0	0	++	0

Certain β-blockers (acebutolol) possess partial agonist activity (Table 6.1). These drugs cause a slight to moderate activation of the β-receptor, even as they prevent access of natural and synthetic catecholamines to the receptor sites. The result is a weak stimulation of the receptor. Mild to moderate partial agonist activity in a β-blocker does not interfere with antiarrhythmic efficacy. Whether partial agonist activity in a β-blocker offers an overall advantage is a matter of controversy. It has been suggested that β-blockers with partial agonism cause a lesser reduction in heart rate and may depress atrioventricular (AV) conduction and left ventricular function less than β-blockers not having this property.

Although β-blocking drugs have similar pharmacotherapeutic effects, their pharmacokinetic properties differ significantly (Table 6.2) in ways that may influence their clinical usefulness in some patients. Among individual drugs there are differences in completeness of gastrointestinal absorption, amount of first-pass hepatic metabolism, lipid solubility, protein binding, extent of distribution in the body, penetration into the brain, concentration in the heart, rate of hepatic biotransformation, pharmacologic activity of metabolites, and renal clearance of the drug and its metabolites.

On the basis of their pharmacokinetic properties, the β-blockers can be classified into two broad categories: those eliminated by hepatic metabolism and those eliminated unchanged by the kidney. Drugs in the first group (e.g., propranolol and metoprolol) are lipid-soluble, almost completely absorbed by the small intestine, and largely metabolized by the liver. They tend to have highly variable bioavailability and relatively short plasma half-lives. In contrast, drugs in the second category (e.g., sotalol and atenolol) are more water-soluble, incompletely absorbed through the gut, and eliminated unchanged by the kidney. They show less variance in bioavailability and have longer plasma half-lives.

EFFECTS OF β-BLOCKERS ON CARDIAC ELECTROPHYSIOLOGY

β-Adrenoceptor blocking drugs have three main effects on the electrophysiologic properties of specialized cardiac tissue. The first and most common effect of all β-blockers results from the specific blockade of the actions of catecholamines on cardiac pacemaker potentials. In drug concentrations causing significant inhibition of adrenergic receptors, the β-blockers produce little change in the transmembrane potentials of cardiac muscle. The anticatecholamine effects of β-blockers can be antiarrhythmic.

The second electrophysiologic effect of β-blockers is one of membrane stabilizing action, also known as "quinidine-like" or "local anesthetic" action. This property is unrelated to inhibition of catecholamine action and is possessed equally by both the D- and L-isomers of the drugs (D-isomers have almost no β-blocking activity). Characteristic of this effect is a reduction in the rate of rise of the intracardial action potential without affecting the spike duration of the resting potential. Associated features include an elevated electrical threshold of excitability, delay in conduction velocity, and a significant increase in the effective refractory period. This effect and its attendant changes have been explained by an inhibition of the depolarizing inward sodium current.

Table 6.2
Properties of Various β-Adrenoreceptor Blocking Drugs Used in Arrhythmias

Drug	Extent of Absorption (% of dose)	Protein Binding (%)	Lipid Solubility	Elimination Half-Life	Predominant Route of Elimination	Active Metabolites	Drug Accumulation in Renal Disease
Acebutolol[a]	≈70	25	Moderate	3–4 hr[a]	RE (≈40% unchanged and HM)[b]	Yes	Yes
Atenolol	≈50	<5	Weak	6–9 hr	RE	No	Yes
Esmolol[b]	NA	55	Weak	9 min	Metabolized by blood esterases	No	No
Metoprolol	>90	12	Moderate	3–4 hr	HM	No	No
Propranolol	>90	93	High	3–4 hr	HM	Yes	No
Long-acting propranolol	>90	93	High	10 hr	HM	Yes	No
Sotalol	≈70	0	Weak	9–10 hr	RE	No	Yes
Timolol	>90	≈10	Weak	4–5 hr	RE U (≈20% unchanged and HM)	No	No

Modified from Frishman WH. Clinical pharmacology of the β-adrenoreceptor blocking drugs. 2nd ed. Norwalk, CT: Appleton-Century-Crofts, 1984. Abbreviation: NA, not applicable; RE, renal excretion; HM, hepatic metabolism.

[a]Acebutolol has an active metabolite with elimination half-life of 8–13 hours.

[b]Ultra short-acting β-blocker available only in IV form.

Sotalol is unique among the β-blockers in that it alone possesses the third effect, class III antiarrhythmic properties, which cause prolongation of the action potential duration, thereby delaying repolarization.

The most important mechanism underlying the antiarrhythmic effect of β-blockers presumably is β-blockade with resultant inhibition of pacemaker potentials. The effect of catecholamines and sympathetic stimulation is an increase in automaticity due to enhancement of phase 4 spontaneous depolarization, an increase in membrane excitability as a result of shortening in refractoriness (phases II and III of the action potential), an increase in membrane conductivity as a result of an acceleration of phase 0 upstroke velocity or rate of membrane depolarization and an increase in delayed afterpotentials. β-Blockers therefore prevent these catecholamine-mediated changes. The contribution of membrane-stabilizing action does not appear to be clinically significant.

All β-blockers are similarly effective at a comparable level of β-blockade. Differences in overall clinical usefulness are related to their other associated pharmacologic properties.

By blocking catecholamine and sympathetically mediated actions, β-blockers slow the rate of discharge of the sinus and ectopic pacemakers and increase the effective refractory period of the AV node by their β-adrenergic blocking actions. They also slow both antegrade and retrograde conduction in anomalous pathways. Because all β-blockers studied thus far cause an increase in AV conduction time, advanced AV block is a potential complication when β-blockers are used. Agents with partial agonist activity (intrinsic sympathomimetic activity [ISA]), such as acebutolol, may provide some protection from the AV conduction impairment induced by blockade.

In high doses, β-blockers can induce sinus node dysfunction and lead to sinoatrial block or sinus arrest. These drugs are therefore best avoided in patients with sick sinus syndrome, a condition that can be exacerbated by β-adrenergic blockade. β-Blockers can also aggravate the sinus node and AV node depressant effects of the calcium blockers diltiazem and verapamil, and should be combined with caution.

THERAPEUTIC USES IN CARDIAC ARRHYTHMIAS

β-Adrenergic blocking drugs have become an important treatment modality for various cardiac arrhythmias (Tables 6.3, 6.4).

Mitral Valve Prolapse

It has been suggested that many of the symptoms associated with mitral valve prolapse are related to a dysfunction of the autonomic nervous system, which is frequently associated with this syndrome. Current therapy is directed at symptomatic relief of this condition. Propranolol appears to be the drug of choice for many of the ventricular arrhythmias, especially in those patients with a prolongation of the Q-T interval.

Table 6.3
Effects of β Blockers in Various Arrhythmias

Arrhythmia	Comment
Supraventricular	
Sinus tachycardia	Treat underlying disorder; excellent response to β-blocker if need to control rate (e.g., ischemia)
Atrial fibrillation	β-blockers reduce rate, rarely restore sinus rhythm, may be useful in combination with digoxin
Atrial flutter	β-blockers reduce rate, sometimes restore sinus rhythm
Atrial tachycardia	Effective in slowing ventricular rate, may restore sinus rhythm; useful in prophylaxis
Ventricular	
PVCs	Good response to β-blockers especially digitalis-induced, exercise (ischemia)-induced, mitral valve prolapse, or hypertrophic cardiomyopathy
Ventricular tachycardia	As effective as quinidine, most effective in digitalis toxicity or exercise (ischemia)-induced
Ventricular fibrillation	Electrical defibrillation is treatment of choice, β-blockers can be used to prevent recurrence in cases of excess digitalis or sympathomimetic amines; appear to be effective in reducing the incidence of ventricular fibrillation and sudden death postmyocardial infarction

From Frishman WH. Clinical pharmacology of the β-adrenoreceptor blocking drugs, 2nd ed. Norwalk, CT: Appleton-Century-Crofts, 1984.

Table 6.4
Recommended Dosages of β Blockers as Antiarrhythmics and as Prophylaxis in Myocardial Infarction (FDA Approved)

Antiarrhythmia	Dosing
Acebutolol	200 mg daily (once or 2 divided doses)
Esmolol	I.V. infusion 500 μg/kg/min for 1 min, followed by maintenance I.V. infusion of 50 μg/kg/min for 4 min. If response is inadequate, repeat sequence with loading I.V. infusion (as above) and 100 μg/kg/min maintenance dose. Sequence is repeated until adequate response is obtained. For SVT, 100 μg/kg/min after loading dose as above[a]
Propranolol	10–30 mg three to four times daily (tablets) 1–3 mg at 1 mg/min (I.V.)
Sotalol	120–240 mg daily (oral)
Myocardial infarction prophylaxis	
Atenolol	5 mg/5 min (parenteral) 50 mg 10 min after last I.V. dose (repeat 12 hr later); 100 mg once daily or 50 mg twice daily (oral)
Metoprolol	5 mg q2 min for 3 doses (I.V.) 50 mg q6h after last I.V. dose for 48 hr, then 100 mg twice daily for at least 3 mo (oral)
Propranolol	180–240 mg daily in divided doses after myocardial infarction
Timolol	10 mg twice daily after myocardial infarction

[a]SVT, supraventricular tachycardia.

Prolonged Q-T Syndrome

Patients who present with a prolonged Q-T syndrome have an abnormality of the activation of the adrenergic sympathetic nervous system, possibly accounting in part for the Q-T prolongation noted on the surface electrocardiogram (ECG). These are individuals who are at great risk for paroxysmal ventricular tachyarrhythmias (VTs) and sudden death. The most effective agents currently are β-blockers, which appear to decrease the frequency of syncopal episodes and may prevent sudden death.

Cardiomyopathy

There are preliminary data suggesting that β-blocker therapy, particularly metoprolol, can be safely used in patients with a dilated cardiomyopathy and congestive heart failure. Preliminary data suggest that β-blocker therapy in these patients is associated with a reduction in cardiac mortality. They may be particularly beneficial in patients who have a persistent sinus tachycardia out of proportion to the degree of left ventricular dysfunction and in the absence of overt congestive heart failure. The reduction in heart rate can improve hemodynamic status by prolonging the diastolic filling period. Additionally, in such patients β-blockade may protect against serious VTs. However, these agents must be used with extreme caution because they could cause a worsening of congestive heart failure and hence have an adverse effect.

ADVERSE EFFECTS

Adverse Cardiac Effects Related to β-Adrenoceptor Blockade

CARDIAC FAILURE

β-Adrenoceptor blockade with any β-blocker may cause congestive heart failure in an enlarged heart with impaired myocardial function where excessive sympathetic drive is essential to maintain it on a compensated Starling curve. Congestive heart failure may also occur if the stroke volume is restricted and tachycardia is needed to maintain cardiac output.

It is possible that an important component of heart failure may be accounted for by increases in peripheral resistance produced by nonselective agents.

ATRIOVENTRICULAR CONDUCTION DELAY AND SINUS NODE DYSFUNCTION

Slowing of the resting heart rate is a normal response to treatment with a β-blocking drug. Drugs with intrinsic sympathomimetic activity (ISA) do not lower the resting heart rate to the same degree as propranolol. However, all β-blocking drugs are contraindicated in patients with sick sinus syndrome unless an artificial pacemaker is present. If there is complete or partial AV conduction defect, use of a β-blocking drug can lead to a serious bradyarrhythmia. Compounds that have ISA can cause less impairment of AV conduction.

β-BLOCKER WITHDRAWAL

An increase in heart rate and blood pressure, resulting in exacerbation of angina, and in some cases acute MI, have been reported after the abrupt cessation of propranolol therapy chronically administered to patients with severe coronary artery disease. This is due to "rebound," and there is a transient increase in receptor sensitivity to catecholamines. This rebound effect has not been as clearly defined with the other β-blocking agents. However, discontinuation of any β-blocker therapy should be done gradually and cautiously in patients with ischemic heart disease.

Adverse Non-Cardiac Effects Related to β-Adrenoceptor Blockade
Effect on Ventilatory Function

The bronchodilator effects of catecholamines on the bronchial β-2 receptors are prevented by β-blockade with nonselective agents. Compounds with ISA and/or β_1-receptor selectivity are less likely to increase airway resistance in asthmatics than propranolol. β_1-receptor selectivity is not absolute, however, and may diminish with higher doses. Therefore, in general, all β-blockers should be avoided in patients with active bronchospastic disease.

PERIPHERAL VASCULAR EFFECTS

Cold extremities and absent pulses have been described in patients receiving β-blockers. β-Blocking drugs with β_1-receptor selectivity or ISA will not affect peripheral vessels to the same degree as propranolol. Raynaud's phenomenon is one of the more common side effects of propranolol treatment and it too is probably related to nonselective β-blockade.

Patients with peripheral vascular disease who suffer from intermittent claudication often report worsening of symptoms when treated with β-blocking drugs.

GLUCOSE METABOLISM

β-Receptor blocking drugs (especially nonselective blockers) may retard recovery from insulin-induced hypoglycemia.

Additionally, β-blockers cause a marked diminution in the manifestations of sympathetic discharge associated with hypoglycemia, and this interference with compensatory responses to hypoglycemia can mask some "warning signs" of this condition.

CENTRAL NERVOUS SYSTEM EFFECTS

Dreams, hallucinations, insomnia, depression, and fatigue can occur during therapy with β-blockers. These symptoms are evidence of drug entry into the central nervous system (CNS), and are especially common with the highly lipid-soluble β-blockers (propranolol, metoprolol) that presumably penetrate the CNS better.

OTHER EFFECTS

Diarrhea, nausea, gastric pain, constipation, and flatulence have been seen occasionally with all β-blockers. Hematologic reactions are rare; rare cases of purpura and agranulocytosis have been described with propranolol.

Adverse Effects Unrelated to β-Adrenoceptor Blockade

β-Blockers have been associated with the development of antinuclear antibodies (ANA).

Symptoms (generally persistent arthralgias and myalgias) related to this abnormality are infrequent (1–1% with both drugs). Symptoms and ANA titers are reversible on discontinuation of treatment (10).

Drug Interactions

β-Blockers may often be administered as part of combined antiarrhythmic therapy or may be one of several agents in a patient's overall therapeutic regimen. They may be used together with digitalis to control the ventricular rate in atrial fibrillation or flutter or to convert to sinus rhythm. Combinations of β-blocking drugs and quinidine have been used to convert atrial fibrillation to sinus rhythm and to maintain sinus rhythm after successful conversion of the rhythm. Because β-blockade appears to be the major factor in the antiarrhythmic effects of β-blockers and the "quinidine-like" (membrane-depressant) action appears negligible, it would seem logical that such combined therapy would have a beneficial additive effect.

SUGGESTED READING

Frishman WH. Beta-adrenergic blocker withdrawal. Am J Cardiol 1987;59:26F–32F.

Frishman WH, Charlap S. The alpha- and beta-adrenergic blocking drugs. In: Parmley WW, ed. Cardiology. Philadelphia: JB Lippincott, 1990: 1–18.

Frishman WH. Comparative pharmacology of beta-adrenergic blockers. In: Deedwania PC, ed. Beta blockers and cardiac arrhythmias. New York: Marcel Dekker, 1992:89–106.

Frishman WH, Murthy VS, Strom JA. Ultra-short-acting β-adrenergic blockers. Med Clin North Am 1988;72:359–372.

Frishman WH, Skolnick AE, Lazar EJ, Fein S. β-Adrenergic blockade and calcium channel blockade in myocardial infarction. Med Clin North Am 1989;73:409–436.

Furberg LD, Hawkins CM, Lichstein E, for the Beta Blocker Heart Attach Trial Study Group. Effect of propranolol in post infarction patients with mechanical or electrical complications. Circulation 1984;69:761–765.

Norwegian Multicenter Study Group. Timolol-induced reduction in mortality and reinfarction in patients surviving acute myocardial infarction. N Engl J Med 1981;304:801–807.

Yusuf S, Sleight P, Rossi P. Reduction in infarct size, arrhythmias, and chest pain by early intravenous beta blockade in suspected acute myocardial infarction. Circulation 1983;67 (suppl 1): 32–41.

7 Amiodarone

Amiodarone is an iodinated benzofuran derivative. Because of its coronary and peripheral dilating properties, the drug was initially developed for the treatment of angina pectoris. In the United States, oral amiodarone is approved to treat patients who have sustained life-threatening ventricular tachyarrhythmias (VTs). In addition to its approved indications, amiodarone has demonstrated effectiveness in the treatment of atrial fibrillation, paroxysmal supraventricular tachycardia, and nonsustained VTs.

BASIC AND CLINICAL ELECTROPHYSIOLOGIC EFFECTS

Amiodarone's basic electrophysiologic and pharmacologic effects are complex (Table 7.1). In Purkinje and ventricular muscle fibers, amiodarone prolongs action potential duration in a time-dependent fashion, with no alteration of resting membrane potential or action potential height. Amiodarone minimally slows the rate of rise of phase IV depolarization (i.e., automaticity is reduced). Because amiodarone prolongs action potential duration, it has been subclassified as a class III antiarrhythmic agent. Amiodarone uniformly lengthens action potential duration at normal and fast heart rates, which differs from other drugs that demonstrate a reverse use-dependent effect on repolarization (i.e., there is more of an effect on repolarization at slower heart rates). Amiodarone blocks cardiac sodium channels and depresses phase 0 in a use-dependent fashion (i.e., the effect on phase 0 is more substantial at faster heart rates).

Amiodarone slows the sinus rate by both depressing the duration of the sinus node action potential and by decreasing the rate of rise of diastolic depolarization (depresses automaticity). The drug prolongs atrioventricular (AV) nodal repolarization and refractoriness.

Amiodarone also has an antisympathetic effect on α- and β-adrenergic responses to sympathetic stimulation or catecholamine infusion. Its α- and β-blocking activity is noncompetitive. It also has significant antifibrillatory actions.

Table 7.1
Pharmacologic Properties of Amiodarone

1. Prolongs action potential duration and refractory period of all cardiac tissue-potassium channel blockade (class III action)
2. Minor decrease in the upstroke velocity of phase 0-sodium channel blockade (class I action)
3. Noncompetitive β-receptor blockade (class II action)
4. Noncompetitive α-receptor blockade
5. Calcium channel-blocking activity (class IV action)
6. May interfere with the effect of thyroxin on the heart
7. Peripheral arterial vasodilatation—reduces peripheral vascular resistance and afterload
8. Coronary artery vasodilatation—increases coronary blood flow
9. Decreases heart rate
10. Mild direct negative inotropic activity

Oral amiodarone's electrophysiologic effects include suppression of sinus node automaticity, prolongation of sinus node recovery times, and slight prolongation of atrial, AV nodal, and ventricular refractoriness. Amiodarone increases the A-H interval and the minimum pacing cycle length associated with 1:1 AV nodal conduction. The drug also prolongs refractoriness and slows conduction in accessory pathway tissue in patients with the Wolff-Parkinson-White (WPW) syndrome.

Many of the effects of the drug are similar to those seen with hypothyroidism. This is an important concern because the drug does contain a substantial amount of iodine (two iodine molecules accounting for 75 mg/200 mg of amiodarone or 38% of its weight).

Electrocardiographic (ECG) effects of amiodarone include reduction in heart rate, which usually is unresponsive to exercise, and other catecholamine-related states. Likewise, atropine fails to alter the rate. Prolongation of the P-R and corrected Q-T intervals are almost universal. In addition, a decrease in T-wave amplitude with T-wave widening and bifurcation and more prominent U-waves can develop. This occurs even in the presence of normal serum potassium levels. It has been suggested that these ECG changes are helpful as a guide to the presence of myocardial tissue levels.

HEMODYNAMIC EFFECTS

Intravenous (i.v.) amiodarone (10 mg/kg) produces a dose-related decrease in left ventricular contractile force. Despite this negative inotropic effect, cardiac output tends to increase secondary to a more pronounced reduction in systemic vascular resistance. In addition, cardiac output may increase secondary to extending the plateau phase of the action potential, i.e., prolonging the corrected Q-T interval (Q-Tc) or time to repolarization, thus facilitating calcium entry and enhancing contractility. This is often seen with the class III antiarrhythmic drugs that prolong repolarization.

In humans with normal left ventricular function, heart rate and arterial pressure decrease and cardiac output increases secondary to a fall in systemic vascular resistance and a reduction in afterload. Several studies have shown no demonstrable change in radionuclide-measured ejection fractions as a result of amiodarone treatment. In patients with underlying left ventricular dysfunction, the drug infrequently depresses ventricular function further, and the provocation of congestive heart failure is uncommon. The reason for this is that a major effect of the drug is peripheral vasodilatation and a reduction in systemic vascular resistance, which offsets its mild negative inotropic actions.

Amiodarone can cause a profound decrease in blood pressure because of marked vasodilatation during cardiac surgery in patients with marked left ventricular dysfunction after cardiopulmonary bypass. Some difficulties in recovering from bypass may necessitate the use of pressor agents to increase systemic vascular resistance.

CLINICAL PHARMACOLOGY

Amiodarone has a large volume of distribution, moderate but erratic bioavailability, and an unusually long half-life (Table 7.2). The drug is highly lipophilic and

Table 7.2
Clinical Pharmacology of Amiodarone

Absorption rate	2–12 hr
Extent of absorption	Poor and slow
Bioavailability	Variable (22–86%)
Peak plasma levels	4–6 hr
Protein binding	96%
Volume of distribution	
Acute	1.3–65.8 L/kg
Steady-state	5.0 L/kg
Elimination	Hepatic and intestinal
Elimination half-life	
Acute	3–21 hr
Chronic	52.6 d
Total body clearance	0.10–0.77 L/min
Metabolites	Mono-N-desethylamiodarone
	Bis-N-desethylamiodarone
	Deiodinated metabolites
Therapeutic plasma level	1.0–2.5 μg/mL

distributes extensively into the various tissues, especially those with high fat content.

Because of its long β half-life (1–3 months) and diffuse and vast tissue distribution (especially to adipose stores), months may be required for blood levels to completely reach equilibrium. Peripheral stores must be saturated before steady-state therapeutic levels are achieved. Peak concentrations of i.v. amiodarone are attained within 30 minutes. The drug undergoes deiodinization as well as hepatic metabolism. The drug is extensively metabolized, and the renal elimination of both amiodarone and desethylamiodarone, its major metabolite, is negligible. Excretion via the hepatic and gastrointestinal routes is minimal. Amiodarone and desethylamiodarone are not dialyzable. Desethylamiodarone appears to have electrophysiologic effects similar to those of the parent compound.

After cessation of long-term oral therapy in humans, the mean elimination half-life of amiodarone ranges from 26–107 days (mean, 52.6 ± 23.7 days), with a mean of 61.2 ± 31.1 days for the desethyl metabolite. Because of the drug's long half-life, plasma levels of amiodarone and desethylamiodarone have been measurable as long as 9 months after the cessation of therapy.

Relationship of Drug Levels to Effect

The prolonged time required to attain equilibrium between tissue and plasma levels has made it difficult to predict the antiarrhythmic effect by using serum amiodarone concentrations. Despite this, mean therapeutic plasma concentrations during long-term treatment are probably in the range of 1.0–2.5 μg/mL.

Dosing

Because of amiodarone's long half-life and large volume of distribution, the ideal loading dose schedule has remained controversial but depends upon the nature and severity of the arrhythmia being treated.

In general, loading doses of 800–1800 mg/day should be used. In patients with acute life-threatening ventricular arrhythmias in whom therapeutic levels need to be attained sooner, either the higher loading dose or a combination of oral and i.v. amiodarone can be administered. Depending on the severity of the arrhythmia, attempts to decrease the dose safely to no more than 400 mg/day should be made so as to minimize side effects. In patients with atrial arrhythmias, lower loading doses (600–800 mg/day) are used, and a maintenance dose of about 200 mg/day is the standard dosage. Serum amiodarone levels may be useful in safely monitoring dose decreases. In children, amiodarone loading doses of 10–15 mg/kg daily, which are then decreased to about 5 mg/kg daily for maintenance, are recommended.

INTRAVENOUS AMIODARONE

Intravenous amiodarone is available for use in life-threatening tachyarrhythmias refractory to other therapies. A combination of i.v. and oral amiodarone given concomitantly has been used in an attempt to attain therapeutic levels more rapidly. The onset of action after a small i.v. dose ranges between 1–30 minutes, and its duration of effect is 1–3 hours. Amiodarone is infused in D_5W with an initial 75- to 150-mg bolus over 10 minutes. A loading infusion of 0.5–1.0 mg/minute is given for 6 hours. Maintenance infusions of 0.25–0.5 mg/minute are then used.

USE IN SUPRAVENTRICULAR ARRHYTHMIAS

EFFICACY IN SUPRAVENTRICULAR TACHYCARDIA

Amiodarone exhibits long-term efficacy in more than 70% of patients with supraventricular tachycardias (SVTs).

Electrophysiologic testing for SVT during amiodarone therapy suggests that lack of suppression of tachycardia induction during serial studies may not be predictive of clinical response. Amiodarone may be effective in many of these patients by causing a marked suppression of the triggering event (premature ventricular or atrial contractions).

EFFICACY IN ATRIAL FIBRILLATION

Amiodarone has been found to be a very effective agent for treating atrial fibrillation. The drug can be completely effective in preventing a recurrence of paroxysmal and chronic atrial fibrillation (AF) in about 70% of patients. In an additional 15–22% of patients, the drug reduces the frequency, rate, or duration of paroxysms. It has been reported that low-dose amiodarone may be effective for preventing recurrent AF.

Little data are available comparing the efficacy of amiodarone to that of other antiarrhythmic agents in treating AF.

Only rarely does amiodarone result in spontaneous reversion of sustained atrial fibrillation to sinus rhythm, but it may prevent paroxysmal arrhythmia. It should be kept in mind that, during the first several weeks of therapy, while amiodarone levels are still increasing, the patient may be at risk for recurrences of paroxysmal arrhythmia. If, after loading of amiodarone, the patient has not reverted to sinus rhythm, electrical cardioversion is used. Amiodarone does not appear to increase the amount of energy needed to cardiovert atrial fibrillation to sinus rhythm.

EFFICACY IN ATRIAL FIBRILLATION ASSOCIATED WITH WPW SYNDROME

Amiodarone has demonstrated efficacy in patients with AF and WPW syndrome. The drug is useful in slowing antegrade conduction of the accessory pathway or prolonging pathway refractoriness. Similar to procainamide, however, amiodarone is rarely effective in significantly prolonging accessory pathway refractoriness when the baseline refractory period is very short, i.e., <270 msec. Amiodarone may be effective in suppressing spontaneous episodes of AF associated with the syndrome because of the drug's effect on the atrial myocardium, as well as its ability to suppress premature atrial contractions and episodes of reentrant SVT that may degenerate into atrial fibrillation.

Because this drug is not protective in all patients, safety should be verified by careful induction of AF during repeat electrophysiologic study.

EFFICACY IN ECTOPIC ATRIAL TACHYCARDIA

Amiodarone appears to be useful in treating ectopic atrial tachycardia. The true efficacy of the agent in this entity is difficult to discern from the literature, however, because many patients with ectopic atrial tachycardia have been analyzed together with patients who have paroxysmal SVT.

USE IN TACHYCARDIA-BRADYCARDIA SYNDROME

Several investigators have reported amiodarone to be effective in suppressing the various SVTs associated with tachycardia-bradycardia syndrome. Amiodarone has certain electrophysiologic effects that warrant cautious use of the drug in this syndrome. The agent may depress sinus node and escape pacemaker automaticity, as evidenced by prolongation of the sinus node recovery time. In addition, it may accentuate block at the level of the AV node.

USE IN POTENTIALLY LETHAL VENTRICULAR ARRHYTHMIAS

Several early studies demonstrated amiodarone to be an effective suppressant of ectopic ventricular beats.

Control of refractory nonsustained VT (NSVT) by amiodarone has been obtained in 56–94% of patients. Amiodarone has been an effective drug for suppressing NSVT in patients with a cardiomyopathy and congestive heart failure (CHF). Data suggest that it may prolong survival. Although few of the studies have been placebo controlled, so the effect of the drug on improving survival and reducing sudden death in this group is still uncertain. Indeed, one recent trial from Argentina reported a reduction in mortality, while a study carried out by the Veterans Administration reported no benefit.

It has been suggested that amiodarone may improve survival in patients with hypertrophic obstructive cardiomyopathy who have serious or potentially serious ventricular arrhythmia. However this remains controversial.

AMIODARONE IN THE MYOCARDIAL INFARCTION SURVIVOR

Survivors of myocardial infarction (MI), especially those with a depressed ejection fraction, are at significant risk for sudden cardiac death. Several studies report that amiodarone is effective for reducing mortality in the post-MI patient.

A metaanalysis of existing data furthermore suggests that amiodarone may reduce mortality in the post-MI setting.

USE IN SUSTAINED VENTRICULAR TACHYARRHYTHMIAS

Amiodarone is extremely effective in preventing recurrent VTs in patients who have survived a cardiac arrest and up to 70% remain free of recurrent arrhythmia for up to 36 months. These data have led some to suggest that empiric amiodarone can be used in this group of patients without the aid of electrophysiologic testing, although this remains controversial.

Amiodarone is an extremely effective agent in treating refractory sustained VT, with 2-year clinical efficacy rates exceeding 60%. Similar to other antiarrhythmic agents, amiodarone is effective in suppressing inducible VT in only 20% of patients. Despite this, higher efficacy rates exist when clinical recurrence is used as an endpoint. Importantly, the efficacy of amiodarone decreases over time and only 40–57% of patients are free of arrhythmia after 5 years of follow-up.

Although amiodarone has been found to be effective in treating sustained VT-VF, there is still a concern that the risk of sudden cardiac death remains high in certain subgroups. In these high-risk groups, implantable cardioverter defibrillator (ICD) therapy may be preferable.

Because of amiodarone's high efficacy in treating sustained ventricular tachyarrhythmias, several trials are ongoing to prospectively compare amiodarone administered empirically to other agents evaluated by noninvasive or invasive testing. There are also studies comparing its efficacy to the ICD.

Despite the low incidence (about 20%) of rendering VT noninducible, electrophysiology studies performed 10–14 days after the initiation of amiodarone may be useful in guiding therapy in patients treated with amiodarone. In patients whose inducible VT can be suppressed, the risk of recurrent symptomatic VT remains low (<20% at 2 years). Interestingly, about 60% of patients will not have a recurrence of VT after 2 years of follow-up, despite persistent inducible VT while they are on amiodarone. Thus, persistent inducibility does not preclude arrhythmia-free follow-up in patients treated with amiodarone. Of more importance, hemodynamic measurements and symptoms during inducible VT appear to be predictive of symptoms during recurrence and may lead to an alteration of antiarrhythmic or nonpharmacologic therapy. Similar to other antiarrhythmic agents, amiodarone slows conduction in the VT circuit and produces a statistically significant prolongation of the VT cycle length. This slowing of the tachycardia rate may result in better hemodynamic tolerance of a recurrent episode of VT in some patients. Combination therapy with class Ia, Ib, and Ic agents may be useful in selected, refractory patients. The combination may suppress the arrhythmia or may cause further slowing of the rate of inducible VT, improving hemodynamics even more than with amiodarone alone.

TOXICITY

Side effects occurring with amiodarone therapy are noted in Table 7.3. The frequency of side effects is dose related and also duration related, increasing over time. Many adverse reactions appear to be more common when serum levels above 2.5 mg/L are maintained. Side effects during long-term treatment with amiodarone are common and occur in 50–80% of patients, although drug discontinuation is only infrequently necessary (10–12%). Minor side effects can usually be eliminated by decreasing the dose. Severe side effects require discontinuation of the drug. Lower maintenance doses of amiodarone appear to be associated with a lower incidence of adverse effects.

OCULAR SIDE EFFECTS

Corneal microdeposits occur frequently in patients treated with amiodarone. These deposits eventually develop into a whorl-like pattern and are localized in the corneal epithelium at the lower third of the cornea. They are usually bilateral and symmetric. Visual symptoms include photophobia, visual blurring, and most

Table 7.3
Side Effects Noted with Amiodarone Therapy

Ocular
  Corneal microdeposits (95%), halo vision, photophobia, visual blurring (6–14%), possible macular degeneration
Dermatologic
  Photosensitivity (25–75%), blue-gray skin discoloration (5–8%), urticaria, rash, hair loss
Gastrointestinal
  Nausea, anorexia, constipation, elevation of liver function tests (50%), hepatitis (3%)
Neurologic
  Sleep disturbances (28%), tremor (30%), peripheral neuropathy (5%), myopathy, headaches (14%), ataxia
Cardiovascular
  Symptomatic bradycardia (6%), AV block, negative inotropy, CHF (4%), proarrhythmia (1%)
Thyroid
  Elevated TSH, T3 and T4 abnormalities (25%)
  Hypothyroidism (1–22%), hyperthyroidism (1–12%)
Pulmonary
  Interstitial pneumonitis (3–7%), postoperative ARDS, cough[a]

[a]ARDS, adult respiratory syndrome.

commonly, halo vision at night when the pupils are dilated and the deposits enter the periphery of the visual field. Microscopic lens opacities and retinopathy have also been described. No permanent visual impairment has been reported. Fortunately, visual symptoms are rare (6–14%). Routine surveillance in patients without visual symptoms is not mandatory.

Dermatologic Side Effects

Photosensitivity with increased propensity to sunburn and erythema is common (25–75%) and does not appear to be dose related. Rarely, swelling of the sun-exposed areas can occur. This effect is minimized by limiting sun exposure and using sun screens, which block A and B ultraviolet light. The development of slate-gray pigmentation has been noted in <10% of patients, although this usually takes several years to develop. It usually occurs in sun-exposed areas and may be dose related. Hair loss has rarely been reported.

GASTROINTESTINAL SIDE EFFECTS

Nausea, anorexia, and constipation can occur and appear to be dose related. They are most often seen during the initial loading period. Constipation is quite frequent when a high maintenance dose of 600 mg/day is used.

Asymptomatic elevation of liver function tests can occur within the first 2 months of therapy. Mild elevation in liver transaminase levels has been noted in 14–50% of patients and is not usually dose-related. Although clinical hepatitis can occur, it appears to be rare (<3%). However, it can be serious, leading to cirrhosis.

NEUROLOGIC SIDE EFFECTS

The most common neurologic side effects are headaches, sleep disturbances and fine tremor of the hands. Peripheral neuropathy with reduced nerve conduction velocities and proximal muscle weakness can occur and appear to be dose related because decreasing the dose can often reverse these effects. Ataxia is not uncommon and may be dose related, being more frequent with initial loading doses. Extrapyramidal symptoms have rarely been noted.

CARDIOVASCULAR SIDE EFFECTS

The most common cardiovascular side effect of amiodarone is symptomatic sinus bradycardia (6%), which may require pacing. This response may be additive if amiodarone is used concomitantly with β-blockers or verapamil. Mobitz I AV block can occur and is dose dependent. Second- or third-degree AV block, intra-ventricular conduction defects, and even asystole have been reported but are rare. Rarely, negative inotropic effects in patients with left ventricular dysfunction may be noted. The long time course of drug action makes it difficult to distinguish a drug-related problem from natural history.

Although amiodarone prolongs action potential duration, and thus the Q-T interval, amiodarone-induced torsade de pointes is rare. The drug can interact with type I antiarrhythmic agents, however, causing a marked increase in Q-T interval and a drug-induced arrhythmia. Hypokalemia is also a factor provoking arrhythmia. Overall, aggravation of arrhythmia is observed in approximately 5% of patients. However, the actual incidence is difficult to establish because of the delayed onset of drug action.

The development of ventricular proarrhythmia is extremely uncommon in patients receiving amiodarone for treatment of SVT. Rarely, incessant atrial flutter may develop in patients treated for paroxysmal atrial fibrillation. Compared to the 5–10% incidence with class Ia or Ic agents, the occurrence of atrial proarrhythmia with amiodarone appears to be low.

THYROID TOXICITY

The cellular electrophysiologic effects of long-term amiodarone administration resemble those of spontaneous hypothyroidism. Amiodarone contains two atoms of iodine (75 mg or 37% of the total molecular weight) as part of its molecular structure. The excessive iodine load delivered to the body may itself create thyroid abnormalities. Because of its similarity to the iodothyronines, thyroid metabolism may be affected. By blocking the peripheral conversion of T4 to T3, amiodarone frequently causes elevated levels of serum T4 and reverse T3. Desethyl-amiodarone can act as an active thyroid hormone antagonist by competitively inhibiting T3 binding to solubilized nuclear thyroid receptors. Increases in reverse T3 occur as a function of dose and duration of therapy and have been used as a guide to monitor the onset of drug efficacy. Although these chemical changes in thyroid function are common, the frequency of clinical hypothyroidism or hyper-thyroidism is lower.

The frequency of amiodarone-induced hypothyroidism ranges from 1–22%. In general, clinical hypothyroidism is much more common than hyperthyroidism. Clinically, hypothyroidism can be easily managed by lowering the dose of amio-darone and adding synthetic thyroid therapy. The frequency of clinical hyperthy-roidism has ranged from 1–12%, averaging <3%. The frequency of amiodarone-induced hyperthyroidism may be environmentally aggravated, as it may be higher in certain geographic areas where the average iodine intake of the population is moderately low. Hyperthyroidism may result in arrhythmia recurrence, as well as the other manifestations of excessive thyroxin. Therapy is difficult because radioactive iodine is not taken up by the gland, and this form of ablation is inade-quate. Long-term therapy with antithyroid drugs may be problematic. Surgical ablation or drug discontinuation is often necessary.

PULMONARY TOXICITY

The most serious lung-related toxicity of amiodarone is pulmonary alveolitis. Clinical features may include dyspnea, a nonproductive cough, and low-grade fever. Diffuse interstitial changes or alveolar infiltrates may be seen radiographically. Histologic evaluation shows accumulation of foamy macrophages in alveolar spaces, hyperplasia of type 2 pneumocytes, and widening of the alveolar septum. The frequency of pulmonary toxicity ranges from 1–17%; however, in most reports the incidence is 3–7%. The true frequency is difficult to determine because many patients have concomitant heart failure or pneumonic changes that may be difficult to distinguish from true pulmonary toxicity. This complication appears to be somewhat dose related, as it is rare to see it when maintenance doses <400 mg/day are used. Pulmonary function tests have not been predictive of this complication, although similar to other drug-induced pulmonary fibrosises, abnormalities of diffusion capacity (>15%) can be helpful in the diagnosis. Treatment requires drug withdrawal with or without the use of steriods.

INTERACTIONS

DRUG-DRUG INTERACTIONS

Amiodarone has been shown to interact with warfarin, digoxin, several antiarrhythmic agents, and phenytoin (by interfering with its metabolism) (Table 7.4). It potentiates the anticoagulant effect of warfarin as early as 4 days. The prothrombin time must be carefully watched and warfarin dose adjusted accordingly. The mechanism of the interaction with antiarrhythmic drugs is unknown. Amiodarone can nonetheless be safely and effectively used in combination with other antiarrhythmic agents or even β-blockers. However, the potential for sinus and AV node conduction abnormalities can be additive with this combination.

DRUG-DEVICE INTERACTIONS

From 40–70% of patients with ICDs take concomitant antiarrhythmic drugs. Amiodarone is the most common drug used in ICD patients. It may cause increases in capture threshold in patients with pacemakers. This agent has been shown to increase the defibrillation threshold (DFT) in several studies when used in com-

Table 7.4
Amiodarone-Drug Interactions

Concomitant Drug	Effect
Warfarin	Increased prothrombin time (2–3 fold)
Digoxin	Doubling of digoxin level
Quinidine, procainamide disopyramide, flecainide	20–35% increase in type I levels
β-blockers, calcium blockers	Additive effects on slowing heart rate and slowing AV nodal conduction
Phenytoin	Increases phenytoin levels
Anesthetic drugs	Hypotension, potentiating bradycardia

Table 7.5
Recommended Laboratory Follow-up During Amiodarone Therapy

Liver function tests	Baseline and every 6 mo (more frequent if progressive rise)
Thyroid function	Baseline and every 6 mo (more frequent for symptoms or progressive rise)
Routine chemistries	Baseline and every 6 mo
Chest x-ray	Baseline and every 6 mo (more frequent for symptoms or abnormalities)
Ophthalmologic exam	Baseline and for symptoms
Pulmonary function test	? Value (optional)[a]
Amiodarone blood levels	? Value
ECG	Baseline, 1 mo, every 6 mo (more frequent for dose change or addition of other drugs)
Ambulatory monitoring	Baseline, 2–4 wk, every 6 mo (more frequent for symptoms, dose change, or addition of other drugs)
Electrophysiologic test	Baseline, 2–4 wk

[a]?, questionable.

bination with an implantable cardioverter/defibrillator. Clinicians should carefully test such patients so that a DFT safety margin exists in all such patients.

SUMMARY

Amiodarone is an extremely effective antiarrhythmic agent, but side effects are frequent, and close, continuous follow-up is essential (Table 7.5).

SUGGESTED READING

Ceremuzynski L, Kleczar E, Krzemlinska-Pakula M, et al. Effect of amiodarone on mortality after myocardial infarction: a double-blind, placebo-controlled pilot study. J Am Coll Cardiol 1992;20:1056–1062.

Gosselink AT, Crijns HJ, Van Gelder IC, Hillige H, Wiesfeld AC, Lie KI. Low-dose amiodarone for maintenance of sinus rhythm after cardioversion of atrial fibrillation or flutter. JAMA 1992;267:3289–3293.

Heger JJ, Prystowsky EN, Jackman WM, et al. Amiodarone: clinical efficacy and electrophysiology during long-term therapy for recurrent ventricular tachycardia or ventricular fibrillation. N Engl J Med 1981;305:539–545.

Herre JM, Sauve NJ, Malone P, et al. Long-term results of amiodarone therapy in patients with recurrent sustained ventricular tachycardia or ventricular fibrillation. J Am Coll Cardiol 1989;13:442–449.

Holt DW, Tucker GT, Jackson PR, Storey GCA. Amiodarone pharmacokinetics. Am Heart J 1983;106:840–846.

Huang SK, Tan de Guzman WL, Chenarides JG, Okike NO, Vander Salm TJ. Effects of long-term amiodarone therapy on the defibrillation threshold and the rate of shocks of the implantable cardioverter-defibrillator. Am Heart J 1991;122: 720–727.

Marcus FI. Drug interactions with amiodarone. Am Heart J 1983;106:924–929.

McKenna WJ, Oakley CM, Krikler DM, Goodwin JF. Improved survival with amiodarone in patients with hypertrophic cardiomyopathy and ventricular tachycardia. Br Heart J 1985;53:412–416.

Singh BN, Nademanee K. Amiodarone and thyroid function: clinical implications during antiarrhythmic therapy. Am Heart J 1983;106: 857–868.

Wellens HJJ, Brugada P, Abdolla AH. Effect of amiodarone in paroxysmal supraventricular tachycardia with or without the Wolff-Parkinson-White syndrome. Am Heart J 1983; 106:876–879.

8 Sotalol and Bretylium

SOTALOL

Pharmacology

Sotalol is available in the United States only as an oral formulation, although it can be administered intravenously and is available in a parenteral formulation in several countries. Its clinical pharmacokinetics have been summarized. After oral ingestion of its tablet formulation, sotalol is virtually completely absorbed and displays no significant first-pass metabolism, resulting in nearly 100% bioavailability when administered on an empty stomach (about 80% bioavailability when given with food). Its apparent volume of distribution is 2 liters/kg. Sotalol shows negligible protein binding.

Circulating sotalol undergoes no significant biotransformation and is eliminated almost entirely (80–90% of dose) by renal excretion. Renal handling of the *d*- and *l*-isomers is identical. Terminal elimination half-life ranges from 10–20 hours, being influenced primarily by renal clearance. The pharmacokinetics of sotalol are unchanged with chronic use. Given sotalol's lack of protein binding and biotransformation, it is not surprising that no clinically significant drug interactions have been described. Both its β-blocker and class III effects are related to plasma concentrations of drug but show separate dose-response curves, with β-blockade reaching maximal effect at lower plasma concentrations than class III effects.

Commercially available racemic sotalol, given orally, has about one-fourth to one-third of the potency of oral propranolol, whereas, given intravenously its potency is one-eighth to one-sixteenth of propranolol's. When its isomers are tested separately, however, the β-blocking actions of sotalol are found to be due almost entirely to the contribution of the *l*-isomer, the *d*-isomer having less than one-fiftieth of the activity of the levocompound.

The clearance of sotalol is reduced in renal insufficiency and in the elderly (also on the basis of age-related reductions in renal clearance). The usual dose of sotalol hydrochloride is 80–160 mg given two to three times daily. Sotalol should be initiated in a low dose (80 mg), with dose increases every 2–3 days as needed. In the presence of renal insufficiency, the dose must be reduced. The clinical pharmacokinetic profile of sotalol is summarized in Table 8.1.

Hemodynamics of Sotalol

Clinical hemodynamic studies have shown less negative inotropic effects than anticipated, based on the degree of β-blockade achieved. Acutely administered intravenous (i.v.) sotalol (mean dose, 0.34 mg/kg), given to patients with cardiac disease undergoing catheterization (N = 24), was shown to reduce heart rate, cardiac index, and left ventricular dP/dT, both at rest and during exercise. Reductions in cardiac index paralleled those in heart rate, leaving stroke volume unchanged.

Table 8.1
Clinical Pharmacokinetic Profile of Sotalol

Rate of absorption (time to peak Cp)[a]	2.5–4 hr
Extent of absorption	90–100%
Bioavailability of absorbed drug	~ 100%
Binding to plasma proteins	0%
Apparent volume of distribution	2.0 ± 0.4 L/kg
Biotransformation	0%
Metabolites	None detected
Total body clearance (with normal renal function)	150 mL/min
Percent of drug eliminated renally (unchanged)	>75%
Plasma elimination half-life (patients)	1.5 (10–20) hr
Therapeutic plasma concentration range[b]	≈ 1–4 µg/mL
Pattern/model of elimination kinetics	First order/2-compartment
Dose proportionality of Cp?	Yes (linear)
Special features	• Water-soluble, little CNS penetration
	• Primary renal elimination
	• Accumulates in renal, not hepatic failure
	• No pharmacokinetic drug interactions[c]

Table prepared from data in Antonnacio MJ, Gomoll A. Pharmacology, pharmacodynamics and pharmacokinetics of sotalol. Am J Cardiol 1990;65:12A; Hanyok JJ: Clinical pharmacokinetics of sotalol. Am J Cardiol 1993; 72:19A.

[a]Cp, Concentration of drug in plasma
[b]Therapeutic Cp range not well established; limited clinical use
[c]Pharmacodynamic interactions are possible.

Left ventricular end diastolic pressure and total systemic resistance increased, whereas pulmonary artery pressure, total pulmonary resistance, and mean arterial pressure showed little change. In patients with acute myocardial infarction (MI) and arrhythmias, i.v. sotalol (40–120 mg) reduced heart rate and mean arterial pressure but did not change pulmonary capillary wedge pressure or systemic vascular resistance. Left ventricular end diastolic volume was unchanged or decreased, and stroke volume remained constant.

Chronic, oral sotalol was evaluated in a double-blind, placebo- and active (quinidine)-controlled, crossover trial in 27 patients with complex ventricular arrhythmias, the majority (85%) with structural heart disease. Sotalol therapy, given as 320–640 mg/day for 4 weeks, was associated with hemodynamic changes. A small reduction in cardiac output was observed, accounted for almost entirely by reductions in heart rate. Systolic blood pressure was also modestly reduced (by 7 and 9 mm Hg, at rest and with exercise). Stroke volume was maintained or increased at rest and with exercise (by 11 and 8 mL/m^2, respectively). Radionuclide ventriculography showed favorable changes in left ventricular ejection fraction at rest (47±13 to 51, ± 15%, P<.002) and with exercise (52±15 to 55, ±14%, P = NS). Sotalol was generally well tolerated and overall did not adversely affect cardiac function. Two patients (7%) developed overt congestive heart failure (CHF) while taking sotalol (versus none on quinidine); these patients had a markedly depressed ejection fraction at rest (18 and 23%) and markedly dilated left ventricular chambers (end diastolic indexes >200 mL/m^2), indicating a subgroup at increased risk of adverse hemodynamic (and proarrhythmic) effects.

In another study, the hemodynamic effects of oral sotalol (mean dose, 160 mg every 12 hours for ≥4 doses) were assessed in 12 patients with life-threatening arrhythmias undergoing electrophysiologic testing. Peak drug effects (2 hours postdose) included a 21 beats/minute (28%) reduction in heart rate and a 0.8 L/minute;pdm2 (24%) decrease in cardiac index, associated with increases in systemic vascular resistance (by 25%), stroke volume (by 8%), and pulmonary capillary wedge pressure (from 6.4–11.8 mm Hg), compared with the drug-free baseline measures. No significant changes in mean arterial pressure, pulmonary artery pressure, or stroke work index were observed in these moderately compromised patients (mean ejection fraction, 37%). One patient discontinued treatment because of worsening heart failure.

Despite its β-blocking effects, sotalol should be used with caution, even in patients with compromised left ventricular systolic function. With acute dosing, negative chronotropic and, to a lesser degree than expected, negative inotropic effects are observed. With chronic dosing, cardiac function is maintained or improves in most patients. Those with markedly reduced function (ejection fractions <25%) and markedly increased end diastolic volumes (>200 mL/m^2) are at greater risk for adverse hemodynamic effects.

Clinical Electrophysiology

Intravenous sotalol lengthens effective refractory periods throughout the heart, including the atrium (+25%), atrioventricular (AV) node (+25%), and right ventricle (+15%) (all with P<.01). It also lengthens sinus node recovery time, Q-T and Q-Tc intervals, and conduction time through the AV node (A-H interval) but not the His-Purkinje system (H-V interval) or ventricle (QRS). These increases in effective refractory periods in atria, ventricles, AV node, and bypass tracts, and prolongation in conduction time in intranodal but not infranodal structures have been replicated in several studies of i.v. sotalol. In still other electrophysiologic studies, these effects were shown to be associated with lengthening of the monophasic action potential in human atria and ventricles.

The electrocardiographic effects of chronic, oral therapy were evaluated in 114 patients with chronic ventricular premature complexes (VPCs) enrolled in a multicenter study of sotalol in daily doses of 320 and 640 mg, given for 4 weeks. Heart rate decreased by an average of 19 beats/minutes (−25%) on a dose of 320 mg/day and by 16 beats/minute (−24%) during 640 mg/day sotalol (P<.001 for each). P-R interval increased slightly (~6%), although significantly (P<.001), with both doses. QRS duration did not change, but Q-T interval increased by an average of 80 msec (~21%) during 320 mg/day and 91 msec (~23%) during 640 mg/day (both, P<.001). Corrected Q-T interval (Q-Tc) showed more moderate increases, averaging 21 (~5%) and 30 msec (~7%) for the two doses (P<.01 for both). Left ventricular ejection fraction was not adversely affected, and in fact increased by 3–4 percentage points during therapy (P<.01).

Indications

VENTRICULAR ARRHYTHMIAS

Two doses of sotalol (320 and 640 mg/day, divided in two doses) were compared with placebo in a 6-week randomized, double-blind, multicenter study in 114 patients with chronic VPCs ($\geq$30/hour). Sotalol significantly reduced VPCs in patients receiving both the lower and higher doses compared with those receiving placebo (by 75 and 85%, respectively, vs. 10%; each P<.001 vs. placebo). Individual efficacy ($\geq$75% VPC reduction) was achieved in 34% of lower dose and 71% of higher dose sotalol patients versus 6% of placebo-treated patients (P<.003, sotalol vs. placebo). Repetitive VPCs were effectively suppressed by both doses of sotalol (80 and 78%, vs. 25% by placebo) (each P<.005). Proarrhythmia (non-life-threatening) occurred in three sotalol and two placebo patients. Nine sotalol patients discontinued therapy because of adverse effects (one on lower and eight on higher dose, P<.02). These data suggest that sotalol is an efficacious antiarrhythmic agent for complex VPC suppression; in a dose of 320 mg/day it was somewhat less effective but better tolerated than in a dose of 640 mg/day.

In a double-blind, placebo-controlled, parallel study, the antiarrhythmic effects of sotalol and propranolol were compared in 172 patients with frequent VPCs (>30/hour). Sotalol was given in a dose of 160 mg twice daily and propranolol in a dose of 40 mg, administered three times daily. Those not achieving efficacy >75% VPC suppression were given higher doses (sotalol = 320 mg twice a day, propranolol = 80 mg three times a day). Overall, sotalol reduced VPC frequency by 80% (274 to 54/hour) and propranolol by 59% (255 to 104/hour) (P<.002, sotalol vs. propranolol). A significantly greater percentage of patients responded to sotalol (56%) compared to propranolol (29%) (P<.001).

In a review of 13 trials in which complex but nonsustained ventricular arrhythmias were treated with sotalol (N = 626 patients), using either placebo (N = 114) or active controls (N = 395 patients), efficacy (>75% VPC suppression) was achieved in a median of 58% of patients and proarrhythmia in only 3.6%. Ejection fraction effects were evaluated in six studies. None showed worsening, and three showed small increases (i.e., 31 ± 8 to 35; ±12%, P<.05).

The initial U.S. experience in patients with sustained ventricular tachycardia (VT) or ventricular fibrillation (VF) included 37 patients. Intravenous sotalol rendered VT or VF noninducible in 15 (45%) patients. Holter monitoring was subsequently performed on oral sotalol. A good (though imperfect) correlation was achieved between Holter and PES-defined efficacy. Long-term therapy was successful more frequently in Holter responders (7 of 11) than nonresponders (two of 10). A number of other small but supportive open studies have also appeared. Subsequently, a multicenter, randomized trial comparing i.v. sotalol with i.v. procainamide (double-blind, prospective protocol) was undertaken in 110 patients. Sotalol suppressed VTs induced with triple extrastimuli in 15 (30%) of 50 patients, whereas procainamide was effective in 10 (20%) of 50 evaluable patients (P = .19).

Oral sotalol was subsequently tested and found to be effective by PES in 8 of 11 responders to the i.v. drug, suggesting a good correlation between response to sotalol given by i.v. and oral routes.

In a European randomized study, sotalol and amiodarone were compared in 59 patients with sustained VT or VF. Therapy was empiric, with dosing guided by clinical tolerance. Of 29 patients assigned to sotalol, one had arrhythmia recurrence, nine were withdrawn (due to adverse effects), and five died (three during therapy). Of 30 randomized to amiodarone, five had recurrences, nine were withdrawn, and four died (each after withdrawal). Thus, in this limited comparison, no clear distinction between the two drugs in response profile was found.

An open-label, multicenter, historically controlled study design was employed to evaluate sotalol in 481 patients with drug-refractory sustained VTs. Therapy was initiated at 80 mg every 12 hours, with dose increments of 160 mg every 3 days as needed, up to a maximum dose of 480 mg every 12 hours. During hospital testing, efficacy determinations by programmed stimulation were made in 269 patients, with 94 (35%) showing complete suppression of inducible VT. Of 109 patients assessed by Holter monitoring, 34 (39%) showed a complete response. Sotalol was discontinued in 26% because of lack of efficacy and in 9% because of adverse effects. Proarrhythmia was observed in 23 patients (4.8%), most commonly in the form of torsade de pointes or an increase in episodes of clinical VT. Only three patients (1%) were forced to discontinue sotalol because of early heart failure.

Of 268 patients entering long-term therapy, the proportions remaining free of arrhythmia recurrence at 12, 18, and 27 months were 76, 72, and 66%, respectively. Of interest, differences in times to arrhythmia recurrence were not significantly predicted by differences in response on PES, Holter monitor, or baseline ejection fraction testing. Of 70 arrhythmia recurrences, only 16 (23%) were sudden death events. Late-onset heart failure occurred in seven (2%) and proarrhythmia in eight (3%) patients during follow-up. No noncardiac organ toxicity occurred during chronic therapy.

A 5-year, prospective study coordinated by the Massachusetts General Hospital was undertaken in 1985 to assess the efficacy and safety of sotalol, guided by electrophysiologic study, in patients with life-threatening VTs refractory to at least one class I antiarrhythmic drug. Of the 161 patients enrolled, 41 had an ejection fraction ≤30%, 87% had coronary artery disease (82% with previous MI), and 132 had baseline and follow-up electrophysiologic studies, performed on a median dose of sotalol of 240 mg/day (range, 160–960). Sotalol therapy suppressed inducible VT at PES in 34% of patients. Chronic sotalol was given to 45 PES responders and 34 others in whom sotalol was believed to be the best therapeutic option. The proportion of these patients free from recurrent VT or sudden death was 79% at 1 year and 67% at 2 years. Recurrence rate was lower in patients with VT suppression at PES than in unsuppressed patients (86 vs. 52% at 2 years). Overall, actuarial survival was 98% at 1 year and 90% at 2 years.

The Electrophysiologic Study Versus Electrocardiographic Monitoring (ESVEM) Trial compared the predictive value for arrhythmia recurrence of these two methods and seven drugs in patients with sustained VT. In ESVEM, 486 patients with a history of aborted sudden death or sustained VT were entered and treated sequentially with up to six class I antiarrhythmic agents (procainamide, quinidine, mexiletine, propafenone, imipramine, and pirmenol) or sotalol, assigned in random order, until a drug predicted to be effective was found. The overall in-hospital response rate was 43% for sotalol and 21–36% for the other six drugs (P = .015). For patients evaluated by the more demanding electrophysiologic method, the response rates were 35% for sotalol versus a range of 10–26% for the other drugs (P< .001). Among in-hospital responders placed on long-term therapy, patients treated with sotalol had lower mortality rates than those treated with class I antiarrhythmics (risk ratio 0.50, P = .004) and lower VT recurrence rates (risk ratio 0.43, P<.001) (uncensored analysis), as well as lower withdrawal rates, both during titration (16% vs. 23–43%, P<.001) and during long-term follow-up (7% vs. 7–32% P = .003). The most commonly used sotalol doses in ESVEM were 320–480 mg/ day. The ESVEM trial suggests that sotalol is generally more effective than class I antiarrhythmic drugs in treating sustained VTs. The design of ESVEM does not allow the effect of sotalol to be compared with either no pharmacologic therapy (no placebo given) or an implantable cardioverter defibrillator (ICD).

Sotalol, which has class II as well as β-blocking effects, was evaluated in a double-blind, placebo-controlled secondary prevention (postinfarction) trial in 1,456 patients in the United Kingdom. Sotalol was used in the higher than recommended initial dose of 320 mg, given once daily. Despite a suggestion of an early slight adverse effect with this large initial dose, overall mortality (at approximately 1 year) tended to be reduced by sotalol. The favorable trend may not have achieved significance because of the relatively small number of patients in this trial or because of a small early adverse effect, perhaps caused by excessive dosage. Another, smaller postinfarction study (TEST, Timolol, Encainide, Sotalol Trial) also suggested an early adverse potential with high-dose sotalol (320 mg twice daily) in early (<1 month) postinfarction patients at high risk (ejection fraction ≤40%, ≥10 PVC/hour, or VT). The study was stopped prematurely after 20 patients had been entered in the sotalol arm, and six either died (N = 4) or suffered proarrhythmic events (N = 2) within 2 weeks of initiating therapy. Thus, it appears likely that sotalol can be given to patients with previous MI without an overall adverse effect on mortality and with the possibility of benefit if started in smaller (≤160 mg/day) doses at >1 month after infarction, but may be associated with adverse potential if given in excessive dosage at early times postinfarction in higher risk patients. Standard β-blockers are thus preferred for routine postinfarction prophylaxis.

Antiarrhythmic therapy is being used increasingly in combination with ICDs to reduce the frequency of serious arrhythmias requiring defibrillation. Some drugs used for these purposes (some class I drugs and amiodarone) may, however, increase this threshold and reduce the efficacy of defibrillation shocks. Sotalol, on the other hand, lowers the defibrillation threshold in experimental animals. One study reported the lowest energy required for defibrillation to be 5.9 ±3.4 J (range, 2–15 J) in 25 patients who received ICDs and were treated with oral sotalol (171 ±58 mg daily). This compared favorably with a nonrandomized comparison group treated with amiodarone (N = 23 patients) that had an average defibrillation threshold of 16 ± 10 J (P<.01). Thus, sotalol may favorably modify VF and enhance defibrillation efficacy. In view of its effectiveness for preventing supraventricular and ventricular arrhythmias, together with its favorable effects on VF thresholds, sotalol may be particularly well suited as adjunctive therapy in patients with ICDs.

SUPRAVENTRICULAR ARRHYTHMIAS

Intravenous and oral sotalol has been evaluated for its ability to terminate and prevent supraventricular tachyarrhythmias, including paroxysmal supraventricular tachycardias (PSVT) and paroxysmal atrial fibrillation and flutter (PAF). In seven open trials, i.v. sotalol (0.4–1.5 mg/kg) converted 46% (47 of 106) of episodes of PSVT or PAF. In six studies, i.v. sotalol (0.6–2.75 mg/kg) prevented the reinduction of sustained PSVT by PES in 59% of patients (44 of 74). Subsequent oral sotalol prevented reinduction of PSVT in 68% of patients in three trials. Sotalol was compared with metoprolol in one study and was found to be more effective than metoprolol in preventing reinduction of PSVT (59% vs. 28%, P<.05). Several clinical studies (open design) evaluated the effectiveness of oral sotalol in a small number of patients. Of 74 patients with resistant PSVT, sotalol was effective in 39%. In a multicenter efficacy and safety study, i.v. sotalol (1.5 mg/kg/10 minutes) and a placebo were compared for their ability to terminate ongoing SVT in 43 patients. Most patients (N = 27) had AV nodal reentrant tachycardia; an additional 11 had AV reentrant tachycardia using an accessory connection. Sinus rhythm was achieved within 30 minutes in 83% of patients who received sotalol as the first drug, compared with 16% of patients receiving placebo (P<.0001). Sotalol was well tolerated, and no proarrhythmic effects were observed.

Postoperative supraventricular arrhythmias (primarily atrial fibrillation [AF]) were reduced from 37% with a placebo to 2% with sotalol in a study of 161 patients. In another study among 429 consecutive patients undergoing coronary bypass grafting, two doses of sotalol were compared with propranolol for prevention of supraventricular arrhythmias. Supraventricular tachyarrhythmia occurred in 11–19% of patients, with a nonsignificant trend favoring sotalol.

An open, parallel-group study in Sweden compared quinidine with sotalol for maintenance of sinus rhythm after cardioversion from chronic AF. At the end of a 6-month treatment period, 52% of patients receiving sotalol compared with 48% receiving quinidine remained in sinus rhythm. In those relapsing, however, heart rate was greater in those treated with quinidine than with sotalol (109 vs. 78 beats/minute), and relapsing patients in the sotalol group were less symptomatic. Sotalol was better tolerated than quinidine, as demonstrated by a lower adverse effect rate and a lower withdrawal rate (11 vs. 26%).

A randomized comparison of sotalol versus propafenone for treatment of AF was performed in 99 patients who had failed an average of two type I agents. Patients were stratified into four groups based on AF pattern (chronic vs. paroxysmal) and left atrial size (large, ≥4.5 cm vs. small,<4.5 cm). The proportion remaining in sinus rhythm after 6 months was compared by the Kaplan-Meier method. Overall, 41% of patients remained in sinus rhythm (range, 34–51%) among the eight treatment-disease subgroups, with no significant differences between drugs. Side effects led to discontinuation in 8% of propafenone and 12% of sotalol patients.

In summary, both i.v. and oral sotalol may be effective in terminating ongoing SVTs or preventing recurrence or reinduction of sustained supraventricular arrhythmias. Trials of prophylaxis for PSVT/PAF have indicated a variable, generally good rate of effectiveness and an acceptable profile of adverse effects, in prevention of recurrence of PSVT and PAF, compared with class Ia and Ic agents (approximately equivalent efficacy), and superior to agents with β-blocker effects alone.

Adverse Effects

Adverse reactions to sotalol are accounted for virtually entirely by those related to β-blocker activity and, in addition, those associated with Q-T prolongation (a result of its class III effects), specifically, torsade de pointes (Table 8.2).

Table 8.2
Summary of Common Adverse Effects of Sotalol[a]

Adverse Effect	Incidence (%)	Patients Discontinued (%)
Cardiac		
Proarrhythmia	4.3	3
Torsade de pointes	2.4	
History of VT/VF	4	
No VT/VF	1–1.4	
Worsened VT (history of VT)	1	
Congestive heart failure	3.3	1
History of VT/VF	4.6	
History of CHF	7.3	
Bradycardia	13	3
Sinus node arrest		≤1
2nd or 3rd degree heart block		≤1
Syncope	5	1
General adverse effects		
Dyspnea	21	3
Fatigue	20	4
Dizziness	20	2
Asthenia	13	2
Light-headedness	12	1
Hypotension	6	2

Data taken from Product information: Betapace® (sotalol HCl). Wayne, NJ, 07470: Berlex Laboratories, 1992.

aAdverse effects given were associated with discontinuations in ≥1% of patients.

During premarketing trials, 3,186 patients with cardiac arrhythmias (1,363 with sustained VT) received oral sotalol, 2,455 for at least 2 weeks. In patients with a history of sustained VT, the incidence of torsade de pointes was 4% and worsening of clinical VT, 1%. In patients with other, less serious, ventricular arrhythmias or supraventricular arrhythmias, the incidence of torsade de pointes was 1% and 1.4%, respectively. The risk of torsade de pointes was greater in women than in men and increased with increasing dosage.

Overall, discontinuation because of unacceptable side effects was necessary in 17% of all patients in clinical trials and 13% of patients treated for at least 2 weeks. The most common adverse reactions leading to discontinuation of oral sotalol were fatigue, 4%; bradycardia, 3%; dyspnea, 3%; proarrhythmia, 3%; asthenia, 2%; and dizziness, 2%. Organ toxic effects likely to be caused by sotalol have not been observed in short- and long-term trials. As with other β-blockers, elevated blood glucose levels and increased insulin requirements may occur.

Sotalol, like other β-blockers, is contraindicated in patients with bronchial asthma, severe sinus bradycardia, second- and third-degree AV block (unless a functioning pacemaker is present), congenital or acquired long Q-T syndromes, uncontrolled CHF, cardiogenic shock, and previous evidence of sotalol hypersensitivity or allergy. In premarketing studies, new or worsened heart failure occurred in 3.3% of 3,257 patients, leading to discontinuation in approximately 1%. The incidence was higher in those with sustained VT-VF (4.6%) or a history of prior heart failure (7.3%). The 1-year incidence of new or worsened heart failure was 3% in patients without and 10% in those with a history of heart failure. Sotalol should not be given to patients with hypokalemia or hypomagnesemia prior to correction of electrolyte imbalance because of the increased potential for exaggerated Q-T prolongation and torsade de pointes. Excessive prolongation of Q-T interval (>550 msec) should be avoided during sotalol therapy because of an increased risk of proarrhythmia. Bradycardia (heart rate consistently <50 beats/minute) was reported in 13% of patients, sinus node arrest or dysfunction in ≤1%, and second- or third-degree AV block in ≤1%. In patients with labile diabetes or a history of episodes of spontaneous hypoglycemia, sotalol, like other β-blockers, may mask premonitory signs of hypoglycemia and hence should be used with caution. Sotalol, in patients with sick sinus syndrome, should be avoided or used with extreme caution. Because sotalol is eliminated mainly via the kidneys, dose modification is necessary with renal impairment.

Pharmacokinetic interactions of sotalol with other drugs have not been described. However, pharmacodynamic interactions with other antiarrhythmic agents (especially those causing lengthening of the Q-T interval), with calcium or other β-blocking agents (negative inotropic/chronotropic interactions), may occur.

D-SOTALOL

d-Sotalol has been shown to increase the VF threshold and reduce experimental VF. The clinical efficacy of i.v. d-sotalol (1–2 mg/kg/10 minutes) and procainamide (1 g/50 minutes) was analyzed in 23 patients with recurrent, sustained

VT refractory to conventional drugs and with inducible, sustained VT. Sustained VT was suppressed in nine patients (39%) and rendered nonsustained in four others. No clinical arrhythmias were observed during oral therapy (mean dose, 430 mg/day) in seven patients treated for an average of 10 months.

The antiarrhythmic properties of i.v. d-sotalol were investigated in 38 patients undergoing electrophysiologic studies for malignant ventricular arrhythmias. For comparison, 17 of these patients were also evaluated following procainamide infusions. (The stimulation protocol utilized two stimulation sites and up to three extra stimuli.) After d-sotalol, VT was no longer inducible in 18 patients (47%), and the rate of VT in inducible patients was reduced from an average of 220 to 160 beats/minutes. Effectiveness was observed both in those with monomorphic (14 of 28) and polymorphic VT (four of 10) and was associated with significant prolongation in effective refractory period and Q-Tc. Of 17 patients given both d-sotalol and procainamide, four responded to procainamide and seven to d-sotalol. Oral d-sotalol (200–800 mg/day) was evaluated in 11 patients for periods of up to 17 months. Nine survived, one died of acute MI, and one had recurrent arrhythmia, and was switched to amiodarone therapy.

The efficacy of i.v. and oral d-sotalol was evaluated in patients with clinical and inducible VT; 73 were tested with the i.v. drug (1.5–2.5 mg/kg), and 33 were also tested on oral therapy (400–600 mg/day). Acute success rate was 41% with i.v. d-sotalol; oral therapy yielded a concordant response in 80% of patients.

BRETYLIUM TOSYLATE

Pharmacology

Bretylium tosylate is an adrenergic neuron-blocking drug possessing complex pharmacology, including indirect effects that arise from its interactions with adrenergic neurons, as well as direct (cardiac membrane) actions. Interaction with adrenergic neurons includes early sympathomimetic activity, caused by norepinephrine release, and subsequent adrenergic neuronal blockade. These actions are a consequence of selective accumulation of bretylium in sympathetic ganglionic and postganglionic adrenergic neurons. The uptake leads to initial norepinephrine release, followed by subsequent inhibition of norepinephrine release caused by depression of adrenergic neuronal excitability, essentially causing a chemical sympathectomy. Its direct effects on cardiac membranes include the proportionate lengthening of action potential and refractory period duration, a class III effect, related to blockade of potassium-carrying ionic channels.

After i.v. injection of bretylium in dogs, serum concentrations decrease in a biexponential fashion, whereas myocardial concentrations increase for up to 6 hours. In parallel with these changes, the ratio of myocardial to serum drug concentrations increase to a maximum of 12 by 12 hours. Thereafter, parallel elimination of the drug from the myocardium and serum are observed, with an elimination half-life of 10.5 hours. In human volunteers, an i.v. injection of bretylium

Table 8.3
Pharmacokinetic Profile of Bretylium

Absorption/bioavailability (oral drug)	20–25% (range, 10–40%)
Bioavailability (I.V. drug)	≈100%
Plasma protein binding	<1%
Apparent volume of distribution (steady-state)	3–7 L/kg
Biotransformation (%)	0%
Metabolites	None detected
Total body clearance (wirth normal renal function)	300–450 mL/min
Percent of drug eliminated renally (unchanged)	90–100%
Plasma elimination half-life (patients)	9–14 hr (range, 4–20)
Therapeutic plasma concentration range[a]	≈ 1–3 µg/mL
Special features	• Water-soluble, little CNS penetration
	• Primary renal elimination: filtration/secretion
	• Accumulates in renal, not hepatic failure
	• No pharmacokinetic drug interactions[b]

Table prepared primarily from data of Anderson JL. In: Messerli F, ed. Cardiovascular drug therapy. Philadelphia: WB Saunders, 1990:1257; Anderson JL: Adrenergic neurone-blocking as class III antiarrhythmic agents: focus on bretylium. In: Singh BW, ed. Control of cardiac arrhythmias by lenghtening repolarization. Mount Kisco, NY: Futura, 1988:315; Anderson JL, Patterson E, Wagner JG, et al. Oral and intravenous bretylium disposition. Clin Pharmacol Ther 1980;28:468; Anderson JL, Patterson E, Wagner JG, et al. Clinical pharmacokinetics of intravenous and oral bretylium tosylate in survivors of ventricular tachycardia or fibrillation, J Cardiovasc Pharmacol 1981;3:485.

[a]Therapeutic Cp range not well established; limited clinical use.
[b]Pharmacodynamic interactions are possible.

leads to serum concentrations 10-fold greater than those observed after oral administration of equivalent doses. Calculated oral bioavailability is variable, averaging only 20–25%. As in animal models, elimination by both routes follows biexponential decay, accounted for entirely by renal clearance. Similar kinetics have been shown to apply to cardiac patients given i.v. bretylium. Disposition is entirely attributed to renal elimination, which averaged 400 mL/minute. Terminal elimination half-life averaged 13.5 hours. Apparent volumes of distribution of bretylium average 3–7 liters/kg. Bretylium is negligibly bound to plasma proteins, has no known metabolites, and is not known to interact directly with other drugs. The pharmacokinetics of bretylium are summarized in Table 8.3.

Hemodynamic Effects

Injections of bretylium cause a biphasic cardiovascular response. Initially, increases in heart rate and blood pressure are observed, a result of norepinephrine release from adrenergic nerve endings. This is followed within 15–30 minutes by reductions in vascular resistance, blood pressure, and heart rate, which are manifestations of sympathetic neuronal blockade, a result of interference with release but not depletion of norepinephrine stores. Bretylium also inhibits norepinephrine reuptake but does not affect postganglionic adrenergic receptor function.

Unlike other antiarrhythmic agents, bretylium does not lead to depression in left ventricular function. Initially, a positive inotropic effect occurs, because of norepinephrine release. Later, contractility returns to, but not below, control levels. In one canine model, however, a deleterious effect of bretylium on hemodynamic recovery from VF was reported, which was ascribed to inhibition of sympathetic nervous system function by bretylium.

Clinical Studies

Early clinical reports of bretylium usage were uncontrolled and involved patients with drug refractory, life-threatening ventricular arrhythmias. In these studies, bretylium was often used as a treatment of last resort for VF. Overall, a beneficial effect of bretylium was reported in 60–70% of patients, with antifibrillatory effects occurring within 10–15 minutes. In contrast, maximal antiarrhythmic activity (suppression of ventricular ectopy or tachycardia) has generally not been observed for several hours. A small number of studies have indicated a limited ability of bretylium to suppress chronic ventricular ectopy and reentrant (monomorphic) VT.

In an important observational study, 27 consecutive patients with resistant VF, attended by a hospital cardiac arrest team, were given bretylium. Successful termination of VF was achieved in 20 (74%) within 9–12 minutes, and 12 (44%) survived to discharge. In a controlled emergency ward study in 59 patients with cardiopulmonary arrest, bretylium was associated with a 35% survival rate, compared with a 6% rate in patients treated with resuscitative measures and other therapies (including lidocaine) alone. The outcome of bretylium treatment, however, was adversely affected by increasing times from cardiac arrest to therapy in another study.

Bretylium was compared with lidocaine in a controlled study in out-of-hospital patients experiencing VF. In this Seattle Heart Watch study, no significant difference was observed in the percentage of patients converting to an organized rhythm (about 90%), the proportion of patients successfully resuscitated (about 60%), and the percentage surviving to hospital discharge. In a similarly designed, randomized Milwaukee paramedic study in 91 patients with refractory VF, conversion to an organized rhythm was observed in 81% of lidocaine-treated versus 74% of bretylium-treated patients; an organized rhythm with pulse was achieved in 56 versus 35%, respectively. Survival to emergency room admission occurred in 23 versus 23%, and survival to discharge in 10 versus 5%.

Bretylium has recently been compared with i.v. amiodarone in a multicenter study of patients with VT-VF refractory to or intolerant of lidocaine and procainamide. Bretylium showed comparable efficacy, measured as time to recurrence and survival, but caused more side effects (e.g., hypotension) than amiodarone.

Bretylium is available only for parenteral administration. Based on clinical trial results, it has been approved and is indicated as a first-line agent for the treatment of VF, especially when occurring after MI. It is also indicated for acute therapy of other life-threatening ventricular arrhythmias (e.g., VT) that have not responded to lidocaine or other first-line agents. Bretylium is not recommended for the suppression of ventricular ectopy.

Indications

Bretylium has not been tested clinically for use in acute supraventricular arrhythmias, although it shows activity in experimental models of atrial flutter and fibrillation. Torsade de pointes ventricular arrhythmia, a polymorphic VT associated with a long Q-T interval, has been treated successfully with bretylium in selected cases and may be considered a second-line drug in patients failing to respond to standard therapies. Bretylium protects the hyperthermic ventricle in some models of induced VF but has not been studied in clinical trials for this indication.

Bretylium has been tested as a prophylactic therapy against VF in acute MI. Its use has been reported to be associated with a low incidence of VF in observational studies, but with a higher incidence of clinically significant hypotension than either lidocaine or no therapy. It is currently not recommended for prophylactic use in patients with acute MI.

Dosage/Administration

Bretylium should be administered in a monitored, critical-care setting. For VF and hemodynamically unstable VT, an initial dose of 5 mg/kg is given undiluted by rapid i.v. injection (Table 8.4). If VF persists, the dosage may be increased to 10 mg/kg and repeated, together with other measures. There is fairly little experience or rationale for using doses >30 mg/kg.

When hemodynamically stable VTs are treated, the dose is 5–10 mg/kg over a period of at least 8 minutes (preferably 15–30 minutes) to prevent nausea and vomiting. Subsequent doses may be given at 1–2-hour intervals if arrhythmia persists or recurs. For maintenance therapy, a diluted solution of bretylium is administered as a constant infusion, generally at a rate of 1–2 mg/minute. Alternatively, a dose of 5–10 mg/kg may be administered by slow injection (i.e., 10–30 minutes) every 6 hours. Intramuscular therapy may be given, if necessary, but i.v. administration is preferred.

Table 8.4
Summary of Bretylium Clinical Indications and Administration

Indications	VF, VT, and related rhythms
Route of administration	Parenteral (i.v. preferred; may also give i.m.)
How supplied	10 mL ampule containing 500 mg bretylium tosylate in water
Dosing	Loading: 5–10 mg/kg; may repeat once or twice if needed for an initial therapeutic response
	Maintenance: 1–3 mg/min infusion, or 5–10 mg/kg every 6 hr

Accumulation of bretylium may occur in patients with advanced renal failure (especially when creatinine clearance is <25 mL/minute). If prolonged administration is required, maintenance dosing should be reduced when infusions are given or injection intervals increased. Dialysis increases bretylium clearance 2-fold. Hepatic dysfunction and heart failure are not known to change the pharmacokinetics of bretylium importantly, except to the extent that renal clearance has changed.

Adverse Effects, Precautions, and Contraindications

Adverse effects of bretylium are primarily related to its modification of adrenergic function. Tachycardia and hypertension may follow the initial catecholamine release reaction but are typically transient. Anxiety, excitement, flushing, substernal pressure, headache, and angina pectoris, as well as occasional increases in ventricular arrhythmias, are other manifestations that may be associated with the initial catecholamine release. Subsequent hypotension (especially postural) frequently accompanies bretylium and may begin within 15 minutes. Hypotension has required drug discontinuation in about 10% of patients. To avoid postural hypotension, patients should remain supine during and until well after administration of the drug until blood pressure stabilizes (which may require 12–48 hours). Less commonly, bradycardia is observed as a result of sympathetic blockade. Asymptomatic hypotension is generally untreated (i.e., systolic pressure >80 mm Hg). Rarely, severe hypotension not responding to postural measures, volume repletion, and drug discontinuation may occur and requires dopamine or norepinephrine infusion; in these cases, cautious dosing should be given, because bretylium may enhance pressor response by causing postdenervation hypersensitivity. Partial pharmacologic reversal of hypotension may be achieved with protriptyline (5–10 mg by mouth every 6–8 hour), a secondary amine antidepressant.

Caution in the use of bretylium is appropriate in patients with severe aortic stenosis, pulmonary hypertension, and other syndromes associated with fixed cardiac output, who may be unable to compensate for peripheral vasodilatation caused by bretylium.

Nausea, vomiting, and/or retching has been reported in about 10% of patients given bretylium, but is usually related to excessively rapid i.v. injections (i.e., <8 minutes). Because bretylium is primarily excreted via the kidney, accumulation may occur in those with advanced renal failure. In these patients, when maintenance therapy is given, infusion doses should be reduced and/or intervals for injections increased. Other occasionally reported adverse reactions to bretylium include diarrhea, flushing, anxiety, dyspnea, diaphoresis, conjunctivitis, and nasal stuffiness. Many of these relate to bretylium's vascular and adrenergic effects.

SUGGESTED READING

Anderson JL. Bretylium tosylate. In: Messerli F, ed. Cardiovascular drug therapy. Philadelphia: WB Saunders, 1990:1257–1268.

Antonnacio MJ, Gomoll A. Pharmacology, pharmacodynamics and pharmacokinetics of sotalol. Am J Cardiol 1990;65:12A–18A.

Campbell RWF, Furniss SS. Practical considerations in the use of sotalol for ventricular tachycardia and ventricular fibrillation. Am J Cardiol 1993;72:80A–87A.

Kehoe RF, Zheutlin TA, Dunnington CS, et al. Safety and efficacy of sotalol in patients with drug-refractory sustained ventricular tachyarrhythmias. Am J Cardiol 1990;65:58A.

Koch-Weser J. Drug therapy: bretylium. N Engl J Med 1979;300:473–479.

Mason JW, for the ESVEM Investigators. A comparison of seven antiarrhythmic drugs in patients with ventricular tachyarrhythmias. N Engl J Med 1993;329:452–459.

Nademanee K, Feld G, Hendrickson JA, Singh PN, Singh BN. Electrophysiologic and antiarrhythmic effects of sotalol in patients with life-threatening ventricular tachyarrhythmias. Circulation 1985;72:555–559.

Sahar DI, Reiffel JA, Bigger JT, Squatrito A. Efficacy, safety, and tolerance of d-sotalol in patients with refractory supraventricular arrhythmias. Am Heart J 1989;117:562–569.

9 Other Antiarrhythmic Agents

CALCIUM CHANNEL BLOCKERS

The role of calcium channel blockers as antiarrhythmic compounds is limited to a reasonably well defined spectrum of ventricular, especially supraventricular, arrhythmias. In such arrhythmias, their utility is essentially in the control of symptoms with little or no impact on prolongation of survival. Not all calcium channel blockers are effective antiarrhythmic agents, and their clinical antiarrhythmic effects can be correlated with their specific electrophysiologic properties.

The selective block of the slow-channel activity results in an increase in the time-dependent refractoriness and conduction in the slow-response dependent fibers. These dual effects characterize the fundamental property of the so-called slow-channel inhibitors as antiarrhythmic agents. Cardiac fibers dependent on slow-channel activity, under either physiologic (autonomic influences on SA and atrioventricular [AV] nodes) or pathologic (ischemia, infarction) conditions, thus become the primary locus of action for calcium antagonists.

ROLE OF SLOW-CHANNEL ABNORMALITIES IN THE GENESIS OF CARDIAC ARRHYTHMIAS

Only those arrhythmias that arise on the basis of abnormal slow-channel function are likely to respond to calcium channel blockers. Recent experimental studies have focused on the role of slow-channel function in the genesis of triggered automaticity in the form of early afterdepolarizations (EADs) as well as delayed afterdepolarizations (DADs). Although EADs are known to be produced by a variety of pathophysiologic interventions, such as hypoxia and acidosis, and experimentally by blocking repolarizing currents (e.g., cesium and aconitine), most commonly they are associated with the use of antiarrhythmic agents that prolong cardiac repolarization. It is likely that at least certain forms of clinical torsade de pointes are caused by an increase in calcium current through the slow channel.

Delayed afterdepolarizations are oscillations that develop at the end of repolarization, which may cause triggered automaticity. This occurs in association with factors that elevate the intracellular level of calcium beyond a certain critical level, as may result from high extracellular concentrations of calcium, high stimulation frequencies, digitalis, and catecholamines.

DADs may also play an important role in myocardial reperfusion arrhythmias, but the clinical relevance of these observations remains to be clarified.

ELECTROPHYSIOLOGIC PROPERTIES OF CALCIUM-CHANNEL BLOCKERS AS THEY RELATE TO THEIR ANTIARRHYTHMIC ACTIONS

The precise relationship between the abnormality of slow-channel activity and the origin of the various types of supraventricular tachyarrhythmias in humans is still unclear.

118

The normal AV node is slow-channel dependent. It may become the site of deranged impulse formation and impulse conduction, the two most significant mechanisms underlying the genesis of cardiac arrhythmias.

Calcium channel blockers block the slow calcium channel in a concentration or dose-dependent fashion. Thus, in fast-channel fibers they have no significant effect on atrial, ventricular, or His-Purkinje refractory periods, nor on conduction velocity. They slow phase 4 depolarization in the S-A and AV nodes, and also slow conduction velocity. The major effect on the refractory period is in the AV node, where both the effective and the functional refractory periods are significantly lengthened in the anterograde as well as in the retrograde directions.

The clinical electropharmacologic and pharmacodynamic effects of calcium antagonists represent a balance of their in vitro actions and those that result from reflex activation of the sympathetic reflexes engendered by their often potent vasodilator actions. The reflex actions induced by the dihydropyridines either nullify or reverse the intrinsic actions on the sinus node. Thus, these agents do not exert measurable effects on the electrophysiologic parameters in man and appear to be devoid of antiarrhythmic actions. In general, the clinical electrophysiologic effects of various calcium antagonists are in accord with their in vitro effects. With regard to diltiazem, verapamil, and bepridil, the net effects are also modified by the noncompetitive sympatholytic effects of these compounds.

The major clinical electrophysiologic actions of various calcium antagonists are summarized in Table 9.1. Undoubtedly the most significant action whereby calcium antagonists exert their salutary effects in arrhythmias is by modulating the electrophysiologic functions of the AV node. The depressant effect on AV nodal

Table 9.1
Clinical Electrophysiologic Effects of Adenosine and Calcium Antagonists

Effects	Verapamil	Diltiazem	Bepridil	Adenosine
Heart rate	↓↑a	↓+	↓+	↓++
QRS	0	0	↑+	0
Q-Tc	0	0	↑++	0
PR	↑++	↑++	↑++	↑++
A-H	↑+++	↑+++	↑++	↑+++
H-V	0	0	↑+	0
Atrial ERPb	±	±	↑+	↓++
AV node ERP	↑++++	↑++++	↑+++	?↑
AV node FRPc	↑++++	↑++++	↑+++	?↑
Ventricular ERP	0	0	↑++	0
His-Purkinje ERP	0	0	↑++	0
Bypass tract ERP	±	±	↑++	?↓
Sinus node recovery time	0d	0d	↑+	?↑
Ventricular automaticity	0	0	↓+	0

a↓, decrease; ↑ increase; ↑↓ equivocal effect; range of change from minimal to large: 0, no effect; ±, variable effect; ?, uncertain effect; ++++, large effect.
bERP, effective refractory period
cFRP, functional refractory period
dProlonged in sick sinus syndrome.

conduction is utilized in the termination of the acute episodes of paroxysmal supraventricular tachycardia (SVT) and in the slowing of the ventricular response in atrial flutter and fibrillation. These agents have no measurable effects on intraatrial, interventricular, or His-Purkinje conduction or refractoriness. Most calcium antagonists as well as adenosine have little or no electrophysiologic effects on ventricular muscle, the exception being bepridil (Table 9.1). There are certain forms of ventricular tachycardias (VTs) that are sensitive to the action of adenosine and calcium channel blockers. These appear to occur on the basis of triggered activity.

CLINICAL PHARMACOLOGY OF CALCIUM CHANNEL BLOCKERS

Verapamil and diltiazem can be given intravenously or orally. Their clinical pharmacology is shown in Table 9.2.

Clinical Use for Arrhythmias

TERMINATION OF SUPRAVENTRICULAR TACHYARRHYTHMIAS

Paroxysmal supraventricular tachycardia (SVT) is a fairly common arrhythmia; it may account for about half of all of supraventricular tachycardias. Experimental and clinical observations suggest that most SVTs arise on the basis of reentry. The least common variety is the automatic form.

Intranodal reentry (AV nodal reentrant tachycardia [AVNRT]) is perhaps the most common form of the clinically encountered SVT and is based on dual pathways in the AV node. The pathways have different anterograde and retrograde conduction velocities. Acute termination of SVT by drug administration is based on the interruption of anterograde or retrograde conduction in the AV node.

Numerous compounds are effective in the acute conversion of SVT when simple vagal maneuvers fail to effect a prompt conversion (Fig. 9.1). Verapamil is accepted as the treatment of choice, except in patients with hypotension and markedly impaired ventricular function. More recently, intravenous (i.v.) diltiazem and adenosine have also been added to the list of very desirable agents for the acute conversion of SVT.

Table 9.2
Clinical Pharmacology of Calcium Channel Blockers Useful for Arrhythmia

	Verapamil	Diltiazem
Dose		
Oral	80–160 mg t.i.d. or q.i.d.	30–120 mg t.i.d. (short acting)
	240–360 mg daily (long acting)	60–180 mg b.i.d. (intermediate acting)
Intravenous	5 mg (bolus) repeated 3–4 times	20–25 mg (bolus) repeated 3–4 times
		5–15 mg per hour (continuous infusion)
Absorption (oral)	90%	90%
Onset of		
action (oral)	30–90 minutes	60 minutes
Half-life	8–12 hours	2–6 hours
Metabolism	Hepatic (first pass effect)	Hepatic (first pass effect)
Metabolites	Minimal activity	Inactive
Interactions	Digoxin, β-blockers, negatively inotropic agents	β-blockers, negatively inotropic agents

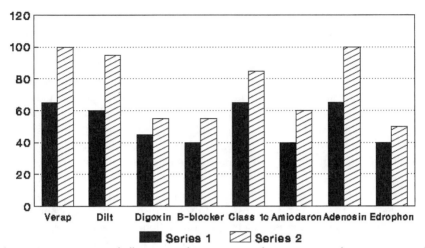

Figure 9.1. Percentage of effectiveness of SVT conversion for i.v. regimens of various compounds. Abbreviations: Verap, verapamil; Dilt, diltiazem; Edrophon, edrophonium; Series 1, lowest efficacy rate; Series 2, highest efficacy rate.

In the largest numbers of patients with SVT, the anterograde limb of the tachycardia circuit is the AV node, the "weakest link" of the reentrant loop; it is most susceptible to the blocking action of i.v. verapamil and diltiazem. This may account for the prompt and predictable reversion of 80–100% of cases of SVT using 3–5 mg (in children) to 10–15 mg (in adults) of verapamil, or 17–25 mg of diltiazem administered intravenously.

When verapamil is given intravenously during an episode of SVT, the onset of its action is rapid; sinus rhythm is restored in most cases in 2–3 minutes, and in some cases within 10 minutes of drug administration. The success rate of conversion of SVT to sinus rhythm by verapamil may be improved to nearly 100% by carotid sinus massage or the addition of 5–10 mg of edrophonium (Tensilon) given in rapid succession after verapamil. Although less experience is available in children, the antiarrhythmic spectrum of verapamil appears similar in children, adults, and in the elderly. Verapamil is less safe in patients with hypotension, impaired ventricular function, especially those with a history of heart failure, and in patients already taking β-blockers.

The effects of i.v. diltiazem are similar to those of verapamil in terms of overall conversion, rapidity of response, and safety, but there is less experience with the drug. The drug is highly efficacious and safe for the acute termination of SVT. The differences between verapamil and diltiazem are clinically insignificant, although diltiazem may exert a less negative inotropic effect. This has not been substantiated in a direct comparative study.

OTHER FORMS OF SUPRAVENTRICULAR TACHYCARDIA

Calcium channel blockers appear to be of limited value in other forms of reentrant and automatic supraventricular tachycardia. There are limited data to indicate their efficacy in sinus nodal tachycardia (due to reentry within the sinoatrial [S-A] node or its adjacent tissue) or in SVT due to intraatrial reentry. Similarly, these agents do not have demonstrated efficacy in the termination of ectopic atrial tachycardia, although paroxysmal atrial tachycardia with block due to digoxin toxicity as well as to other causes may convert to sinus rhythm following oral doses of verapamil. The exact mechanism mediating such a beneficial response is not known.

The role of calcium antagonists for acute treatment or prophylaxis of multifocal atrial tachycardia (MAT) is unclear. Verapamil may be effective in controlling MAT, and such a disorder of rhythm may be a triggered arrhythmia.

Available data suggest that, in contrast to the extreme potency of the i.v. drug, the oral formulation (given 80–120 mg t.i.d. or q.i.d.) may not have comparable efficacy in preventing recurrences of SVT during chronic administration. It has been suggested that it might be possible to select responders to long-term verapamil therapy by programmed electrical stimulation. However, relatively little data are available to indicate how successful such an approach might be.

The role of calcium antagonists in the oral prophylaxis of orthodromic AV reentrant tachycardia (AVRT) occurring in a preexcitation syndrome remains to be defined, but inasmuch as they prolong AV nodal refractoriness, they are likely to be of value at least in some patients. In contrast, because they have no significant effect on the refractoriness of the bypass tract, they are less likely to terminate antidromic AVRT; nevertheless, the theoretical possibility exists that they may, in large doses, terminate the arrhythmia by inhibiting retrograde AV nodal conduction.

It must be emphasized that in patients with atrial flutter and atrial fibrillation (AF) complicating preexcitation, agents that shorten the effective refractory period of the bypass tracts (e.g., digitalis) and those that lengthen it over the AV node (digitalis and β-adrenoceptor blocking drugs) will augment the ventricular response and may possibly precipitate ventricular fibrillation. Calcium antagonists that increase AV nodal refractoriness (e.g., verapamil, diltiazem, and other class I agents) fall into the latter category. Published data, however, pertain only to verapamil.

Calcium antagonists do not predictably terminate atrial flutter or AF. However, they do have the propensity to convert atrial flutter to AF in a small number of patients. It is presumed that this is because of the shortening of the atrial effective refractory period.

Certain calcium antagonists impede conduction over the AV node. This property also been used to control the ventricular response in atrial flutter and AF; however, reliable data exist for verapamil, and new data have recently been added for diltiazem.

The clinical value of orally administered verapamil is in controlling ventricular response in chronic AF, regardless of etiology. It should be noted that verapamil tends to reduce both the resting as well as the exercise-induced increases in heart rate in the setting of AF, whereas the major effect of digoxin is on the resting rate. It is important to also note that when digoxin and verapamil are used together, their depressant effect on the AV node may combine. Because a significant interaction occurs between the two compounds, the net effect may be unexpectedly exaggerated, necessitating careful monitoring of serum drug concentration versus response. On the other hand, recent data have suggested that in many patients verapamil may replace digoxin for the control of the ventricular response in atrial flutter and AF.

Such a beneficial effect undoubtedly results from the direct action of the calcium antagonist on the AV node in addition to the sympatholytic action of the compound. The use of verapamil in this context will be imprudent if there is a significant impairment of ventricular function or a history of clinical heart failure occurring independently of the arrhythmia.

Diltiazem (240–360 mg/day) is also effective for controlling the ventricular response in atrial flutter and AF when combined with digoxin. A significant reduction in resting, as well as exercise heart rate, is attained by both doses of the drug, but there is a higher incidence of side effects at the higher dose. The lower dose of diltiazem, when combined with digoxin, is an effective and safe regimen in the control of the ventricular response in atrial flutter and AF. At present, there are little data on the effects of diltiazem used alone in this setting.

Neither verapamil nor diltiazem prolong the effective refractory period in the atria. Thus, they are unlikely to contribute to the maintenance of sinus rhythm in patients converted chemically or electrically to sinus rhythm. Data suggest that they are ineffective in this setting.

A single i.v. dose of verapamil has been found to be of diagnostic value in differentiating atrial flutter with 2-1 AV conduction from SVT, when these two arrhythmias are not readily distinguished electrocardiographically. If the rhythm is atrial flutter, the AV block increases immediately after i.v. verapamil, thus revealing the true nature of the arrhythmias. Diltiazem exerts similar effects.

CALCIUM ANTAGONISM AND VENTRICULAR ARRHYTHMIAS

The role of calcium antagonists in ventricular arrhythmias is less well defined. The effects of these drugs in cases for VT or VF resulting from transient coronary artery spasm are well substantiated, but such cases are uncommon. Calcium antagonists are poor suppressants of premature ventricular contractions (PVCs) in patients with structurally normal hearts or those with heart disease. As a class, they have a clinically insignificant antiarrhythmic effect in hypertrophic cardiomyopathy, dilated cardiomyopathy, or mitral valve prolapse. They have no impact on arrhythmia mortality in these conditions.

It is generally agreed that as a class, calcium channel blockers have a limited role in the treatment of patients with VT or VF in the setting of organic heart disease, except in the case of patients in whom coronary artery spasm is the immediate cause of the arrhythmia. They do not suppress nonsustained VT, nor do they prevent the inducibility of VT/VF after programmed electrical stimulation. Neither conduction nor refractoriness of the ventricle or His-Purkinje system is lengthened by slow-channel blockade.

In the setting of myocardial infarction (MI), verapamil is known to suppress PVCs. Successful control of polymorphous VT by verapamil was also recently reported. However, these are uncontrolled studies, which raise the possibility but do not provide conclusive proof that calcium antagonism by verapamil might be effective in controlling ventricular tachyarrhythmias.

Several recent reports have suggested that exercise-triggered VT having the morphologic pattern of left bundle branch block and right axis deviation might respond predictably and promptly to i.v. verapamil. Such an arrhythmia may occur in patients without identifiable cardiac disease. At present, it is not clear whether the VT in question is caused by an automatic focus or by triggered automaticity; nor is it known whether the observed response to i.v. verapamil in a small series of patients is a property unique to the drug or a common property of all type I calcium antagonists.

In young patients without demonstrable cardiac disease, sustained VT that sometimes occurs has the morphologic pattern of right bundle branch block with left axis deviation. This arrhythmia appears to be a distinct clinical entity. Interestingly, in most cases the VT in these patients responds to i.v. verapamil, whereas β-blockers or class I antiarrhythmic agents either fail or exert only a partial response. The precise mechanism for the arrhythmia is not known.

Calcium channel blockers might have a potential role in the prevention of torsade de pointes, but clinical data are not convincing for their effectiveness. It is possible that the well-documented beneficial effects of i.v. magnesium are due, at least in part, to calcium antagonism.

IMPACT OF CALCIUM CHANNEL BLOCKERS ON ARRHYTHMIA MORTALITY

There are compelling reasons for calcium channel blockers to exert a favorable effect on sudden death by ameliorating ischemia in the survivors of acute MI. However, this has remained a theoretical possibility that has not been validated. The effects on mortality have varied somewhat, depending on the agent being tested, although the difference between any of the test calcium channel blockers and placebo has not been significantly different. The overall data from a recent metaanalysis are summarized in Figure 9.2. No agent was found to unequivocally and decisively decrease mortality, a finding that is in sharp contrast to the widely appreciated effects of β-blockers. When the data for the five calcium channel blockers are pooled, an unfavorable trend in total mortality is seen.

The issue with verapamil is less clear, but the drug has not been found to increase mortality in any subset of patients. Data suggest benefit from verapamil; however, this is confined to patients without a history of congestive cardiac failure. In those with a history of heart failure, no benefit is found. Diltiazem exerts no significant effect on mortality; there is no benefit in patients without evidence of pulmonary congestion on chest x-ray, while there are excess deaths in the group with pulmonary congestion.

Routine prophylaxis of the postinfarct patients with calcium channel blockers does not appear justified.

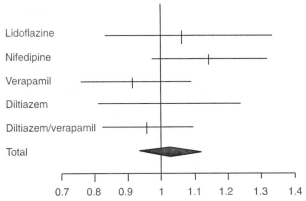

Figure 9.2. Typical odds rates ± 95% confidence intervals. Metaanalytic data from controlled clinical trials with calcium channel blockers in survivors of acute myocardial infarction. The typical odds of death by each drug are shown. The horizontal lines indicate 95% confidence intervals. Portions to the left of the vertical line indicate reduced risk with treatment; portions to the right indicate increased risk. The size of the horizontal lines correspond to the number of events in each category of trial. No agent seemed to reduce mortality, although the effect of heart rate-lowering agents (diltiazem or verapamil) indicates a trend that might be favorable in some subsets of patients. See text for details. (From Held PH, Yusuf S. Impact of calcium channel blockers on mortality. In: Singh BN, Dzau VJ, Vanhoutte PM, Woosley RL, eds. Cardiovascular pharmacology and therapeutics. New York: Churchill Livingstone, 1993:525–533.)

Adverse Reactions and Contraindications to the Use of Calcium Antagonists

The most common side effect during i.v. drug administration is the transient decrease in blood pressure. More serious side effects have, however, been reported: persistent hypotension, bradycardia, and rarely ventricular asystole. In most such cases, the patients had been on chronic β-blocking therapy before verapamil was given. Because the negative inotropic actions and depressant effects on impulse generation of β-antagonists and of calcium antagonists (especially verapamil and diltiazem) are additive, hypotension, bradycardia, and asystole are predictable side effects when these drugs are administered in combination. However, in general, side effects that occur in this setting may be reversed by i.v. atropine (only partially effective), isoprenaline, and particularly i.v. calcium (10–20 mL of 10% solution); temporary ventricular pacemaker therapy may also be used in recalcitrant cases. Dizziness, headache, fatigue, blurred vision, flushing, and minor degrees of block may occur when the diltiazem is given in a daily dosage between 240–360 mg and verapamil in a dosage of 320–480 mg. In the latter case, constipation is the dominant side effect. Prolongation of the P-R interval, i.e., a first-degree block, occurs in a proportion of patients given chronic oral therapy with verapamil, its congeners, or diltiazem. Advanced grades of heart block are unusual, unless antecedent conduction system disease is present. The development of clinically evident cardiac failure in patients with normal ventricular function is very uncommon. If the left ventricular ejection fraction is severely depressed and the patient has clinical congestive heart failure (CHF), or when the drug is given concomitantly with β-blocking drugs in patients with more than mild impairment of myocardial performance, manifest cardiac failure may ensue.

In general, the main contraindications to the use of calcium antagonists are the presence of advanced heart failure, unstable heart block, disease of the conduction system, including the sick sinus syndrome, and low blood pressure states such as cardiogenic shock. However, in situations in which heart failure is related to a persistent rapid atrial tachyarrhythmia, a prompt reversion to sinus rhythm by a calcium antagonist may lead to an improvement in the degree of cardiac decompensation. This is particularly likely to occur in patients with SVT. It must be stressed that in patients with wide QRS tachycardias (supraventricular vs. ventricular in origin), it is generally imprudent to use i.v. verapamil or diltiazem in attempts to revert the arrhythmia. In practice, wide QRS tachycardias are uncommonly of supraventricular origin, and those that are of ventricular origin rarely convert to sinus rhythm in a predictable manner. If conversion does not occur, an alarming decrease in blood pressure may ensue. Similarly, in cases of atrial flutter or AF complicating the Wolff-Parkinson-White (WPW) syndrome, i.v. verapamil and diltiazem are contraindicated. In this setting, AV block that results from the use of these compounds may increase the ventricular response over the bypass tract to dangerous rates, with the likelihood of the development of VF.

Of particular importance is the necessity to avoid the combined use of verapamil or diltiazem and β-adrenoceptor-blocking drugs in patients with overt or marginal hemodynamic dysfunction.

This consideration also holds for their use individually or in combination in patients with the sick sinus syndrome and impaired conduction. In these cases, β-blockers and calcium antagonists may, however, be used for the prophylactic treatment of tachyarrhythmias if a demand ventricular pacemaker is first inserted. Clearly, the same precaution also applies to combination therapy with digoxin. However, unless there is evidence of impaired conduction, prior digitalization is not a contraindication to the use of i.v. verapamil or diltiazem.

DIGOXIN

The two primary indications for the use of digoxin are to improve myocardial contractility in patients with CHF and to manage arrhythmias involving the AV node, that is, to slow the rapid ventricular response in atrial flutter or AF or to terminate AVNRT.

CLINICAL PHARMACOLOGY

ADMINISTRATION AND DOSING

The 36–48-hour half-life of digoxin is relatively long, and institution of an oral maintenance dose of 0.25–0.50 mg/day will result in a steady-state serum and tissue concentration after 4–5 half-lives in patients with normal renal function. If a therapeutic effect is needed in a short period of time, a loading dose of 0.5–1.5 mg is required. An i.v. loading dose will result in an appreciable electrophysiologic effect in 15–30 minutes with a peak effect in 1.5–4 hours. An oral loading of digoxin will produce a similar initial effect in 1–2 hours with a peak effect in 4–6 hours. The final maintenance dose of digoxin may be adjusted based on the therapeutic response and the patient's renal function, as well as guidance by serum drug levels.

METABOLISM AND EXCRETION

The rate of absorption of digoxin after oral ingestion is variable. The bioavailability of most oral preparations averages 67–75%, with the bioavailability of the encapsulated gel form of digoxin approaching 100%. The rate of absorption in individual patients may vary because of the presence of food in the gastrointestinal tract, delayed gastric emptying, or malabsorption syndromes. Finally, various drugs have been shown to affect the absorption of digoxin. Bacterial flora in the gastrointestinal tract and its alteration with antibiotics may result in biotransformation of digoxin and alteration in its absorption. Most of digoxin is excreted unchanged by the kidney. Renal excretion is proportional to glomerular filtration. Hence, serum digoxin levels rise in proportion to the degree of decline in creatinine clearance. A small amount of tubular secretion and reabsorption of digoxin occurs, which also may become significant in patients with decreased renal blood flow such as those with prerenal azotemia. On the other hand, acute vasodilator therapy has been shown to increase renal clearance of digoxin in CHF and may require an increase in dose to maintain therapeutic drug levels. Neither dialysis nor cardiopulmonary bypass significantly alters serum drug levels of digoxin because of the extensive protein binding properties of digoxin. However, dialysis may predispose a patient to electrolyte abnormalities that increase the risk of toxicity.

DRUG INTERACTIONS

Quinidine decreases the rate of elimination of digoxin and may result in as much as a 2-fold rise in serum digoxin drug levels (Table 9.3). Although the mechanism is unknown, it is most likely related to displacement of digoxin from tissue-binding sites by quinidine as well as reduction in the renal clearance of digoxin. Verapamil and amiodarone have also been shown to increase serum drug levels of digoxin. Diuretics affect the serum digoxin level by decreasing glomerular filtration and may also predispose to digoxin toxicity via electrolyte disturbances.

MONITORING SERUM DIGOXIN CONCENTRATIONS

The ratio of toxic to therapeutic effect of digoxin is small, and the need to find the maximum tolerated dose of digoxin is decreased with the availability of newer agents demonstrated to be effective for the treatment of heart failure and others very effective in controlling the ventricular rate during AF. Thus, digoxin may be beneficial in the treatment of these modalities—especially in combination therapy with other agents—without serum drug concentrations that approach levels increasing the risk of digoxin toxicity. Studies have shown that the mean serum

Table 9.3
Drug Interactions with Digoxin

Drug	Mechanism of Interaction	Alteration in Concentration
Cholestyramine Antacids Kaolin-pectate Neomycin Sulfasalazine PAS	Absorption of digoxin	↓
Erythromycin Tetracycline	↑ Intestinal metabolism by altering gut flora	↑
Quinidine	Displacement of tissue-binding sites, reduced renal clearance	↑
Amiodarone Verapamil Spironolactone	↓ Renal and nonrenal clearance	↑
Nicardipine	Unknown	↑
Indomethacin	↓ Renal clearance	↑

Adapted from Marcus Fl. Pharmacokinetic interactions between digoxin and other drugs. J Am Coll Cardiol 1985;5:82A–90A.

concentration of digoxin in patients without toxicity is 1.4 ng/ml and that the positive inotropic effect of the drug is maximal at concentrations of 1.5–2.0 ng/ml.

It should be recognized that the time course for uniform tissue distribution after oral digoxin administration is at least 5–6 hours. Serum digoxin concentration obtained less than 5–6 hours after ingestion will not reflect steady-state serum concentration.

ELECTROPHYSIOLOGIC EFFECTS

The predominant electrophysiologic effect of digoxin is mediated via the autonomic nervous system. Digoxin acts both centrally and peripherally to enhance vagal tone. Studies have shown that excitation of baroreceptors in the carotid sinus and aortic arch may occur and that digoxin may also sensitize the autonomic ganglion to acetylcholine and potentiate end-organ responsiveness to acetylcholine. The effects of digoxin on the sympathetic nervous system are not as well defined. Although at therapeutic levels digoxin may have an antiadrenergic effect, there are data to suggest that as drug levels approach toxicity there may be an actual enhancement of efferent sympathetic discharge in the central nervous system (CNS), resulting in the release of catecholamines. The increase in adrenergic activity with toxic concentrations of digoxin may play a role in potentiating some of the tachyarrhythmias seen in this setting. The effect of digoxin on the sinus node is mediated entirely by its cholinergic antiadrenergic effects, resulting in minimal slowing of rate. The most marked electrophysiologic effect of digoxin in the heart is on the AV node. AV nodal conduction is slowed, and the AV nodal refractory period is prolonged. Studies comparing the innervated and denervated heart have shown that prolongation of AV nodal refractoriness is mediated predominantly through the enhancement of vagal tone with less of an antiadrenergic or direct effect.

Studies examining the effects of digoxin on atrial tissue have yielded conflicting results. At therapeutic concentrations, digoxin has minimal electrophysiologic effects on the atria as a whole, but the atrial tissue that is innervated by the vagus is affected and exhibits a reduction in refractoriness and increased conductivity. Because vagal innervation is sparse and heterogeneous, these digoxin-related changes result in an increase in heterogeneity. His-Purkinje and ventricular tissue are not affected by digoxin, unless the serum concentration approaches toxicity. At high levels digoxin abbreviates phase II, shortens action potential duration, and accelerates repolarization, hence shortening the Q-T interval. There is evidence that in some ventricular tissue there is vagal innervation and digoxin may have antiarrhythmic actions.

ELECTROCARDIOGRAPHIC EFFECTS

In the therapeutic range of serum digoxin concentrations, very few electrocardiographic effects are observed. Sinus rate and atrial P wave duration are typically unchanged. A slowing of the sinus rate during digoxin administration is typically observed only in those patients with significant underlying sinus node dysfunction or those with CHF, in whom improved left ventricular function results in a reduction in sympathetic tone and a decrease in heart rate. P-R interval prolongation during normal sinus rhythm is also not significant unless underlying AV nodal disease is present. QRS duration is not influenced by digoxin. Digoxin produces characteristic changes in the ST segment. ST scooping and flattening of the T wave are characteristic of the electrocardiographic changes produced by digoxin (Fig. 9.3). These changes have been described as typical digoxin effects and do not represent a toxic manifestation of digoxin.

Use of Digoxin in the Management of Arrhythmias

ATRIAL FIBRILLATION

Patients with AF (acute, chronic, or paroxysmal) and depressed left ventricular systolic function should be treated with digoxin. Digoxin may also be helpful in controlling the ventricular rate in patients with chronic AF at rest, when vagal tone is high and further enhanced by digoxin; however, digoxin's effectiveness during exercise may be limited because this is a time of sympathetic stimulation and catecholamine excess that offsets the vagal effect of digoxin. Indeed, in most studies digoxin has no beneficial effect on blunting exercise heart rate. Conversely, it is clear that the addition of a calcium antagonist or β-blocker to digoxin results in ventricular rate control in patients not only at rest but during exercise, again provided that severe left ventricular dysfunction is not present. In acute AF, rapid digitalization is frequently performed for controlling the ventricular response as well

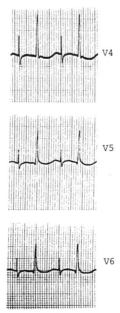

Figure 9.3. Example of ECG from patient on digoxin. The patient has an atrial pacemaker. Noted is a long "P-R" interval (i.e., from pacer stimulus to QRS complex) of 0.28 seconds. The ST segments are "scooped," typical of digoxin effect.

as for potentially facilitating the conversion to normal sinus rhythm. If the goal of therapy is to slow ventricular response, digoxin may be a reasonable therapeutic option. However, it likely has no role for the reversion of AF inasmuch as it has no direct effects on atrial myocardium. Data, however, are limited. There does not appear to be a difference in the rates of conversion to sinus rhythm between the placebo- and digoxin-treated groups. Thus, digoxin should not be used in acute AF when the intent is to convert the rhythm to normal sinus rhythm.

AFTER CORONARY ARTERY BYPASS GRAFTING

Patients undergoing coronary artery bypass graft surgery (CABG) are at high risk for postoperative supraventricular arrhythmias. The use of digoxin after surgery as a prophylactic agent has been proposed. Two recent metaanalyses examine this issue and concluded that the use of β-blockers either alone or in combination with digoxin were effective in decreasing the incidence of postoperative supraventricular arrhythmias. They also concluded that neither digoxin nor verapamil alone reduced the likelihood of supraventricular arrhythmias postoperatively. Based on these observations, one can conclude that the role of digoxin in the prevention of supraventricular arrhythmias after coronary artery bypass graft surgery is limited to combination therapy in conjunction with β-blockers, if at all.

SUPRAVENTRICULAR TACHYCARDIA

The role of digoxin in the management of acute episodes of AVNRT without preexcitation is limited because of its delayed onset of action. The use of digoxin is contraindicated in patients with asymmetrical septal hypertrophy with dynamic outflow obstruction because of these patients' sensitivity to variations in myocardial contractility. Digoxin is also contraindicated in patients with documented or suspected AV accessory pathways. In these patients, digoxin can potentially accelerate conduction via the accessory pathway. This occurs as a result of slowing or blockade of impulse conduction via the AV node, eliminating the modulating effect of the impulse on ventricular refractoriness and reducing the degree of retrograde concealed conduction via the accessory pathway, as well as shortening the accessory pathway refractoriness.

VENTRICULAR ARRHYTHMIA

It is well established that there is vagal innervation of the ventricle and that these fibers are in close proximity to the Purkinje fibers. It has been reported that vagal stimulation will reduce the automaticity of ventricular myocardium and will raise the ventricular fibrillation threshold of both normal and ischemic myocardium, preventing ventricular fibrillation. Unfortunately, however, the clinical efficacy of digoxin for patients with sustained ventricular tachyarrhythmias has not been documented. Thus, the antiarrhythmic effects of digoxin on ventricular arrhythmias should not be considered of clinical importance at this time.

DIGOXIN TOXICITY

FACTORS PREDISPOSING TO DIGOXIN TOXICITY

Whenever digoxin is being administered, special care should be given to ensure that the patient's potassium, magnesium, and calcium levels are all within normal ranges. Hypokalemia may inhibit digoxin excretion by the kidney through inhibition of tubular secretion of digoxin, thereby leading to potentially toxic levels of the drug. Additionally, hypokalemia increases the binding of digoxin at the tissue level and can potentiate the development of toxicity at normal serum digoxin concentrations. Low magnesium levels may also predispose a patient to digoxin toxicity.

The tachyarrhythmias associated with digoxin excess are thought to be caused by one of two mechanisms. The first is an increase in intracellular calcium concentration and in turn the development of delayed afterdepolarizations. Elevated serum calcium levels may, in theory, predispose to the tachyarrhythmias noted with digoxin excess. A second mechanism for digoxin toxic arrhythmia is activation of the sympathetic nervous system. This results in the enhancement of ectopic pacemakers and hence the development of tachyarrhythmias resulting from enhanced automaticity.

With the diminution of the glomerular filtration rate, there is a reduction in the elimination of digoxin. Every other day or even less frequent dosing may be sufficient to maintain a therapeutic concentration of the drug. Digoxin toxicity frequently results from failure in dose modification with renal insufficiency.

The geriatric patient appears to be at increased risk for the development of digoxin toxicity. Factors such as the age-related decline in the glomerular filtration rate; an increased number of concurrent medications; and more severe cardiac, pulmonary, and renal disease all require careful adjustments in the dosage and close monitoring of serum digoxin concentrations to avoid toxicity.

Patients with acute or chronic lung disease manifesting as hypoxia, hypercapnia, or cor pulmonale have been shown to have excessive sensitivity to digoxin therapy and are prone to arrhythmias caused by digoxin toxicity at low concentrations of the drug.

Hyperthyroidism decreases digoxin levels because of an increased metabolic rate and renal clearance. At the same time the clearance of digoxin is impaired in patients with hypothyroidism. Although patients who are hyperthyroid tolerate high digoxin levels, those who are hypothyroid and who have myxedematous myocardial changes are extremely sensitive to digoxin, and even low levels may result in toxicity.

NONCARDIAC MANIFESTATIONS OF DIGOXIN TOXICITY

Noncardiac manifestations of digoxin toxicity are listed in Table 9.4. Anorexia is frequently an early symptom of toxicity and may be followed by nausea and vomiting. These effects are not mediated by a direct irritant effect on the gastrointestinal tract, but by the interaction of digoxin with chemoreceptors located in the area postrema of the medulla.

Headache, malaise, weakness, neuralgic pain, disorientation, and seizures may all occur in digoxin toxicity. Alterations in color perception and other visual symptoms such as scotomata and halo vision have been reported.

MECHANISMS AND MANIFESTATIONS OF CARDIAC TOXICITY

Excess digoxin produces two major electrophysiologic effects. The first is a direct and/or vagally mediated slowing of conduction and block in the sinus node

Table 9.4
Noncardiac Manifestations of Digoxin Toxicity

Anorexia
Nausea and vomiting
Headache
Malaise
Neuralgic pain
Disorientation
Alterations in color perception
Scotomata
Halo vision

(sinus exit block) and AV node. This may result in slowing of the sinus rate, sinus pauses, and AV conduction disturbances. The second major electrophysiologic effect of digoxin excess is an enhanced abnormal automaticity and triggered activity in atrial muscle, the AV junction, the His-Purkinje system, and ventricular muscle. Although still controversial, most evidence suggests that triggered activity is the arrhythmia mechanism responsible for tachycardias associated with digoxin excess in humans, although enhanced automaticity is also important.

Certain tachyarrhythmias are more specific for digoxin intoxication (Table 9.5). Accelerated junctional rhythms, especially in the setting of AF, are often caused by digoxin toxicity. Abrupt regularization of the ventricular response of AF suggests the development of an accelerated junctional rhythm or tachycardia and should make one suspect the presence of digoxin excess (Fig. 9.4). The classic arrhythmia is a nonparoxysmal atrial tachycardia with block (Fig. 9.5). The P waves are upright in the inferior leads. The AV block, due to the enhanced vagal effect of the drug, may be transient and may be variable. It should be remembered that not all atrial tachycardias with block are caused by digoxin toxicity, as block may be seen whenever there is underlying AV nodal disease or when other AV nodal blocking agents are used. Finally, fascicular tachycardias (so-called "bidirectional" tachycardia) usually represents a digoxin toxic rhythm. The fascicular tachycardia will characteristically have a narrow right bundle branch block QRS pattern (≤ 0.12 seconds) and either right or left axis deviation or a beat-to-beat alternating axis in the frontal plane (Fig. 9.6). In some cases there may be alternation of a full right and left bundle branch block. This may also result from a junctional tachycardia with conduction alternating between right and left bundles (Fig. 9.7). Of note, the basis for the conduction system disturbance may not be digitalis excess.

In addition, the bradyarrhythmias associated with digoxin toxicity are not specific for this abnormality. Acute ischemia, chronic cardiac disease states, other pharmacologic agents, and hyperkalemia can produce similar electrophysiologic and electrocardiographic effects.

As a result of the inhibition of sodium-potassium transport, acute ingestion of large quantities of digoxin can result in severe hyperkalemia with associated electrocardiographic and possibly life-threatening hemodynamic sequelae. Although hyperkalemia is common in acute massive digoxin toxicity, it is uncommon in the setting of subacute intoxication, unless there is marked renal insufficiency.

Table 9.5
Tachyarrhythmias Specific for Digoxin Toxicity

Atrial tachycardia with variable atrioventricular block
Accelerated junctional rhythm (regularization of atrial fibrillation)
Fascicular tachycardia

From Marchlinski FE, Hoor BG, Callans DJ. Which cardiac disttubances should be treated with digoxin immune Fab (ovine) antibody? Am J Emerg Med 1991;9(suppl 1):24–28.

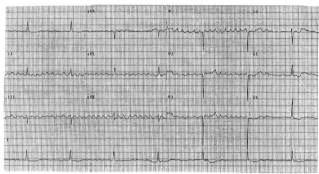

Figure 9.4. Regularization of R-R intervals caused by digoxin toxicity in a patient with AF. There are coarse fibrillatory waves, well seen in leads II, III, aVF, and V1–V3. The R-R intervals are completely regular, resulting from digoxin-related complete blockade of AV conduction and the development of an escape junctional rhythm.

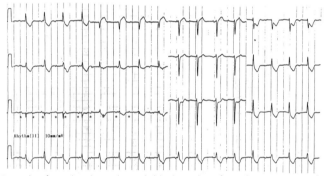

Figure 9.5. Example of atrial tachycardia with block resulting from digoxin toxicity (digoxin level 3.2). Noted is distinct atrial activity at a rate of 160. The P waves are small, diminutive, and upright in the inferior leads. They are from an ectopic atrial focus. Also observed is dissociation of the P waves from the QRS complexes. The ventricular rate is regular at 100 and the QRS complexes are narrow. The diagnosis is atrial tachycardia with complete heart block and an escape junctional rhythm. Also noted is ST segment depression and "scooping" changes caused by digoxin.

TREATMENT OF DIGOXIN TOXICITY

STANDARD TREATMENT

Rhythm abnormalities without hemodynamic compromise, such as ectopic beats or first-degree AV block, frequently respond simply to temporary cessation of digoxin therapy. Adjunctive or alternative therapy for treatment of brady-arrhythmias includes the use of atropine or temporary ventricular demand pacing. Adjunctive or alternative therapy for tachyarrhythmias includes phenytoin for the management of paroxysmal atrial tachycardia with variable block and lidocaine for

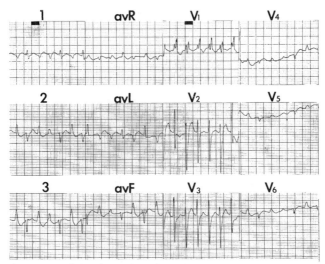

Figure 9.6. Characteristic "fascicular" tachycardia with relatively narrow (<120 msec) RBBB pattern in V1 and beat to beat shift in the QRS axis seen in lead 2. (From Marchlinski FE, Hoor BG, Callans DJ. Which cardiac disturbances should be treated with digoxin immune Fab (ovine) antibody? Am J Emerg Med 1991;9(suppl 1):24–28.)

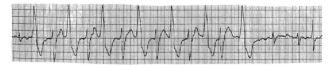

Figure 9.7. Example of bidirectional tachycardia as a result of digoxin toxicity in a patient with underlying AF. There is complete heart block and the development of an escape junctional rhythm. Seen are frequent episodes of an accelerated but regular rhythm that has wide QRS complexes. This is a junctional tachycardia with alternating conduction via the right and left bundle branches, a result of digoxin toxicity.

the management of fascicular or ventricular arrhythmias. Electrocardioversion in digoxin toxicity is to be avoided because of an increased risk of precipitating VT and VF. If direct current countershock is required emergently, lower energy levels should be used. This happens because of the increased myocardial excitability that may be augmented and exposed with any electrical stimulation of the heart.

It is important to note that life-threatening hyperkalemia may occur in the setting of acute severe digoxin toxicity or chronic digoxin toxicity with associated renal failure. In general, calcium administration should be avoided in this situation to avoid the potentiation of digoxin toxic tachyarrhythmias. Acute management includes the administration of sodium bicarbonate, glucose, and insulin, sodium polystyrene sulfonate (Kayexalate), and digoxin-specific antibody Fab fragments. Digoxin-immune Fab (ovine) antibody therapy has been shown to be extremely effective in reversing cardiac and noncardiac manifestations of severe digitalis intoxication.

DIGOXIN-SPECIFIC ANTIBODY

Before the administration of digoxin-specific Fab antibody fragments, several factors should be considered. Any arrhythmia that results in definite hemodynamic compromise or the threat of hemodynamic compromise should be treated aggressively with appropriate supportive measures and digoxin-specific antibody fragments. Ingestion of more than 3 mg of digoxin or serum digoxin concentrations greater than 5 ng/ml may be an indication to administer digoxin-specific Fab fragments even before serious arrhythmias become manifest, especially in the elderly patient with significant structural heart disease.

Another consideration in deciding to use the antibody fragment therapy is the adequacy of the patient's renal function and therefore the anticipated time course for reversal of the toxic manifestations of digoxin. Although many bradyarrhythmias can be treated with temporary pacing, prolonged periods of temporary pacing may be required because of anticipated delays in digoxin excretion due to renal dysfunction. One should consider instituting therapy with digoxin-immune Fab antibody fragments if a prolonged period of temporary pacing is anticipated. Keep in mind that the time to response of bradyarrhythmias and tachyarrhythmias to digoxin-immune antibody fragments is usually less than 1 hour.

Additional factors that may need to be considered include the reason digoxin was being administered and alternative forms of therapy to replace the therapeutic effects of digoxin. Fortunately, allergic reactions to the digoxin Fab antibody fragments rarely have been noted. However, patients with a history of severe allergies, especially to antibiotics, may be at increased risk for an allergic response to the antibody fragments.

ADENOSINE

INDICATIONS

At present, the only approved use of adenosine for arrhythmia management is as an i.v. agent for the acute termination of episodes of SVT in which the AV node is involved. Several other uses of adenosine in patients with arrhythmias have been proposed, including diagnostic use in patients with tachycardias of uncertain mechanisms and in the evaluation of patients with WPW syndrome and certain catecholamine-mediated sustained VTs.

PHYSIOLOGY

Adenosine is a key intermediate in cellular metabolism. Two major pathways exist for adenosine production in myocardial cells (Fig. 9.8). Adenosine monophosphate (AMP) may be dephosphorylated to adenosine by 5′-nucleotidases that are found both on the cell membrane and in the cytosol. Adenosine may also be produced by the reversible degradation of S-adenosylhomocysteine (SAH) by the enzyme SAH hydrolase. During periods of hypoxia or ischemia, intracellular adenosine formation using both of these pathways is enhanced.

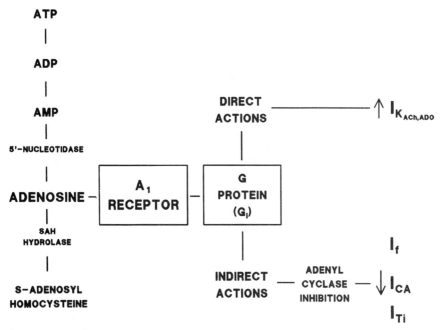

Figure 9.8. Production and electrophysiologic effects of adenosine.

Adenosine receptors are present on the extracellular surface of cardiac cells. The adenosine-induced increase in K⁺ conductance shortens action potential duration, causes hyperpolarization, and decreases contractility in atrial myocytes. These direct effects of adenosine on K⁺ channels may also be demonstrated in cells in both the sinus and AV nodes.

Indirect actions are mediated by antagonism of catecholamine-stimulated adenylate cyclase activity and a resultant decrease in intracellular cyclic AMP accumulation.

Adenosine's elimination half-life in humans has been difficult to measure accurately because it is so rapid, but is estimated to be in the range of 0.5–5 seconds. The physiologic and clinical consequences of this are several: (*a*) adenosine secreted endogenously by one organ has only local effects with little potential for action on a distant organ; (*b*) the effects of an intravenously administered bolus dose are seen only during its first pass through the circulation; and (*c*) direct steady-state electrophysiologic effects are difficult to achieve with adenosine administration.

ELECTROPHYSIOLOGIC ACTIONS

In cells in the region of the sinus node, adenosine produces both direct and indirect effects. The direct increase in K⁺ conductance results in hyperpolarization and a decreased rate of spontaneous sinus node discharge. Catecholamine-stimulated increases in sinus node rate are also blocked by adenosine. Conduction within the sinus node complex is also inhibited, and S-A exit block has been observed in vitro.

When bolus doses of adenosine are administered there is a transient slowing of sinus rate. Thereafter, autonomic reflexes are activated, and a brief period of sinus tachycardia is usually observed. In patients with severe autonomic nervous system dysfunction, only bradycardia is observed.

Adenosine causes an increased K^+ conductance and produces a dramatic shortening of the atrial action potential duration, hyperpolarization, inhibition of automaticity, and a decrease in contractility. Conduction in atrial tissue is not affected at concentrations that depress automaticity. Catecholamine-mediated changes in atrial electrophysiology will be blocked, and suppression of abnormal automaticity in atrial tissue has been documented in vitro and may be seen during clinical studies.

In the AV node, adenosine markedly decreases AV nodal conduction, decreases the duration and amplitude of the action potential, and depresses the maximum rate of rise of the action potential.

The effects of adenosine on tissues below the AV node are more variable. Adenosine suppresses escape rhythms in some but not all animals with induced AV block. Isoproterenol-induced acceleration of these rhythms are, however, blocked. Adenosine has little direct effect on the action potential of isolated ventricular myocytes but does block isoproterenol-induced changes.

CLINICAL USE OF ADENOSINE

Adenosine is cleared from the circulation after intravascular administration extremely rapidly, and most of the effects resulting from its receptor-mediated actions are produced during its first passage through the circulation.

Intravenous bolus injection of adenosine in patients during normal sinus rhythm results in a transient (usually <10 sec) sinus slowing, followed by a period of sinus tachycardia that lasts from 10–30 seconds (Fig. 9.9). During atrial pacing at a constant cycle length, adenosine produces transient first-, second-, or third-degree AV block within the AV node. Ventriculoatrial conduction may also be inhibited.

In patients with spontaneous or electrically induced AV block, adenosine has little direct effect on the cycle length of His-Purkinje or ventricular escape rhythms. Only small increases in cycle length are observed when adenosine is given after propranolol administration. Adenosine, however, does inhibit isoproterenol-induced increases in rate in these lower pacemakers. Atrial fibrillation is more easily induced by closely coupled atrial extrastimuli after adenosine administration.

Adenosine has mixed actions in patients with accessory pathways. When adenosine is injected during atrial pacing, the most common response is an increase in the electrocardiogram (ECG) manifestations of preexcitation (Fig. 9.10). In some patients, particularly those with left-sided accessory pathways and relatively rapid AV nodal conduction, adenosine may "unmask" preexcitation that could not previously be diagnosed with certainty.

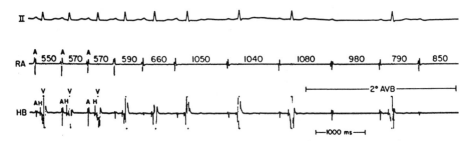

Figure 9.9. Effects of adenosine administered during normal sinus rhythm. The tracings are ECG lead II and bipolar right atrial (RA) and His Bundle (HB) electrogram. Adenosine (112.5 µg/kg) produces a transient increase in sinus cycle length and second-degree AV nodal block. (From DiMarco JP, Sellers TD, Berne RM, West GA, Belardinelli L. Adenosine: electrophysiologic effects and therapeutic use for terminating paroxysmal supraventricular tachycardia. Circulation 1983;68:1258.)

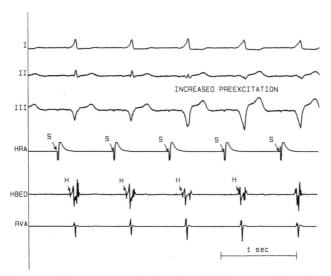

Figure 9.10. Increased preexcitation with adenosine. By blocking AV nodal conduction, adenosine increases the preexcitation pattern on the surface ECG.

EFFECTS ON SVT

Adenosine usually terminates SVT by blocking conduction in the AV node in AVNRT (Fig. 9.11). In AV nodal reentry, block usually occurs during slow pathway conduction, but fast pathway block may also be seen.

Because adenosine is removed from the circulation so rapidly, bolus doses administered at short intervals do not produce cumulative effects. In addition, the onset of any demonstrable effect may appear over a fairly wide range of dosages.

In the largest series reported to date, 92% of patients had their arrhythmias terminated using a two-dose sequence of 6 mg followed, if necessary, by 12 mg.

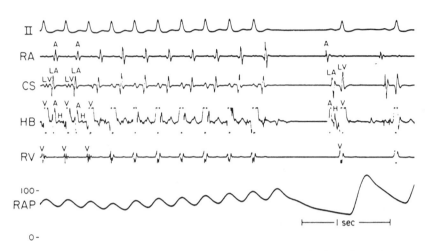

Figure 9.11. Termination of AVNRT by adenosine. The tracings are ECG lead II, right atrial (RA), coronary sinus (CS), His Bundle (HB) and right ventricular (RV) electrograms, and a radial artery pressure (RAP) and begin 18 seconds after an injection of 7.2 mg of adenosine. Note that the tachycardia terminates by block during anterograde conduction in the AV node. Sinus rhythm with normal blood pressure is then observed. (From DiMarco JP, Sellers TD, Lerman BB, Greenberg ML, Berne RM, Belardinelli L. Diagnostic and therapeutic use of adenosine in patients with supraventricular tachyarrhythmias. J Am Coll Cardiol 1985;6:420. Reprinted with permission from the American College of Cardiology.)

Consistent with the known pharmacokinetics of the drug, termination has usually been reported to occur within 30 seconds after drug injection, presumably during the first pass of the drug through the cardiac circulation.

Adenosine and verapamil have equivalent efficacy and the majority of patients can be safely and effectively treated with either agent. Minor side effects are more commonly seen after adenosine than with verapamil, but clinically significant reactions are uncommon with both agents. Adenosine appears to be safer than verapamil in neonates and infants, age groups in which verapamil may rarely produce hemodynamic collapse. No studies comparing adenosine to diltiazem are as yet available.

In patients with poor venous access, the bolus effect of adenosine will be difficult to achieve. Adenosine frequently causes transient dyspnea and is potentially a bronchoconstrictor. Thus, it should probably be avoided in patients with bronchospasm. If reinitiation of tachycardia occurs after an initial termination with adenosine, the less abrupt onset of action seen with the calcium channel blockers may be advantageous. Adenosine may be preferred in patients who are hypotensive at presentation. If the diagnosis of the mechanism of the arrhythmias is uncertain, the relative lack of hemodynamic effects from adenosine (if the arrhythmia does not terminate) make it a safer choice than verapamil or diltiazem.

EFFECTS IN OTHER ATRIAL ARRHYTHMIAS

Adenosine at usual doses does not terminate atrial flutter or AF. However, at the time of peak effect, atrial activity may be more easily recognized during the period of AV block. This may help in the diagnosis of some arrhythmias where atrial activity is difficult to identify on the standard ECG (Fig. 9.12). Tachycardias resulting from other types of intraatrial reentry will show similar responses after adenosine administration. Adenosine will produce a transient termination in the incessant long R-P' tachycardia in patients with the permanent form of junction reciprocating tachycardia, but the arrhythmia will resume within a few seconds. Automatic atrial and junctional tachycardias will occasionally respond to adenosine with a pause in ectopic firing, usually followed by resumption of the initial rhythms.

DIAGNOSIS OF WIDE COMPLEX TACHYCARDIAS

Several groups of investigators have proposed that adenosine injection be used as a diagnostic maneuver in patients who present with a wide complex tachycardia whose mechanism is unknown. There are some potential risks to this approach, however. Adenosine shortens the atrial action potential duration and may facilitate AF induction if atrial premature beats are introduced. This could produce dangerously rapid rates in patients with preexcitation. In preexcited patients already in AF, higher ventricular rates postinjection could be observed as the result of either

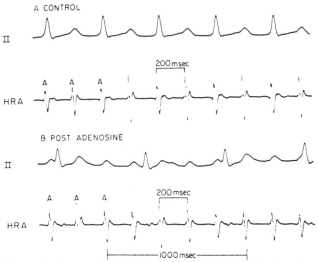

Figure 9.12. Effects of adenosine during atrial flutter. The tracings are labeled as in Figure 9.9. Atrial activity could not be definitely defined on this or any other surface ECG lead. The atrial recording shows atrial flutter. After adenosine, atrial activity at the same cycle length is now visible on the surface tracing. (From DiMarco JP, Sellers TD, Lerman BB, Greenberg ML, Berne RM, Belardinelli L. Diagnostic and therapeutic use of adenosine in patients with supraventricular tachyarrhythmias. J Am Coll Cardiol 1985;6:422. Reprinted with permission from the American College of Cardiology.)

decreased AV nodal conduction, leading to less concealed retrograde penetration or from the reflex increase in adrenergic tone seen after adenosine injection. In most types of VT, no electrocardiographic effects will be seen on the surface ECG.

VENTRICULAR TACHYCARDIA

One form of VT does appear to be adenosine-sensitive. Several groups have described patients without structural heart disease who had recurrent sustained VT that could be reliably terminated by adenosine injection. The clinical arrhythmias in these patients were usually exacerbated or precipitated by exercise or stress. Most patients did not have identifiable structural heart disease. At the time of electrophysiologic study, initiation either required or was facilitated by isoproterenol infusions. Programmed ventricular stimulation could reproducibly initiate and terminate the arrhythmias, and they could also be initiated with rapid atrial pacing. The site of origin was most commonly found in the right ventricular outflow tract, but left ventricular sites were also possible. Adenosine, verapamil, programmed stimulation, and in a less reliable fashion, vagal maneuvers could also reliably terminate individual episodes of tachycardia.

SIDE EFFECTS

Side effects of adenosine are frequently seen, occurring in almost 40–60% of patients with SVT treated with the drug. The most commonly reported adverse reactions are flushing, dyspnea, and chest pressure. These reactions are typically described as mildly or moderately uncomfortable and usually subside within less than a minute. Because adenosine produces effects on AV nodal conduction for only a few seconds, there is no long-lasting protection from recurrence or initiation of a repeat episode of tachycardia. Other arrhythmias such as isolated or repetitive ventricular premature beats, sinus bradycardia, and transient AV block have also been reported to occur at the time of tachycardia termination. These arrhythmias are usually of no clinical significance. More serious arrhythmia, however, can occur. A few patients have been reported to develop AF after adenosine injection.

Adenosine might precipitate AF with dangerously rapid rates in patients with WPW syndrome. Thus, facilities for cardioversion should always be available when adenosine is used for patients known or suspected to have this condition. Pauses and ventricular ectopy may occur after adenosine administration, particularly if unnecessarily large doses are used. In patients who are susceptible to bradycardia-dependent arrhythmias, torsade de pointes has been observed. It would be prudent to use adenosine with caution in any patient with a long Q-Tc interval at the time of presentation.

CONTRAINDICATIONS

There appear to be few contraindications to the use of adenosine. Therapeutic concentrations of methylxanthines, such as theophylline, will completely antagonize the effects of adenosine, so the drug is ineffective in patients on this and sim-

ilar drugs. Dipyridamole blocks adenosine transport back into cells and potentiates the effects of any given dose. If adenosine is to be used in a patient receiving
dipyridamole, much smaller doses should be used, with a starting dose of 0.5 mg
or less. Adenosine has the potential for producing long pauses that may lead to
bradycardia-dependent polymorphic VTs. Patients with known long Q-Tc syndromes should receive adenosine only with great caution.

SUGGESTED READING

Akhtar M, Tchou P, Jazayeri M. Use of calcium-
channel entry blockers in the treatment of cardiac arrhythmias. Circulation 1989;80(suppl
IV):31–39.

Antman EM, Smith TW. Pharmacokinetics of
digitalis glycosides. In: Smith TW, ed. Digitalis
glycosides. Orlando: Grune & Stratton, 1985:45.

Belardinelli L, Linden J, Berne RM. The cardiac
effects of adenosine. Prog Cardiovasc Dis
1989;32:73–97.

Betriu A, Chaitman BR, Bourassa MG, et al.
Beneficial effect of intravenous diltiazem in the
acute management of supraventricular tachyarrhythmias. Circulation 1983;67:88–94.

Cohen JJ, Tucker KJ, Abbott JA, et al.
Usefulness of adenosine in augmenting ventricular preexcitation for noninvasive localization of
accessory pathways. Am J Cardiol 1992;69:
1178–1185.

DiMarco JP. Electrophysiology of adenosine. J
Cardiovasc Electrophysiol 1990;1:340–348.

DiMarco JP, Miles W, Akhtar M, et al.
Adenosine for paroxysmal supraventricular
tachycardia: dose ranging and comparison with
verapamil in placebo-controlled, multicenter trials. Ann Intern Med 1990;113:104–110.

Falk RH, Knowlton AA, Bernard SA, Gotlieb
NE, Battinelli NJ. Digoxin for converting
recent-onset atrial fibrillation to sinus rhythm.
Ann Intern Med 1987;106:503–506.

Garratt C, Linker N, Griffith M, Ward D, Camm
AJ. Comparison of adenosine and verapamil for
termination of paroxysmal junctional tachycardia. Am J Cardiol 1989; 64:1310–1316.

Marcus FI. Pharmacokinetic interactions between
digoxin and other drugs. J Am Coll Cardiol
1985;5:82A–90A.

Smith TW. Digitalis: mechanisms of action and
clinical use. N Engl J Med 1988;318:358.

10 Aggravation of Arrhythmia by Antiarrhythmic Drugs

DEFINITION OF ARRHYTHMIA AGGRAVATION

A number of types of proarrhythmia have been recognized and are listed in Table 10.1. A major concern with the definition of proarrhythmia relates to a distinction between what is drug effect versus what is attributed to the expected random variability of arrhythmia frequency or occurrence. The development of a new arrhythmia as a result of an antiarrhythmic drug is clearly proarrhythmia (Fig. 10.1). However, a change in frequency, duration, length, rate, and stability of preexisting arrhythmia may be problematic because it may be unclear if it represents a true drug effect, is related to the natural history of the arrhythmia, or is the result of random variability.

Proarrhythmia is probable if a significant change in the arrhythmia occurs in temporal relation to the initiation of drug therapy or change in dose. It has been reported that arrhythmia aggravation usually occurs within several days of beginning a drug or increasing the dose, depending on the drug used and its pharmacokinetics.

INCIDENCE OF PROARRHYTHMIA IN PATIENTS WITH VENTRICULAR ARRHYTHMIA

Several studies have reported that arrhythmia aggravation can occur with the use of any antiarrhythmic agent in patients being treated for the suppression of ventricular arrhythmia (Table 10.2).

Table 10.1
Definition of Arrhythmia Aggravation

1. Worsening or a change of a preexisting arrhythmia
   a. Statistically significant increase in the frequency of ventricular premature beats, couplets, runs of nonsustained ventricular tachycardia, episodes of sustained ventricular tachyarrhythmia
   b. Conversion from nonsustained to sustained ventricular tachyarrhythmia
   c. Arrhythmia that is more difficult to terminate
   d. Arrhythmia that becomes incessant and cannot be terminated
   e. Ventricular tachycardia at a more rapid rate and that is associated with hemodynamic instability
   f. Arrhythmia that is more easily inducible during electrophysiologic study (i.e., requires fewer extrastimuli to be induced)
2. Development of a new arrhythmia
   a. Sustained monomorphic ventricular tachycardia
   b. Polymorphic ventricular tachycardia
   c. Torsade de pointes
   d. Ventricular fibrillation
   e. Supraventricular tachyarrhythmia
3. Bradyarrhythmia
   a. Depression of sinus node function
   b. Abnormalities of atrioventricular nodal function

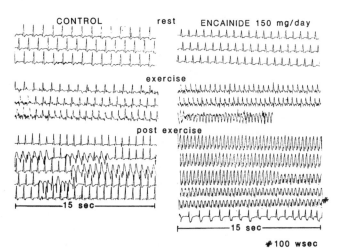

Figure 10.1 Example of arrhythmia aggravation. The patient presented with symptoms of presyncope due to documented runs of NSVT. During baseline exercise test runs of NSVT occurred in the postexercise period. After 5 days of encainide therapy, exercise testing provoked sustained ventricular tachycardia that required cardioversion.

Table 10.2
Incidence of Arrhythmia Aggravation

	Noninvasive (%)	Invasive (%)
Amiodarone	4	6–30
Beperdil		8
Bethanidine		22
Cibenzoline	9	21
Disopyramide	6	5
Encainide	15	37
Ethmozine	11	14–28
Flecainide	4–12	15–33
Indecainide	19	32
Lidocaine		16
Lorcainide	8	9–24
Mexiletine	1–7	
Procainamide	9	7–21
Propafenone	5–8	15
Quinidine	1–15	5–20
Tocainide	8	5
Verapamil		18

aSummary of studies in literature

The incidence of proarrhythmia is low in patients without a history of serious arrhythmia, and is greater in patients presenting with a sustained ventricular tachyarrhythmia (VT).

When electrophysiologic methods are used to evaluate drug effect, the reported incidence of proarrhythmia is higher (Table 10.2). Although most studies of proarrhythmia report the development of a new or worsened tachyarrhythmia, a bradyarrhythmia may also occur and may be potentially serious. Unfortunately, the incidence of this is not known. Because many of the antiarrhythmic drugs may have a depressive effect on the automaticity of the sinus node, sinus pauses or sinus arrest may occur (Fig. 10.2).

Also commonly seen with antiarrhythmic drug therapy is depression of atrioventricular (AV) nodal conduction, resulting in the development of high-grade (second- or third-degree) AV block (Fig. 10.3). As with sinus node dysfunction, the incidence is unknown. This is generally the result of a direct slowing of impulse conduction through this structure and a prolongation of its refractoriness. Less often seen is heart block due to conduction slowing in the bundle of His or within the distal bundle branches, although the development of a bundle branch block with antiarrhythmic drugs is not uncommon. Not infrequently such AV or His-Purkinje conduction block is observed only at higher heart rates. This is because the class I antiarrhythmic agents, especially the Ic drugs, have a property of "use dependency"; that is, their depressive effect on impulse conduction becomes progressively more profound as the heart rate increases. Although not certain, it is likely that such conduction abnormalities are more common in patients with advanced heart disease who have underlying disease of the pacemaker tissue and conduction system.

ARRHYTHMIA AGGRAVATION IN PATIENTS TREATED FOR ATRIAL ARRHYTHMIA

Proarrhythmia caused by antiarrhythmic drugs in patients receiving therapy for an atrial arrhythmia may involve a new or worsened atrial arrhythmia or the provocation of a ventricular arrhythmia. Proposed criteria are

1. Atrial tachycardia with or without AV block (e.g., digitalis toxicity);
2. Conversion of paroxysmal atrial fibrillation (AF) to atrial flutter;
3. Increased frequency of paroxysmal AF;
4. Conversion from paroxysmal to sustained AF;

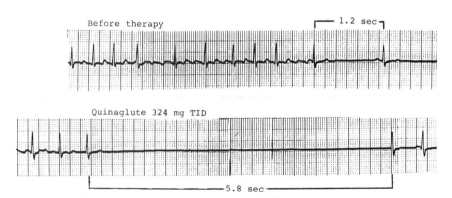

Figure 10.2. Example of drug-induced sinus node dysfunction. The patient presented with episodes of paroxysmal AF, which terminated spontaneously with resumption of sinus rhythm after a 1–2-second pause. After therapy with quinidine gluconate, episodes of AF continued, but after termination there was a 5.8-second pause ended by a junctional beat, indicating sinus node depression.

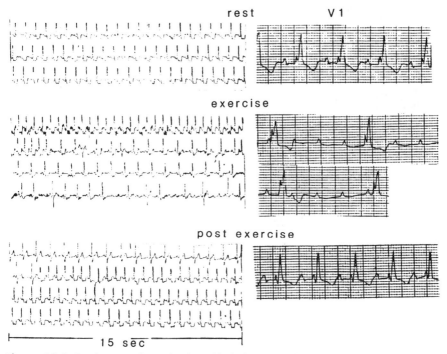

Figure 10.3. Development of complete heart block during antiarrhythmic drug therapy. At baseline the patient had a borderline first-degree AV block and a right bundle branch block that was unaltered by exercise. An exercise test was repeated during therapy with a class Ic agent given as treatment for AF. As the sinus rate increased, there was an abrupt reduction in the ventricular rate. The ECG documented complete heart block. After exercise, sinus rate slowed and normal AV conduction was restored.

5. New, incessant supraventricular tachycardia;
6. Acceleration of ventricular rate during a supraventricular tachyarrhythmia due to (a) enhanced AV nodal conduction, (b) slowing of atrial rate, reducing concealed AV nodal conduction (Fig. 10.4), (c) conversion of AF to atrial flutter, (d) preferential conduction down an accessory pathway (Fig. 10.5);
7. Conduction abnormalities, including (a) AV nodal block, (b) sinus node dysfunction; and
8. New VTs, including (a) torsade de pointes (Fig. 10.6), (b) monomorphic or polymorphic VT, (c) ventricular fibrillation (VF).

Unfortunately, the incidence of any form of proarrhythmia in patients treated for atrial arrhythmias is uncertain. Still, the incidence is generally accepted to be low and it most often occurs in patients with underlying structural heart disease.

Perhaps the most frequently reported form of ventricular arrhythmia aggravation in patients with atrial arrhythmia is torsade de pointes (Fig. 10.6), which occurs with class Ia agents (quinidine, disopyramide, or procainamide) or class III drugs (particularly sotalol). Torsade de pointes is defined as a polymorphic VT, with a changing QRS axis ("twisting of points") associated with Q-T interval prolongation and initiated by a long, followed by a short, R-R interval. Torsade de pointes usually occurs in conjunction with bradycardia. Although quinidine-induced Q-T prolongation and torsade are often dose related, these may be seen when drug dose and blood level are low; hence, they represent an idiosyncratic reaction. Torsade de pointes has been observed with disopyramide and procainamide,but the incidence is unknown. Sotalol, a β-blocker with class III activity, has also been reported to cause dose-related Q-T prolongation and torsade de pointes.

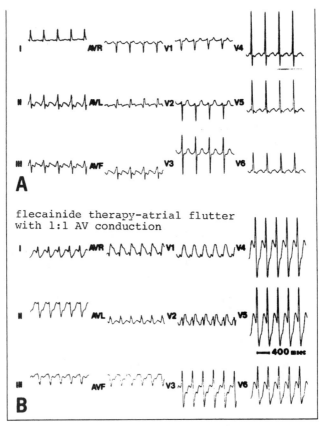

Figure 10.4. Atrial flutter with 2:1 AV conduction (A) converted to flutter with 1:1 AV conduction (B). As a result of therapy with flecainide, the atrial flutter rate slows, permitting 1:1 AV conduction. Note that during drug therapy the QRS complexes are widened or aberrated, the result of use-dependent effects of this agent. (From Crijns HJ, Van Gelder K, Lie KI. Supraventricular tachycardia mimicking ventricular tachycardia during flecainide treatment. Am J Cardiol 1988;62:1303–1306.)

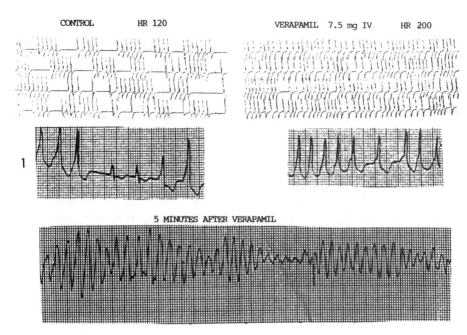

Figure 10.5. Arrhythmia aggravation in a patient with Wolff-Parkinson-White syndrome. The patient presented with AF. (Note the preexcited or aberrated QRS complexes alternating with normal complexes). After therapy with intravenous verapamil, the ventricular rate increases markedly and all of the QRS complexes are widened or preexcited. Several minutes later the patient developed VF. (From Falk RH. Proarrhythmic responses to atrial antiarrhythmic therapy. In: Falk RH, Podrid PJ, eds. Atrial fibrillation: mechanisms and management. New York: Raven Press, 1992:283–305.)

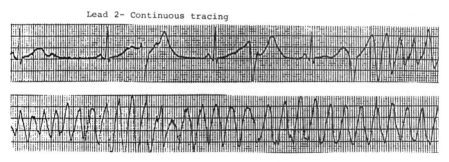

Figure 10.6. Example of torsade de pointes. The patient presented with AF and received therapy with quinidine. Several hours after reversion there were multiple episodes of self-terminating polymorphic ventricular tachycardia associated with significant Q-T prolongation, i.e., torsade de pointes. Note that the arrhythmia is initiated by a sequence of long-short R-R intervals: the long interval is a result of a postextrasystolic pause, then a sinus beat, which is followed by a short R-R interval, a result of another premature ventricular beat.

Although it is clear that in patients with supraventricular tachyarrhythmias the antiar-rhythmic drugs may provoke a new VT, this must be distinguished from rate-related aberration of ventricular conduction during supraventricular tachycardia, which presents as a wide complex tachycardia and can be confused with VT (Fig. 10.4). The widened QRS complex results from the use-dependent effects of the antiarrhythmic agents, par-ticularly the class Ic agents, which cause more pronounced slowing of impulse conduc-tion and hence prolongation of ventricular depolarization at higher heart rates.

There may be an acceleration in ventricular rate as a result of antiarrhythmic agents, such as in a preexcitation syndrome, particularly Wolff-Parkinson-White syndrome (Fig. 10.5). Drugs that block the AV node, specifically digoxin, β-blockers, or calcium channel blockers, may produce an enhancement of conduction along the accessory pathway and an acceleration in ventricular rate.In such patients the precipitation of VF has been reported (Fig. 10.5). More problematic is the diagnosis of an atrial proar-rhythmic event, largely because of the great random variability and unpredictability of such arrhythmias. The incidence of such proarrhythmia is unknown. One definite example of a drug-induced atrial arrhythmia is a nonparoxysmal ectopic atrial tachycar-dia with or without AV block that results from digoxin toxicity.

RISK FACTORS FOR ARRHYTHMIA AGGRAVATION

Torsade de pointes is associated with marked prolongation of the Q-T interval and T-wave abnormalities (i.e., reduction in its amplitude and development of notching, the result of a U wave) as a result of some drugs, there are no other changes on the surface electrocardiogram (ECG) that predict other types of arrhythmia aggravation. It has been reported that factors associated with this com-plication are significantly reduced left ventricular systolic function, a history of clinical congestive heart failure, sustained VT as the presenting arrhythmia, and underlying ischemia, as strongly suggested by the results of the Cardiac Arrhythmia Suppression Trial. It is important to note that aggravation of arrhyth-mia with one drug does not predict this complication with any other drug, even if it is of the same subclass, although this issue remains controversial.

TREATMENT OF ARRHYTHMIA AGGRAVATION

The first step in the therapy of drug-induced aggravation of arrhythmia is recog-nition and discontinuation of the implicated agent. Despite this measure, there may be multiple recurrences of arrhythmia that require suppressive therapy. In some cases lidocaine or procainamide may be an effective agent, although it must be remembered that the addition of another antiarrhythmic agent may result in further toxicity. As with the acute therapy of any sustained tachyarrhythmia, cardioversion or defibrillation is generally effective and may be necessary if the tachyarrhythmia produces significant hemodynamic impairment. If there is symptomatic bradycardia as a result of a marked slowing of impulse conduction, a temporary pacemaker is indicated. The use of β-blockade as a therapy for reversing arrhythmia aggravation with the class Ic drugs, particularly flecainide, has been reported.

Drug-induced Q-T prolongation and resulting torsade de pointes are particularly important. Most often the cause is quinidine, but other class Ia drugs may be implicated. In many cases, serum potassium is low and should be repleted. When quinidine is the causative agent, it is helpful to lower the blood level of free quinidine acutely, which can be achieved by alkalization of the serum with sodium bicarbonate or lactate. This enhances the protein binding of free quinidine. Because torsade is a result of excessive bradycardia and prolongation of repolarization, reversing these may be accomplished with an infusion of a catecholamine such as isoproterenol or by overdrive pacing. The administration of intravenous magnesium is highly effective therapy for drug-induced torsade de pointes. This drug should be administered to all patients, although it may be particularly beneficial when other methods of therapy fail to prevent recurrence of the arrhythmia.

Aggravation of arrhythmia as a result of digoxin toxicity represents an important and not infrequent problem. Although discontinuance of the drug is imperative, digoxin has a long half-life, and proarrhythmia may persist for an extended period of time. Phenytoin has been reported to be effective, particularly when abnormalities of conduction are present. In some situations, especially when there is an increase in atrial or ventricular ectopy, β-blocker may be effective. This is because one of the responsible mechanisms is enhanced automaticity resulting from an increase in central sympathetic neural traffic. Lidocaine may also be helpful in suppressing ventricular ectopy. Recently available are digoxin-specific antibodies that rapidly bind to digoxin and lower the blood level acutely, reversing their toxic effect. When digoxin toxicity manifests as a symptomatic bradyarrhythmia caused by conduction abnormalities, prophylactic pacing or an infusion of isoproterenol an effective therapy.

SUGGESTED READING

Coplen SE, Antman FM, Berlin JA, Hewitt P, Chalmers RC. Efficacy and safety of quinidine therapy for maintenance of sinus rhythm after cardioversion. A meta analysis of randomized control trials. Circulation 1990;82:1106–1116.

Minardo JD, Heger JJ, Miles WM, Zipes DP, Prystowsky EN. Clinical characteristics of patients with ventricular fibrillation during antiarrhythmic drug therapy. N Engl J Med 1988;319:257–262.

Poser R, Lombardi F, Podrid PJ, Lown B. Aggravation of arrhythmia induced with antiarrhythmic drugs during electrophysiologic testing. Am Heart J 1985;110:9–16.

Roden DM, Woosley RL, Primm K. Incidence of clinical features of the quinidine associated long QT syndrome. Implications for patient care. Am Heart J 1986;111: 1088–1093.

Slater WS, Lampert S, Podrid PJ, Lown B. Clinical predictors of arrhythmia worsening by antiarrhythmic drugs. Am J Cardiol Coll 1988;61:349–353.

Velebit V, Podrid PJ, Cohen B, Graboys TB, Lown B. Aggravation and provocation of ventricular arrhythmia by antiarrhythmic drugs. Circulation 1982;65:886–894.

11 Pacemakers

PACEMAKER CODES AND MODES

Implantable pacemakers vary widely in their modes of operation. Pacemaker systems may be single channel, limited to either the atrium or ventricle, or they may be dual chamber. They may sense and pace one chamber, sense one chamber and pace the other, sense one and pace both, or sense and pace both. Pacemaker codes were designed to indicate pacemaker function so that, despite the model pacemaker or pacemaker name, the mode of operation will be known (Fig. 11.1).

The latest code, a result of a joint approach of NASPE and British Pacing and Electrophysiology Group (NBG), requires four positions for completeness, and in the case of antitachycardia devices, five positions.

NBG CODE

Table 11.1 lists generic pacemaker codes and explains their positions. The letter O indicates the absence of any antitachycardia function. The second letter P is for output at the microjoule or traditional pacing level, and the third letter S is for output of one or more joules and is an abbreviation of "shock." The fourth letter D is a combination of pacing and shock, i.e., P + S, in anticipation of devices soon to be available.

The NBG code has been designed to emphasize simplicity and thus maximize its utility, while avoiding specific description of techniques that may soon be obsolete. To provide a code for a pacemaker that has been programmed to the OFF mode, i.e., entirely inactive, the letter O has been allowed in each of the five positions.

Position I designates the chamber(s) paced. A stands for atrium, V for ventricle, D if both atrium and ventricle are paced, and O if the unit is shut down and no pacing is to occur.

Position II designates the chamber(s) sensed. If the atrium alone is sensed, the letter A is used, if the ventricle, V. If both atrium and ventricle are sensed, the letter D is used. O indicates that the pacemaker is insensitive to incoming signals.

Position III designates the response to a sensed signal. I indicates that pacemaker output is inhibited by a sensed event; T, that a stimulus is triggered by a sensed event; and D, that a stimulus may be triggered by a sensed event in one chamber and inhibited by a sensed event in the other.

The letter O in this position indicates that there is no mode of response to the lack of sensitivity indicated by the O in position II.

Position IV describes two different device characteristics: the degree of programmability and the presence or absence of a rate modulation mechanism. The letters are hierarchal, from the absence of function in this channel to the most complex. The assumption is that the next higher level will incorporate all of the features of all lower levels. The letter O in this position indicates that the device is not programmable and does not provide rate modulation. The letter P indicates

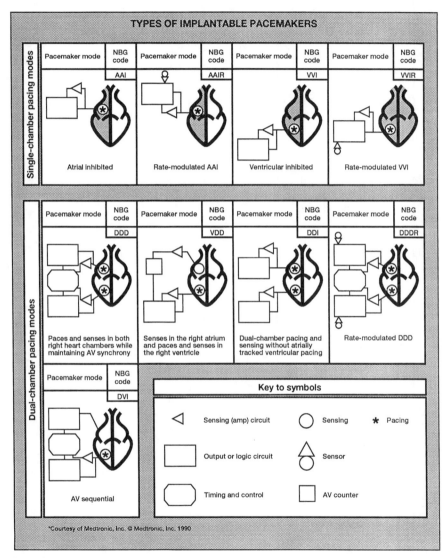

Figure 11.1. A graphic depiction of varying pacing modalities.

Table 11.1
NASPE/BPEG Generic (NBG) Pacemaker Code[a]

Position	I	II	III	IV	V
Category	Chamber(s) paced	Chamber(s) sensed	Response to sensing	Programmability, rate modulation	Antitachyarrhyhmia function(s)
	O, none	O, none	O, none	O, none	O, none
	A, atrium	A, atrium	T, triggered	P, simple programmable	P, Pacing (antitachyarrhythmia)
	V, ventricle	V, ventricle	I, inhibited	M, multiprogrammable	S, shock
	D, dual (A + V)[b]	D, dual (A + V)[b]	D, dual (T + I)[c]	C, communicating (telemetry)	D, dual (P + S)[c]
	S, single chamber[e]	S, single chamber[e]		R, Rate modulation	

[a]NASPE/BPEG, North American Society for Pacing and Electrophysiology/British Pacing and Electrophysiology Group.
[b]Atrial and ventricular
[c]Dual (atrial/ventricular) and inhibited
[d]Pacing and shock
[e]Manufacturer's designation only

simple programmability, almost always in practice signifying change in rate or output or both. *M* indicates multiprogrammability, i.e., more than two functions.

The addition of telemetry allows the use of the letter *C*, which is the abbreviation for "communicating." The degree of programmability refers to antitachycardia features as well as (and even in the absence of) antibradycardia pacing. Nearly all pacemakers being manufactured at this time are multiprogrammable and most have some telemetry capabilities as well.

The last letter in this position is *R* (rate modulation), which indicates sensor-driven variation of the antibradycardia escape interval in response to a physiological or nonphysiological stimulus other than the atrium. Commercially available rate-modulated pacemakers utilize sensors that detect activity or acceleration, changes in temperature, or variations in intrathoracic impedances to estimate minute ventilation. Other sensors undergoing investigation include those measuring dp/dt, stroke volume, preejection interval, oxygen saturation, and evoked potentials.

Position V indicates the presence of one or two antitachycardia functions activated manually or automatically in an implanted device when a tachycardia is anticipated or has occurred. *O* once again indicates the absence of any such capability; *P* indicates a pacing modality utilized to terminate tachyarrhythmias at a level of electrical output of a cardiac pacemaker, i.e., in the microjoule range. *S* indicates a shock to terminate the tachyarrhythmia, i.e., at the level of joules or several orders of magnitude above pacer output. The letter *S*, used previously to indicate "single chamber," has been redefined for position V but this should offer little confusion. If the device is capable of pacing level and shock level output either simultaneously and/or successively, the letter *D* indicates both pacing and sensing (i.e., P + S).

PACING MODE SELECTION

The most widely utilized single chamber-pacing modes include atrial inhibited pacing (AAI), rate-modulated AAI pacing (AAIR), ventricular inhibited pacing (VVI), and VVIR (rate-modulated VVI pacing). Dual-chamber pacemakers provide for the potential of sensing and pacing both chambers while maintaining atrioventricular (AV) synchrony, i.e., DDD pacing. Other dual chamber modes include those that do not involve atrial pacing (VDD), those that provide for dual-chamber pacing without atrially tracked ventricular pacing (DDI), and rate-modulated DDD pacing (DDDR). A brief discussion of the clinical uses of each of these pacing modes is provided in the following paragraphs.

AAI pacing is most appropriate for patients with symptomatic sinus brady-arrhythmias and intact AV conduction (Fig. 11.2). Patients with chronotropic insufficiency, i.e., inadequate heart rate response to activity or stress, may be best managed with AAIR pacing. In the United States, many appropriate candidates for AAI pacing receive DDD pacemakers because of concerns about atrial lead stability or long-term AV conduction integrity.

VVI pacing is ideal for patients with persistent AV block and atrial dysrhythmias or in those where the maintenance of AV synchrony is felt to be less important

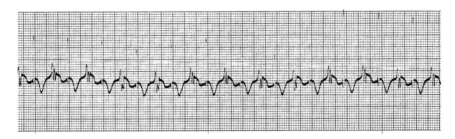

Figure 11.2. AAI. Atrial paced rhythm at 100 beats/minute. AV conduction is intact and each paced atrial event is followed by a native QRS.

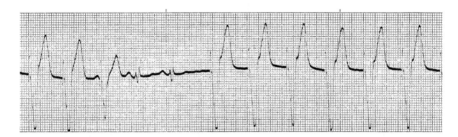

Figure 11.3. VVI. Ventricular paced rhythm at 90 beats/minute. Spontaneous ventricular events inhibit the ventricular output.

(Fig. 11.3). Patients with persistent atrial flutter/fibrillation, infirm or inactive patients, and those in whom follow-up will be difficult are good candidates for this basic mode of pacing. VVIR pacing is recommended for subsets of patients who are active and would benefit from rate response during routine daily activities. The presence of intact retrograde ventriculoatrial conduction, which may be determined at the time of pacemaker implant, is a relative contraindication to VVI pacing because of the risk of "pacemaker syndrome." This syndrome refers to the constellation of signs and symptoms related to the adverse hemodynamic and electrophysiologic consequences of single-rate ventricular pacing. The symptoms may range from vague dizziness and palpitations to overt hypotension and low output state.

DDD is the mode of choice in patients with AV block, with intact atrial function, especially if retrograde conduction is present (Fig. 11.4). Patients with sinus node dysfunction and questionable AV conduction should also be considered for DDD pacing. The DDDR mode is indicated in physically active patients with chronotropic incompetence. Retrospective data strongly support the notion that AV synchrony be preserved during pacing whenever possible, so as to reduce the risk of atrial fibrillation (AF), stroke, and congestive heart failure (CHF). Thus, VVI should be reserved for the finite circumstances outlined earlier.

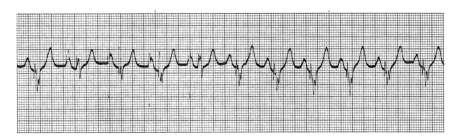

Figure 11.4. DDD. Dual-chamber paced rhythm, atrial and ventricularly inhibited and atrially triggered. Lower rate limit programmed to 85. The patient's spontaneous atrial rate is close to the lower rate limit. Thus, atrially tracked ventricular pacing is alternating with dual-chamber paced rhythm.

AUTOMATIC MODE CHANGE

Rate-modulated pacemakers, as discussed earlier, employ sensors to help determine the desired pacing rate. These sensor-derived rates can be utilized in algorithms for differentiating between rapid physiologic and pathologic atrial rhythms. Such sensor-driven algorithms have been implemented in some DDDR devices to automatically switch from DDDR to VVIR during pathologic tachycardias so a satisfactory pacing rate can be provided without inappropriate tracking of atrial activity.

ANTITACHYCARDIA THERAPY MODES

The various methods may be divided into three general categories:

1. Suppression of arrhythmias through "overdrive pacing" or prevention of pause-dependent tachyarrhythmias. Standard antibradyarrhythmic devices and pacing modes are often sufficient to achieve this limited goal;
2. Termination of tachyarrhythmias via one of several pacing methods. The delivery of single extrasimuli, short bursts, or complex autodecremental techniques are all potential options in many of the available devices; and
3. Termination of tachyarrhythmias through provision of a shock. At this time, such therapy is used only for managing malignant ventricular arrhythmias. A standard nonprogrammable implantable cardioverter-defibrillator is coded *OOOOS*. A device with telemetry, antibradycardia and antitachycardia pacing, and shock capabilities is referred to as *VVICD*.

PACING FOR BRADYARRHYTHMIAS: IMPLANTATION, INDICATIONS, AND SELECTION OF PACING MODE

PACING HARDWARE AND ELECTRONICS

A pacing system consists of the pulse generator, which contains the power supply (lithium-iodine cells) and electronic circuitry, encased in a titanium or stainless steel housing. One- or two-lead electrodes allow passage of current from the pulse generator to the endocardium (Fig. 11.5).

The electrical configuration of a lead may be unipolar or bipolar. In both systems, the cathode is the electrode tip. In a unipolar configuration, the anode is the metal housing of the pulse generator. In bipolar systems, the anode is a ring electrode located a few centimeters proximal to the cathode. The major difference between unipolar and bipolar configurations lies with sensing. The longer separation between the anode and cathode in unipolar systems creates a large antenna. Sensing of intracardiac signals is superior with unipolar systems (generally unimportant clinically) but at the cost of greatly enhanced susceptibility to external interference. Oversensing of muscle myopotentials and environmental signals (e.g., electromagnetic interference) is much more likely with unipolar systems (Fig. 11.6). Oversensing may result in inappropriate inhibition or triggering.

INDICATIONS FOR PERMANENT PACEMAKER IMPLANTATION

Indications for permanent pacemaker implantation may be grouped into six general categories: (*a*) acquired AV block; (*b*) conduction disorders postmyocardial infarction; (*c*) chronic fascicular block; (*d*) sick sinus syndrome; (*e*) hypersensitive carotid sinus syndrome; and (*f*) other circumstances where pacing may be beneficial from a hemodynamic, symptomatologic, or possible survival standpoint (Table 11.2).

PACING IN ACQUIRED AV BLOCK

Current recommendations regarding the need for pacing in AV block consider not only symptomatology but also the site of block.

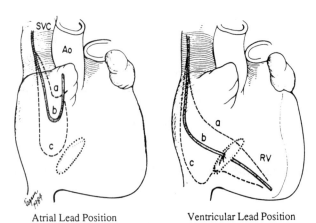

Atrial Lead Position   Ventricular Lead Position

Figure 11.5. Schematic of appropriate lead positioning during dual-chamber pacemaker implantation. For both the atrial and ventricular leads, b represents correct lead positioning. Position a is too taut, and in position c there is excessive lead. With deep inspiration, both leads should approximate position a.

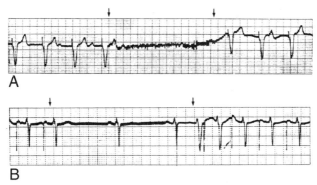

Figure 11.6. Examples of the inhibition of pacemaker output by the sensing of inappropriate signals. A. Pectoral muscle myopotentials cause temporary inhibition of output from a unipolar VVI pacemaker. B. Use of an electric razor inhibits the output from an AAI device. The arrows mark the onset and termination of the inhibitory signal.

First-degree AV block, which may or may not reflect AV nodal disease, has a benign natural history. Pacing is rarely indicated, except in the unusual circumstance where normalization of the P-R interval confers significant hemodynamic benefit.

The natural history of second-degree type I AV block (supra-Hisian) in patients without organic heart disease is similarly benign. Pacing is generally not warranted, unless the patient is symptomatic secondary to the slow ventricular rate.

Type II second-degree AV block has a much higher incidence of progression to complete heart block, and the patient is more frequently symptomatic. Pacing is recommended in the setting of symptomatic bradycardia, although, given the natural history, many clinicians implant pacemakers regardless of symptomatology. Type I AV block at the intra-Hisian or infra-Hisian levels is believed to have the same natural history as type II AV block, and guidelines for pacing are the same.

Survival is greatly improved in symptomatic patients with complete heart block who undergo pacemaker implantation. Although no similar longitudinal study has been done for asymptomatic patients with complete heart block, pacing is generally recommended (particularly with an escape rhythm less than 40 beats/minute).

Pacemakers have been used in patients with AF and rapid ventricular rates who undergo AV nodal or His bundle ablation to create complete heart block. By disrupting conduction to the ventricles, His bundle ablation allows the ventricular rate to be controlled by a VVIR pacing system. Patients with AF or flutter and high-grade AV block with symptomatic bradycardia warrant pacing as well.

Prior to permanent pacemaker implantation, it is important to rule out reversible causes of AV block, particularly Lyme disease, medications and drug toxicity, ischemia, and electrolyte abnormalities. If a patient with symptomatic bradycardia requires medications that suppress an escape rhythm, the drug should be continued and a pacemaker implanted.

The indications for permanent pacing in acquired AV block are listed below.

Table 11.2
Summary of Indications for Permanent Pacemaker Implantation

	Class 1	Class 2	Class 3
Acquired AVB[a]	1. CHB-symptomatic or asymptomatic with slow escape 2. Symptomatic second degree AVB 3. AF with high-grade AVB	1. Asymptomatic transient CHB or CHB with escape rate ≥40/min 2. Asymptomatic type II second degree AVB	1. First degree AVB 2. Asymptomatic type I supra-Hisian second degree AVB
Post-MI	Transient or persistent advanced AVB or CHB and associated IVCD	Persistent advanced AVB without IVCD	1. Transient AVB with LAHB or without IVCD 2. LAHB without AVB 3. BBB with or without first degree AVB
Bifascicular block	1. Symptomatic BFB with intermittent CHB 2. BFB and intermittent	1. Syncope and BFB without documented CHB but no other cause of syncope identified 2. BFB and HV ≥100 msec 3. BFB and pacing-induced infra-Hisian block	1. Asymptomatic fascicular block without AVB 2. Asymptomatic fascicular block with first degree AVB
Sick sinus syndrome	Symptomatic sick sinus syndrome	Symptomatic sick sinus syndrome without documented bradyarrhythmia	Asymptomatic sick sinus syndrome
Hypersensitive carotid sinus syndrome	Syncope and 3-sec pause invoked by CSM	1. History of syncope and 3-sec pause invoked by CSM 2. Syncope and bradycardia induced by HUT responsive to temporary pacing	Asymptomatic and 3-sec pause invoked by CSM
Other (see text)	1. Symptomatic bradycardia postcardiac transplantation 2. Selected patients with congenital heart block	1. ?Medically refractory HOC 2. ?Selected patients with DCMP 3. Medically refractory AF (following His bundle ablation)	

Adapted from Dreifus LS, Fisch C, Griffen JC, et al. Guidelines for implantation of cardiac pacemakers and antiarrhythmic devices. A report of the American College of Cardiology/American Heart Association Task Force on Assessment of Diagnostic and Therapeutic Cardiovascular Procedures (Committee on Pacemaker Implantation). J Am Coll Cardiol 1991;18:1–13.

[a]AVB, atrioventricular block; CHB, complete heart block; BFB, bifascicular block; CSM, carotid sinus massage; HUT, head-up tilt test; AF, atrial fibrillation; HOC, hypertrophic obstructive cardiomyopathy; DCMP, dilated cardiomyopathy; IVCD, intraventricular conduction delay; LAHB, left anterior hemiblock; BBB, bilateral bundle branch block; AF, atrial fibrillation.

I.   Class I (general agreement that the pacemaker should be implanted)
    I.a. Complete heart block, permanent or intermittent, associated with:
        I.a.1. Symptomatic bradycardia;
        I.a.2. Congestive heart failure;
        I.a.3. Medications that are necessary but suppress escape rhythms;
        I.a.4. Asystole ≥3 seconds or an escape rate <40/minute in asymptomatic patients;
        I.a.5. Confusional states that clear with temporary pacing;
        I.a.6. Following His bundle ablation;
    I.b. Symptomatic second-degree AV block, regardless of the type or site of block;
    I.c. AF or flutter with high-grade or complete heart block and bradycardia associated with any of the above conditions. The bradycardia must not result from negatively dromotropic drugs, such as digoxin, β-blockers, or calcium channel blockers;
II. Class II (pacemaker frequently used but diversity of opinion with regard to necessity);
    II.a. Asymptomatic transient or permanent complete heart block with ventricular rates faster than 40/minute;
    II.b. Asymptomatic type II second-degree AV block or intra/infra-Hisian type I AV block;
III. Class III (pacemaker not necessary);
    III.a. First-degree and asymptomatic type I (supra-Hisian) second degree AV block.

PACING AFTER MYOCARDIAL INFARCTION

The incidence of complete heart block complicating an acute myocardial infarction (MI) is approximately 6% and occurs twice as frequently in inferior/posterior infarctions as it does in anterior infarctions. Patients with an MI and complete heart block have higher in-hospital mortality, with a worse prognosis in anterior than inferior infarcts. The increased acute mortality is a reflection of more extensive myocardial necrosis and a higher incidence of left ventricular failure. In contrast, long-term survival appears not to be significantly different in patients who develop complete heart block compared to their unafflicted counterparts.

Heart block in inferior infarctions may occur from high vagal tone (via the Bezold-Jarisch reflex), from ischemia in the AV node, or result directly from anti-ischemic medications with negative dromotropic properties. AV block in inferior infarctions is almost always nodal in origin and usually transient. Permanent pacing is rarely warranted.

Unlike other indications for pacing, those following MI are prophylactic and do not depend on the presence of symptoms. Acutely, the indications for temporary pacing during an infarction may be different.

The indications for permanent pacing post-MI are class I, transient or persistent advanced AV block or complete heart block and associated IVCD; class II, persistent advanced AV block without IVCD; class III, (a) transient AV block with LAHB or without associated IVCD; (b) LAHB without AV block; and (c) bundle branch block with or without first-degree AV block.

PACING IN BIFASCICULAR BLOCK

It is extremely unlikely for unifascicular block to progress directly to complete heart block given that the two remaining pathways to the ventricle manifest normal conduction. Prophylactic pacing is therefore not warranted in isolated RBBB, LAHB, or LPHB. Bifasicular block, with one remaining nondiseased pathway, might be expected to be more precarious. Actually, however, the rate of progression to complete heart block is quite low. The annual incidence of heart block is 1.0–1.5% per year.

Three risk factors have been identified: (a) a prolonged H-V interval, (b) pacing-induced infra-Hisian block, (c) the presence of syncope.

The P-R interval is a nonspecific marker of conduction disease and may be prolonged in AV nodal and distal conduction disease. Its presence does not identify patients with bifascicular block who are at higher risk for developing complete heart block. A more specific measurement of distal conduction is the H-V interval. Based on several observations, the implantation of permanent pacemakers is recommended in patients with bifascicular block and an H-V interval ≥100 (Table 11.3).

It is worthwhile noting that although the progression to complete heart block in patients with bifascicular block is low, these patients have higher total mortality and incidence of sudden death compared to patients with normal conduction. Bifascicular block is a marker of associated heart disease (most commonly coronary artery disease), which exists in 75% of patients. Total cumulative mortality rates of 35% at 5 years and 52% at 7 years, and sudden death rates of 17% at 5 years and 27% at 7 years have been reported. Most sudden deaths are due to MIs or tachyarrhythmias, with a minority due to bradyarrhythmias.

The indications for pacing in bifascicular block are: class I, (a) symptomatic bifascicular block with intermittent complete heart block, and (b) bifascicular or trifascicular block and intermittent asymptomatic type II second-degree AV block; class II, (a) syncope and bifascicular or trifascicular block, where complete heart block

Table 11.3
Rate of Progression to High-Grade AV Block in Patients with Chronic Bifascicular Block Over a 3-Year Period

HV Interval	% Total Population	Progression to (%) High-Grade AV Block
<55	31	4
55–69	32	2
70–100	32	10
≥100	5	24

Adapted from Scheinman MM, Peters RW, Sauve MJ, et al. Value of the AV interval in patients with bundle branch block and the role of the prophylactic permanent pacing. Am J Cardiol 1982;50:1316–1322.

has not been documented but no other cause for syncope can be identified; (*b*) bifascicular block with H-V interval >100 msec; and (*c*) bifascicular block and pacing-induced infra-Hisian block; class III, (*a*) asymptomatic fascicular block without AV block, and (*b*) asymptomatic fascicular block with first-degree AV block.

PACING IN SICK SINUS SYNDROME

Sick sinus syndrome is the most common indication for pacemaker implantation. It is a disorder of sinoatrial impulse formation and conduction, resulting in both bradyarrhythmias and tachyarrhythmias. The AV node is involved in approximately 15% of patients at the time of diagnosis, and AV block develops in about 2–3% of patients per year. Pacing in sick sinus syndrome improves symptomatology but has not been shown to improve survival. Numerous retrospective analyses have reported a reduction in mortality and in the incidence of AF, CHF, and thromboembolism in patients with atrial pacing (AAI or DDD) compared to ventricular pacing (VVI) (Table 11.4).

The indications for pacing in sick sinus syndrome are: class I, sick sinus syndrome with documented symptomatic bradycardia (generally heart rates <lt>40 or pauses >3 seconds), which may result from necessary medications; class II, sinus node dysfunction with symptoms consistent with bradyarrhythmias but without documentation of the culprit bradyarrhythmia; and class III, asymptomatic sinus node dysfunction or sinus node dysfunction with symptoms that are not associated with bradyarrhythmias.

PACING IN HYPERSENSITIVE CAROTID SINUS SYNDROME AND
NEUROCARDIOGENIC SYNCOPE

Hypersensitive carotid sinus syndrome is characterized by syncope resulting from bradycardia and/or a decrease in systemic blood pressure due to carotid sinus stimulation. There are two types of responses: (*a*) cardioinhibitory, which is vagally mediated and associated with bradycardia/asystole and SA or AV block; and (*b*) vasodepressor type due to a decrease in peripheral resistance and hypotension. The cardioinhibitory type is most common (60–80%), although mixed types do occur.

Hypersensitivity to carotid stimulation is defined as sinus arrest or AV block of more than 3 seconds (cardioinhibitory) and/or a fall in systolic blood pressure of 50 mm Hg (vasodepressor type) during carotid sinus massage. In patients with symptomatic hypersensitive carotid syndrome of the cardioinhibitory type, pacing significantly decreases the recurrence of symptoms. Patients with the mixed type may or may not receive benefit from pacing; patients with pure vasodepressor type usually do not. Asymptomatic patients, no matter the type, should not receive pacemakers.

Neurocardiogenic syncope, formerly referred to as vasodepressor syncope, occurs as an abnormal response to upright posture. Peripheral vasodilatation leads to an increase in myocardial inotropy and an excessive activation of cardiac mechanoreceptors, resulting in reflex sympathetic inhibition and increased parasympathetic tone. The associated

Table 11.4
Comparison of Morbidity and Mortality in Ventricular Versus Atrial Pacing[a]

Study	No. of Patients		Atrial Fibrillation (%)		CHF (%)		Thromboembolic Events (%)		Mortality (%)	
	VVI	AAI/DDD[b]	VVI	AAI/DDD	VVI	AAI/DDD	VVI	AAI/DDD	VVI	AAI/DDD
Rosenqvist (1986, 1988)	79	89	47	7	37	15			23	8
Santini, 1990	125	214	47	7			8	2	30	14
Sasaki, 1991	34	41	44	17			20	0	35	12
Feuer, 1989	70	61	25	11	21	2			15	7
Sutton, 1986	651	410	22	4	26	27				

[a]All studies are retrospective.
[b]AAI/DDD, AAI or DDD pacemakers.

hypotension and/or bradycardia may result in syncope. The presentation is highly variable, and upright posture is not a prerequisite to neurocardiogenic syncope. Permanent pacing plays a very limited role in the treatment of neurocardiogenic syncope.

The indications for pacing in hypersensitive carotid sinus syndrome and neurocardiogenic syncope are: class I, recurrent syncope with symptoms and asystole longer than 3 seconds invoked by carotid sinus massage, in the absence of any medications that inhibit SA or AV conduction; class II, (a) recurrent syncope with hypersensitive cardioinhibitory response, and (b) syncope with bradycardia induced by head-up tilt with or without isoproterenol in which a temporary pacemaker clearly documents the benefits of a permanent pacemaker; class III, asymptomatic patients with hypersensitive cardioinhibitory response.

NEWER INDICATIONS FOR PERMANENT PACING

The indications for pacing are continually expanding. Areas where pacing may have an important future role include (a) hypertrophic cardiomyopathy, (b) dilated cardiomyopathy, (c) cardiac transplantation, (d) congenital AV block, and (e) AF with medically refractory ventricular response. In medically refractory obstructive hypertrophic cardiomyopathy, dual-chamber pacing has been shown to improve hemodynamics and symptomatology. There is preliminary evidence that dual-chamber pacing with a short AV delay may be beneficial in idiopathic dilated cardiomyopathy as well.

Following cardiac transplantation, permanent pacemaker implantation is performed in 4–7% of patients. Sinus node dysfunction is the most common arrhythmia (40%), followed by junctional bradycardia (24%). AV block occurs infrequently. The preferred mode of pacing following cardiac transplantation is disputable.

Congenital AV block has traditionally been considered to have a benign natural history without the need for permanent pacing. Usually, the QRS is narrow, and the site of block is in the AV node. Recent evidence suggests that there is a subpopulation of patients with congenital heart block who are at risk for complications such as syncope, sudden death, or the need for a pacemaker. Permanent pacemakers should be considered when congenital AV block is associated with (a) symptoms, (b) mean junctional rate <50, (c) exercise intolerance or inadequate heart rate response to exercise, (d) cardiomegaly and/or decreasing LV function, (e) increased Q-T interval, and/or (f) complex ventricular ectopy.

Traditionally, ventricular pacing in patients with chronic AF has been reserved for patients with symptomatic bradycardia. In the era of radiofrequency ablation, however, pacemaker implantation in conjunction with AV nodal or His bundle ablation is an effective means of rate control. Atrial pacing may stabilize the atria and prevent further paroxysms of AF as well as further deterioration to chronic AF, although data are very limited.

INDICATIONS FOR TEMPORARY TRANSVENOUS PACING

Indications for temporary pacing can be classified by intent. These include pacing (*a*) as therapy for bradyarrhythmias, (*b*) as prophylaxis against anticipated bradyarrhythmia, (*c*) for hemodynamic benefit, and (*d*) as therapy for tachyarrhythmias. Temporary pacing during an acute MI may be performed for bradyarrhythmias, prophylaxis, and/or hemodynamic benefit and will be considered as a separate group.

TEMPORARY PACING FOR BRADYARRHYTHMIAS

Any indication for permanent pacing is an appropriate indication for temporary pacing if the patient is hemodynamically unstable and/or if permanent pacing is not imminently available. These include acquired AV block, sinus node dysfunction, and hypersensitive carotid sinus syndrome.

Prior to permanent pacemaker implantation, it is important to rule out reversible causes of AV block, particularly Lyme disease, medications, drug toxicity, ischemia, and electrolyte abnormalities. If a patient is receiving a nonessential medication that may be responsible for the bradyarrhythmia, it may be appropriate to withhold the medication and utilize temporary pacing until the heart block subsides. A permanent pacemaker may not be necessary.

PROPHYLACTIC TEMPORARY PACING

Patients without bradyarrhythmias but who are at high risk for bradyarrhythmias may require temporary transvenous pacing during procedures or during the administration of medications. The development of complete heart block in patients with bundle branch block is low. This holds true when such patients undergo surgery as well.

The development of complete heart block in patients with preexisting bundle branch block during the administration of antiarrhythmic agents is unusual but can occur. The incidence of complete heart block in asymptomatic patients is so low, however, that the routine use of prophylactic temporary pacing is not indicated, except in unstable patients.

PACING FOR HEMODYNAMIC BENEFIT

Although temporary pacing improves cardiac output in any patient with significant bradyarrhythmias, at times pacing is instituted chiefly to improve hemodynamics, such as in patients following cardiac surgery. Any patient may show hemodynamic and symptomatic improvement with dual-chamber pacing, but the restoration of AV synchrony is especially important to patients with complete heart block and right ventricular infarction. Sinus bradycardia is common following cardiopulmonary bypass. Epicardial pacing provides the increased heart rate needed to augment cardiac output.

AV synchrony is essential in patients with right ventricular infarction and AV block. With right ventricular infarction, the chamber becomes noncompliant and more sensitive to changes in preload. As the right ventricle dilates, intrapericardial pressure increases and restricts left ventricular filling. The loss of atrial systole further impairs left ventricular filling. VVI pacing and loss of AV synchrony are therefore poorly tolerated. With atrial synchronous or AV sequential pacing, systolic arterial pressure improves by approximately 20–50% and cardiac output by 30–50%, compared with VVI pacing.

TEMPORARY PACING FOR TACHYARRHYTHMIAS

Pacing may be effective for suppression of drug-induced torsade de pointes, a polymorphous ventricular tachycardia associated with prolonged repolarization and bradycardia. Appropriate therapy after withdrawal of the precipitating agent is isoproterenol infusion and/or rapid pacing to increase the heart rate. Both therapies increase heart rate, which shortens the Q-T interval and decreases the dispersion of repolarization. Atrial or ventricular pacing may be utilized, but ventricular pacing is preferred. Temporary pacing may also be used to pace-terminate recurrent episodes of sustained monomorphic ventricular tachycardia. Overdrive pacing may also suppress episodes of sustained monomorphic ventricular tachycardia.

TEMPORARY PACING DURING MYOCARDIAL INFARCTION

The incidence of complete heart block complicating acute MI is approximately 5–6%. Complete heart block occurs almost twice as frequently in inferoposterior infarctions than anterior infarctions. Patients developing complete heart block are more likely to suffer severe complications such as cardiac arrest, cardiogenic shock, and pulmonary edema and have higher cardiac fatality rates. The increased morbidity and mortality reflect more extensive myocardial necrosis and/or poor right and left ventricular performance. Death is infrequently a direct result of bradyarrhythmias and is more likely to occur from cardiogenic shock and ventricular tachyarrhythmias. Thus, in terms of mortality benefit, the role of pacing is controversial.

Complete heart block or higher grade AV block occurs in 8–19% of patients with inferior MI. Increased vagal tone that results from the Bezold-Jarisch reflex, ischemia of the AV node area due to impairment of blood flow from collaterals (usually septal perforators), or negatively dromotropic antiischemic medications are generally responsible. The occurrence of high-grade AV block in the setting of inferior infarction follows a bimodal time course. High-grade AV block in the first 6 hours occurs suddenly, is of short duration, and is atropine-responsive. It is most likely vagal in origin. High-grade AV block occurring after 6 hours is generally gradual in onset (i.e., preceded by first-degree AV block), of longer duration, less likely to be atropine-responsive, and more likely to result from ischemia.

Mobitz I and high-grade AV block in the setting of inferior infarction are usually supra-Hisian in origin and are associated with a narrow complex escape rhythm. The escape rate is usually stable and atropine-sensitive. Temporary pacing is not generally required (unless the patient is symptomatic from severe bradycardia). Type I second-degree AV block with a wide QRS may be nodal in origin or may represent conduction block in the contralateral bundle branch or His bundle; temporary pacing should be considered.

Two subsets of patients with inferior infarcts warrant temporary pacing. Patients with right ventricular involvement and high-grade AV block have noncompliant ventricles, and their hemodynamics improve with AV sequential pacing. Alternating Wenckebach AV block may occur during an acute inferior infarction and is characterized by progressive prolongation of the P-R interval during 2:1 AV block until two or more P waves are blocked. Two levels of block occur in the AV node—one producing 2:1 block and the other causing Wenckebach periodicity. These patients have a higher incidence of high-grade AV block, hemodynamic deterioration, and death. Isoproterenol and atropine do not improve conduction (and may exacerbate block secondary to the increased atrial rate), and pacing is indicated.

Mobitz II or higher-grade AV block in patients with anterior wall infarctions is usually associated with bundle branch block and is localized to the His-Purkinje system. It reflects severe myocardial necrosis and is associated with poor left ventricular function and high morbidity. Temporary pacing is warranted but may not improve survival.

The incidence of new bundle branch block and/or bifascicular block in acute infarction is approximately 12%. The most frequent conduction disorder is LBBB (38%), followed by RBBB/LAHB (34%), isolated RBBB (11%), and RBBB/LPHB (10%).

A risk score involves totaling the number of conduction risk factors (worth one point each). These include first-degree AV block, second-degree AV block (types I and II), LAHB and LPHB, and RBBB and LBBB. The progression to complete heart block is dependent on the total risk score. In the absence of risk factors (0 points), 1.2% of patients developed complete heart block, whereas with three or more risk factors (≥3 points) there is a 36.4% incidence of complete heart block (Table 11.5). Prophylactic pacing is recommended in patients with a risk score of 3 or more and no pacing in patients with a risk score of 0 or 1. In the intermediate group with a risk score of 2, consideration should be given to the location of the infarction. Complete heart block in the setting of anterior infarction is frequently associated with a slow, unreliable escape rhythm, in contrast to inferior infarcts. In the former group, transvenous temporary pacing may be preferable, whereas the prophylactic use of a transthoracic pacemaker may be more suitable in the latter group.

ISSUES IN SELECTION OF A PACING PRESCRIPTION

Prior to deciding upon the appropriate pacemaker for a given patient, an understanding of the hemodynamic value of AV synchrony and rate responsiveness is essential.

Table 11.5
Electrocardiographic Risk Factors Used to Predict the Occurrence of Complete Heart Block during Acute Myocardial Infarction and Recommendations for Therapy

Electrocardiographic Risk Factors (1 pt each)	CHB Risk Score	Incidence of CHB (%)	Therapeutic Recommendation
1st AVB	0	1.2	No pacing
2nd AVB, type 1	1	7.8	No pacing
2nd AVB, type 2	2	25.0	P_a, $T_i{}^a$
LAHB	≥3	36.0	Pacing
LPHB			
RBBB			
LBBB			

Adapted from Lamas, GA, Muller JE, Turi ZG, et al. A simplified method to predict occurrences of complete heart block during acute myocardial infarction. Am J Cardiol 1986;57:1213–1219.

$^a P_a$, temporary transvenous pacing for anterior infarction; T_i, temporary transthoracic pacing for inferior infarction.

HEMODYNAMICS AND AV SYNCHRONY

Fixed rate ventricular pacing (asynchronous or inhibited modes) increases the heart rate and thus cardiac output. The optimal rate varies by patient, but for most lies between 60–70 beats/minute. At rest, cardiac output generally does not increase with faster paced rates because of a compensatory decrease in stroke volume.

PACEMAKER SYNDROME

Although fixed rate ventricular pacing provides a normal heart rate and improves cardiac output, it has several major disadvantages. These include (a) a lack of AV synchrony; (b) the potential for VA conduction; and (c) the presence of a fixed heart rate with limited ability to increase cardiac output during exercise.

The lack of AV synchrony may have multiple consequences. At rest, properly timed atrial contractions contribute to approximately 20% of the cardiac output, which is lost without AV synchrony. AV valvular regurgitation occurs if the ventricles contract when the valves are open.

In patients with ventricular pacing, VA conduction may occur. The AV node or an accessory pathway acts as the retrograde circuit. VA conduction may be intermittent or persistent and may occur in the presence of antegrade AV block. With retrograde conduction, atrial contraction occurs immediately following ventricular contraction. The AV valves are closed, and atrial contraction leads to venous regurgitation. Large A waves are visible in the neck and on hemodynamic tracings. Right atrial, pulmonary artery, and pulmonary capillary wedge pressures become elevated. Cardiac output and systemic pressure decrease.

The clinical sequelae from the low cardiac output and/or elevated venous pressure associated with ventricular pacing have been termed the pacemaker syndrome. Symptoms include near or frank syncope, easy fatiguability, dizziness, dyspnea, orthopnea, paroxysmal nocturnal dyspnea (PND), and a sensation of throat fullness. Physical exam may reveal hypotension, rales, cannon A waves, murmurs of tricuspid and/or mitral regurgitation, palpable liver pulsations, and peripheral edema. The pacemaker syndrome most commonly occurs with VVI and VVIR pacing modes but has been described with dual-chamber pacing.

AV SYNCHRONY

The benefit of AV synchrony cannot be overstated (Fig. 11.7). Properly timed atrial contraction increases cardiac output by augmenting ventricular filling via the Starling principle. Coordination of AV closure minimizes valvular regurgitation. Contraction against closed AV valves does not occur, averting its deleterious hemodynamic consequences. AV synchrony is most important to patients with diastolic dysfunction and noncompliant ventricles (e.g., aortic stenosis, hypertrophic cardiomyopathy).

AV INTERVAL

Merely establishing AV synchrony with dual-chamber pacing improves cardiac output compared to ventricular pacing. But maximization of cardiac output requires optimizing the timing of atrial and ventricular contraction. AV intervals of 100–200 msec produce the highest cardiac output in most patients, although the interpatient variability is great.

The optimal AV interval differs, whether the P wave is sensed or paced. Because of latency between the atrial stimulus and eventual atrial depolarization, the AV interval following a paced atrial event should be programmed longer than the AV interval following a sensed atrial event. Prolonging the AV interval after atrial pac-

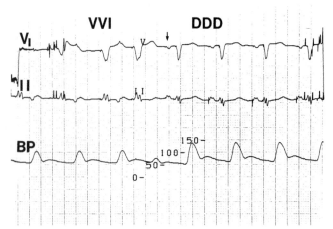

Figure 11.7. A dramatic improvement in systemic arterial pressure occurs following reprogramming from VVI to DDD modes (arrow). In the VVI mode ventriculoatrial conduction is evident. Excessive stimuli on the extreme right and left are programming artifacts.

ing by approximately 50 msec generally allows for equivalent AV intervals during AV sequential and AV synchronous pacing.

A potential drawback to a short AV interval is ventricular activation via a paced beat from the right ventricular apex. The benefits of spontaneous ventricular depolarization are not clear. Shortening the AV delay in paced patients and altering the sequence of ventricular activation does not decrease, but actually increases, cardiac output.

A long AV interval preserves battery life by allowing for spontaneous AV conduction. In programming the AV interval, preserving battery life must be weighed against the hemodynamic benefit of an optimal AV delay. Most patients, except perhaps for those with diastolic dysfunction, are best served by longer AV delays, native ventricular activation, and increased battery longevity.

CHRONOTROPIC INCOMPETENCE

The ideal rate sensor is the sinoatrial node. When an insufficient heart rate is due to AV block and a slow escape rhythm, restoration of AV synchrony with dual chamber pacing restores chronotropic competence. However, a significant number of paced patients have ineffective sinus nodes and are unable to appropriately increase their heart rate during exercise. The diagnosis of such chronotropic incompetence is made during exercise testing and is defined as the inability to increase the heart rate at peak exercise to at least 70–85% of the maximum predicted heart rate.

PACEMAKER THERAPY IN THE MANAGEMENT OF TACHYARRHYTHMIAS

METHODS OF ANTITACHYCARDIA PACING

Tachycardia termination has been extensively achieved in a variety of reentrant supraventricular tachycardias and recurrent sustained ventricular tachycardia.

A variety of pacing methods are available for acute and chronic application using external or implantable pacing devices (Table 11.6). These techniques are typically classified into three general categories, namely, underdrive pacing, overdrive pacing, or extrastimulus methods. Underdrive pacing typically employs asynchronous stimulation at a cycle length longer than the tachycardia cycle length. Thus, the pacing stimuli emerge at varying points during the tachycardia cycle length.

Overdrive pacing generally refers to stimulation at a rate above the spontaneous tachycardia rate. This is to be discriminated from overdrive pacing for suppression of ectopic beats. In the latter method, a range of demand pacing rates is employed for suppression of ectopic activity for purposes of prevention of tachycardia. Rapid overdrive pacing employs two or more pacing stimuli in a train. Interstimulus interval can be constant as in burst pacing or variable (Fig. 11.8).

When the coupling intervals of successive stimuli of the burst are reduced by an equal interval in successive termination attempts, this is referred to as a scanning burst or concertina-accordion pacing.

Table 11.6
Methods of Antitachycardia Pacing

1. Underdrive
2. Overdrive
    Burst
    Fixed
    Variable
    Ramp
    Incremental
    Decremental
    Ultrarapid
3. Programmed extrastimuli
    Scanning
    Centrifugal
    Self-searching

Variable overdrive pacing methods are generally classified under ramp pacing. In a ramp technique, the interstimulus interval progressively increases or decreases within the train. These have also been referred to as tune-down/tune-up ramps or alternatively decremental/incremental ramps. On occasion the pacing rate within a single ramp-pacing burst may both accelerate and decelerate. This is referred to as a changing ramp. The interval between the last sensed cardiac beat and the first ramp-pacing beat is progressively decremented in successive attempts. This is referred to as scanning burst pacing with ramp pacing.

The third major category is the use of programmed extrastimuli for tachycardia reversion. In this method, the timing of one or more pacing stimuli is exactly and independently programmed to achieve penetration of the reentrant circuit. Sequential attempts may increment or decrement the coupling interval by a predetermined small interval (extrastimulus scan), or the timing interval between the first pacing stimulus and the last tachycardia beat can increment or decrement in successive attempts (centrifugal scan).

EVALUATION AND FOLLOW-UP OF PATIENTS FOR ANTITACHYCARDIA PACING

Evaluation of a candidate for antitachycardia pacing involves careful assessment of the clinical history to determine the frequency and hemodynamic stability of tachycardia episodes. Immediate onset of hemodynamic compromise eliminates the possibility of using manually triggered pacemakers and emphasizes the need for rapid arrhythmia reversion. The use of rapid pacing modes in a patient with significant angina pectoris may precipitate an ischemic episode. Exercise testing to assess the maximum sinus rate is valuable in defining the programmed sensing rate.

Spontaneous recordings of tachycardia on a definitive drug regimen are often valuable for the same purpose. Ambulatory ECG monitoring provides information regarding the number of episodes of nonsustained and sustained tachyarrhythmias observed during the recording period as well as the variations in native sinus rate. This information is also used in programming the detection rate for pacing therapy.

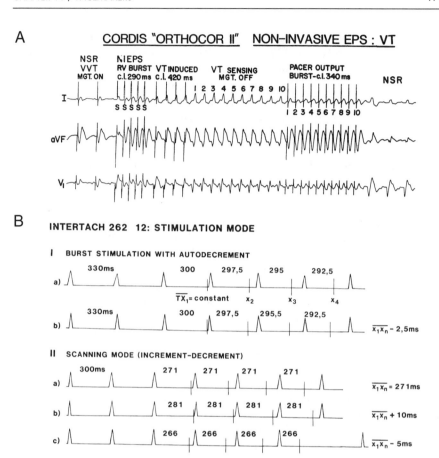

Figure 11.8. Noninvasive electrophysiologic study in a patient with a Cordis model 284A anti-tachycardia pacemaker. A. Noninvasive induction VT with right ventricular burst pacing is shown on the left panel of the recording. VT is induced with a cycle length of 420 msec, and the magnet is removed. The tachycardia is sensed for 10 beats, and the pacemaker delivers a burst at a cycle length of 340 msec for 10 beats. Termination to sinus rhythm is noted. C.L., cycle length; MGT, magnet; NIEPS, noninvasive electrophysiologic study; NSR, normal sinus rhythm; RV, right ventricle; VVT, triggered ventricular mode. (From Klein H, et al. Diagnostic evaluation of the prospective antitachycardia device patient. In: Saksena S, Goldschlager N, eds. Electrical therapy for cardiac arrhythmias. Philadelphia: WB Saunders, 1990:439.) B. Schematic representation of the selected tachycardia termination modes during noninvasive testing under different conditions. Both forms include an adaptive change of the burst cycle length. After detection of tachycardia, autodecremental burst pacing is initiated (Ia). The cycle length within the burst will automatically be decreased by a programmable amount of 2.5 msec. If unsuccessful, the burst will be repeated with the same cycle length (Ib). In case of tachycardia persistence, the consecutive incremental-decremental scanning sequence will be activated. In the scanning mode, all the intervals of a single burst have the same msec value (IIa). In the next steps, the cycle length is first incremented by a programmed amount of 10 msec (IIb) and then decremented by a preset value of 5 msec (IIc). (From Jung W, et al. Clinical results of chronic antitachycardia pacing in supraventricular tachycardia. In: Luderitz B, Saksena S, eds. Interventional electrophysiology. Mount Kisco, NY: Futura, 1991:197.)

Electrophysiologic evaluation is an essential part of patient assessment. Electrophysiologic studies should be performed in the absence of antiarrhythmic drug therapy using standard techniques and after the final drug regimen is established. At the preimplant electrophysiologic study, repeated arrhythmia induction and reproducible arrhythmia termination need to be demonstrated. In most patients at least 20 episodes of induced arrhythmia should be reproducibly terminated by the selected mode.

Efficacy of Pacing Modes for Acute Termination of Tachyarrhythmias

Single atrial extrastimuli and bursts of atrial pacing are effective in the termination of paroxysmal supraventricular tachycardia. Repeated attempts at pace termination can induce AF, particularly when rapid atrial pacing techniques are used. Pacing techniques are generally contraindicated in patients with short antegrade refractory periods for accessory pathways. Sudden death due to ventricular fibrillation (VF) induced by AF has been reported in patients with implanted antitachycardia pacemakers for interruption of supraventricular tachycardia. An antegrade effective refractory period of <300 msec has been suggested as a contraindication to pacing therapy.

Ventricular stimulation techniques may also be used for termination of AV reentrant tachycardia. Single ventricular extrastimuli commonly terminate these tachycardias by preexciting the atrium, with subsequent block of the retrograde atrial impulse in the AV nodal-His-Purkinje system.

The likelihood of achieving tachycardia termination is also increased by the use of multiple extrastimuli or pacing bursts. The possibility of inducing VT and VF ipso facto remains a constant concern. Therefore, ventricular stimulation techniques have been largely used for acute termination of AV reentrant tachycardia in the electrophysiology laboratory. Chronic use of this pacing modality is not recommended at present.

Pacing techniques have also been used for the termination of AV nodal reentrant tachycardia. The reentrant circuit in AV nodal reentrant tachycardia utilizes electrophysiologic pathways in the AV junction. Intraatrial reentrant tachycardia and atrial flutter are also amenable to pacing termination (Fig. 11.9).

Common atrial flutter with slower rates (type a) is more suitable for pacing termination. Flutter cycle lengths below 250 msec are less likely to revert by pacing techniques. The most effective mode is burst atrial pacing. Induction of AF can be an important limitation of this technique. Long-term experience with antitachycardia pacing in atrial flutter is limited to a few reported series.

Devices that are currently available for tachycardia termination utilizing antitachycardia pacing vary widely for atrial and ventricular application. Several antitachycardia pacemakers that were available for chronic use in supraventricular tachyarrhythmias were also utilized initially for ventricular application on a standalone basis. However, because of the perpetual risk of tachycardia acceleration, these were utilized almost exclusively with concomitant implantation of a cardioverter-defibrillator for backup shock therapy in patients with ventricular tach-

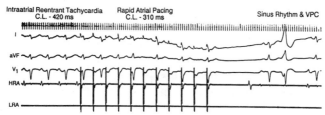

Figure 11.9. Termination of intraatrial reentrant tachycardia by rapid atrial pacing bursts. Atrial tachycardia is interrupted by a pacing train of 11 beats at 73% of tachycardia cycle length. This was reproducibly demonstrated in this patient. C.L., cycle length; HRA, high right atrium; LRA, low right atrium; VPC, ventricular premature contraction. (From Saksena S, et al. Electrophysiologic mechanisms underlying management of supraventricular tachycardia by electrical stimulation. In: Saksena S, Goldschlager N, eds. Electrical therapy for cardiac arrhythmias. Philadelphia: WB Saunders, 1990:384.)

yarrhythmias. More recently, third-generation cardioverter-defibrillator devices now incorporate both antibradycardia and antitachycardia pacing in a hybrid multiprogrammable unit.

Prevention of Tachycardias

Tachycardia prevention by pacing techniques has been most widely employed for the temporary or permanent treatment of drug-resistant supraventricular tachycardia. While fixed-rate atrial or ventricular pacing is occasionally employed, particularly in patients with concomitant sinus node disease and bradycardia-dependent atrial flutter/fibrillation or supraventricular tachycardia, dual chamber pacing is used with greater success. Prevention of AV reentrant tachycardia induction by introducing an atrial premature beat after the supraventricular tachycardia initiating beat has also been reported.

Prevention of atrial flutter by electrical stimulation techniques has been analyzed. Atrial flutter often coexists in the bradycardia-tachycardia syndrome. Rate support by atrial pacing may be useful in tachycardia prevention in selected instances. Reducing atrial ectopy by overdrive pacing could theoretically reduce the trigger mechanism for atrial flutter. More commonly, atrial flutter recurs but with reduced frequency. Concomitant antiarrhythmic drug therapy is usually required for prolongation of atrial refractoriness and suppression or atrial ectopic activity. These preventive approaches are also used in patients with paroxysmal AF or chronic AF after electrical conversion attempts. Electrical stimulation is also occasionally effective for overdriving or preventing ectopic atrial tachycardia or intraatrial reentrant tachycardia. Drug or ablative therapy is the primary treatment in these disorders.

Tachycardia prevention for VT has been widely discussed, but clinical experience with this approach is quite limited. One major clinical scenario where pacing techniques can be effective is drug-induced torsade de pointes due to prolongation of repolarization (i.e., the Q-T interval). Overdrive atrial or ventricular pacing with temporary leads at rates from 90–150 beats/minute may reduce dispersion of refractoriness and homogenize repolarization. This may in turn prevent the triggers or alter the substrate or affect both mechanisms for the genesis of the arrhythmia.

Tachycardia prevention with implantable pacemakers on a chronic basis has been largely limited to prevention of atrial tachyarrhythmias. Individual reports of a few patients carefully selected for this approach have appeared in the literature. However, this approach has lost its appeal because of the availability of catheter ablation techniques for chronic therapy of paroxysmal reentrant supraventricular tachycardia. It is now largely used for the treatment of bradycardia-dependent tachyarrhythmias such as atrial flutter/fibrillation.

NONINVASIVE CARDIAC PACING WITH AN EXTERNAL PACEMAKER

Advantages of the External Pacemaker

A transthoracic external pacing system can be used for the maintenance of heart rate until a temporary transvenous pacemaker, if required, can be inserted under nonemergency circumstances. Additionally, such an external pacing system would be of importance for out-of-hospital emergency situations where a transvenous pacemaker is not available by emergency personnel. The external pacemaker is now available as a therapeutic tool and has been demonstrated to be an effective and safe.

External Pacemaker Characteristics

The currently available external pacemaker units differ with regard to pulse duration used, which is usually fixed and ranges from 20–40 msec, although in a few devices the pulse duration is programmable. The waveform is usually monophasic and rectangular although other waveforms are used by some devices. The current output is generally programmable and can be adjusted from 0–210 ma, usually in 5–10 ma steps. The pacing rate is also programmable and ranges from 30–180 beats/minute. The threshold necessary for pacing depends upon the individual patient. It has been reported that the pacing threshold is not altered by certain cardiac drugs such as verapamil or propranolol, although the effects of other drugs have not been established. These units are capable of antibradycardia pacing, tachycardia termination, and defibrillation, and they provide clear, electrocardiographic monitoring that can be used with or without actual pacing. It is now well established that the external pacemaker stimulates and paces the ventricle (Fig. 11.10).

Hemodynamic Effects of the External Pacemaker

With the external pacemaker there is a small decrease in systemic vascular resistance, an increase in left ventricular end-diastolic pressure, but no significant change in cardiac index. It is noteworthy that, with external pacing, there is simultaneous right and left ventricular contraction. This is in contrast to transvenous

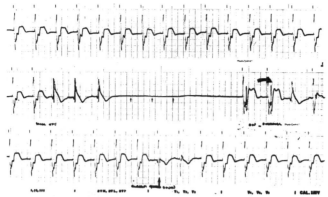

Figure 11.10. Recording from a patient undergoing external pacing. Top panel shows successful pacing with 100% ventricular capture. In the middle panel, the energy output of the device is reduced to below threshold and there is no ventricular capture (beats 3–5). When the external pacemaker is turned off, there is no spontaneous ventricular activity, although small P waves (arrows) are seen. Pacing is reinstituted thereafter (bottom panel). (From Falk RH. Noninvasive external cardiac pacing. In: El Sherif NA, Samit P, eds. Cardiac pacing and electrophysiology. 3rd ed. Philadelphia: WB Saunders, 1991:675–684.)

pacing, in which there is abnormal septal movement suggestive of a left bundle branch block due to pacing from the right ventricle. During external pacing, septal movement is normal, suggesting that the external pacemaker does not alter the normal ventricular contraction pattern.

Clinical Application of External Pacemaker

Although originally proposed and developed as a therapy for symptomatic bradycardia, the external pacemaker is also used to terminate supraventricular and ventricular tachyarrhythmias, for external defibrillation, and as a prophylactic "standby" for high-risk patients.

TREATMENT OF BRADYCARDIA

The external pacemaker is a highly effective approach for the treatment of symptomatic bradycardia resulting from complete AV block or sinus node dysfunction; implanted or temporary pacemaker dysfunction; hyperkalemia; or from drugs that impair sinus and AV nodal function, such as β-blockers, calcium channel blockers, or digoxin. It may be especially helpful when pharmacologic therapy for increasing the heart rate (i.e., atropine, isoproterenol, or epinephrine) is ineffective, contraindicated, or associated with risk.

The external pacemaker is also a reasonable approach in patients who are at high risk for the development of asymptomatic bradycardia. This includes post-MI patients with evidence of conduction system disease, patients with symptoms such as syncope who are suspected of having bradycardia or heart block, patients with an MI receiving thrombolytic therapy, or patients with bradycardia or conduction system disease who require drugs that may worsen these conditions.

CARDIAC ARREST

The external pacemaker is indicated and is of benefit when there is loss of consciousness or hemodynamic impairment as the result of a bradycardia, especially if a pulse is initially obtained indicating tissue perfusion and viable myocardium. The external pacemaker has a significant advantage over transvenous pacing in this situation, as it is quick and simple to use. However, results in patients with a pulseless cardiac arrest due to bradycardia or asystole have been less impressive. A number of studies have reported that transcutaneous pacing with an external pacemaker results in electrical capture rates of 40%, while mechanical capture is documented in only 20% of patients, even when used early during cardiopulmonary resuscitation (Fig. 11.11). However, in most of these studies survival was nevertheless very poor, mainly because in these patients bradycardia and asystole are usually the result of a cardiac arrest of long duration and generally indicate the presence of irreversible myocardial damage.

The external pacemaker does not result in improved survival or hospital discharge, even when considering early response and prompt initiation of pacing, initial presence or absence of a pulse or blood pressure, or nature of the presenting arrhythmia. Thus, external pacing has limited usefulness in the setting of an out-of-hospital cardiac arrest, even if due to a bradyarrhythmia or asystole, especially when pharmacological therapy has been ineffective. Survival is determined by the amount of myocardial damage resulting from the cardiac arrest. In those with asystole, the heart is severely damaged and is most likely inexcitable.

TERMINATION OF VENTRICULAR OR SUPRAVENTRICULAR TACHYCARDIA

In the electrophysiology laboratory, overdrive or underdrive pacing is an effective approach for the acute termination of both ventricular and supraventricular tachycardias. The external pacemaker using underdrive pacing is of limited benefit for terminating rapid VT but is more effective when it delivers asynchronous overdrive pacing for slower VT. The arrhythmia terminates in 70–90%. The external pacemaker is effective for terminating AV reentrant tachycardia (80% response) or an AV nodal reentrant tachycardia (50% response). The mean pacing current

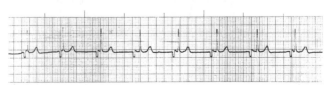

Figure 11.11. Example of noncapture of the external pacemaker. Seen is a negative pacemaker stimulus artifact, which fails to capture and stimulate the ventricle. Native QRS complexes are seen. (From Falk RH. Noninvasive external cardiac pacing. In: El Sherif NA, Samit P, eds. Cardiac pacing and electrophysiology. 3rd ed. Philadelphia: WB Saunders, 1991:675–684.

needed is high and often >100 ma. The external pacemaker is of limited value for terminating atrial flutter. One potential complication is acceleration or worsening of arrhythmia.

Side Effects of External Pacemaker

The external pacemaker is generally safe for use in patients and, like other forms of pacing, does not result in any myocardial damage. It is unlikely for VT or VF to occur, even though an occasional stimulus may be delivered during the vulnerable period, i.e., on the apex of the T wave, even if during ischemia. A major limitation to the use of the external pacemaker is the degree of discomfort resulting from the delivery of stimuli to the chest wall. The external pacemaker causes skeletal muscle and cutaneous nerve stimulation. The discomfort level is related to the amount of energy that is necessary to capture and pace the heart. Above a level of 50 ma, there is substantial discomfort, especially when the pacemaker is used for any prolonged period of time.

SUGGESTED READING

Bernstein AD, Brownlee RR, Fletcher R, Gold RD, Smyth NPD, Spielman SR. Report of the NASPE mode code committee. PACE 1984;7: 395-402.

Brignole M, Menozzi M, Lolli G, Bottoni, Gaggioli G. Long-term outcome of paced and nonpaced patients with severe carotid sinus syndrome. Am J Cardiol 1992;69:1039-1043.

Danforth J, Goldschlager N. Indications for cardiac pacing. In: Saksena S, Goldschlager N, eds. Electrical therapy for cardiac arrhythmias. Philadelphia: WB Saunders, 1990:91- 107.

den Dulk K, Bertholet M, Brugada P, et al. Clinical experience with implantable devices for control of tachyarrhythmias. PACE 1984;7:548.

Dhingra RC, Palileo E, Strasberg B, et al. Significance of the HV interval in 517 patients with chronic bifascicular block. Circulation 1981;64:1265-1271.

Dreifus LS, Fisch C, Griffin JC, et al. Guidelines for implantation of cardiac pacemakers and antiarrhythmia devices, July 1991. A report of the American College of Cardiology/ American Heart Association Task Force of Diagnostic and Therapeutic Cardiovascular Procedures (Committee on Pacemaker Implantation). J Am Coll Cardiol 1991;18:1-13.

Estes NAM, Deering TF, Manolis AS, Salem D, Zoll PM. Noninvasive transcutaneous cardiac pacing for termination of sustained supraventricular and ventricular tachycardia. In: Birkui PJ, Trigano JA, Zoll PM, eds. Noninvasive transcutaneous cardiac pacing. Mount Kisco, NY: Futura, 1993:131-145.

Fananapazir L, Cannon RO, Tripoli D, Panza JA. Impact of dual-chamber permanent pacing in patients with obstructive hypertrophic cardiomyopathy with symptoms refractory to verapamil and β-adrenergic blocker therapy. Circulation 1992;85:2149-2161.

Feuer JM, Shanding AH, Messenger JC. Influence of cardiac pacing mode on the long-term development of atrial fibrillation. Am J Cardiol 1989;68:1376-1379.

Hindman MC, Wagner GS, JaRo M, et al. The clinical significance of bundle branch block complicating acute myocardial infarction. 2. Indications for temporary and permanent pacemaker insertion. Circulation 1978;58:689-699.

Levy S. Role of pacing in treatment of supraventricular tachycardia. In: Josephson ME, Wellens HJJ, eds. Tachycardias: mechanisms, diagnosis, treatment. Philadelphia: Lea & Febiger, 1984:223.

Parsonnet V, Bernstein AD, Lindsay B. Pacemaker-implantation complication rates: an analysis of some contributing factors. J Am Coll Cardiol 1989;13:17-21.

12 Catheter Ablation of Cardiac Arrhythmia

SUPRAVENTRICULAR ARRHYTHMIA

The principle of catheter ablative therapy was introduced in 1982, when both Scheinman et al. and Gallagher et al. reported the results of closed-chest ablation of the atrioventricular (AV) junction with direct current shocks to control refractory supraventricular arrhythmias. The disadvantages of the direct current approach are now well recognized and comprise the induction of fairly large lesions, the risk of barotrauma and of rupturing thin-walled structures, the lack of graded energy delivery, and the need for general anaesthesia. These drawbacks are not present when alternating current in the radiofrequency range (usually 300–750 kHz) is used instead of direct current. Radiofrequency energy achieves its effect by tissue desiccation, and the initial clinical experience using this modality has been extremely promising.

Tachycardias Involving Accessory AV Connections

A residual muscular connection between atrium and ventricle (formerly known as Kent's bundle) is a congenital disorder that may precipitate paroxysmal episodes of seriously symptomatic reentrant tachycardia. These anomalous pathways of AV conduction lie along the mitral and tricuspid valve rings (parietal pathways) or within the septum. They may have bidirectional conduction properties or, in about 25% of patients, conduct only in the retrograde direction ("concealed" accessory pathways). Pathways capable of antegrade conduction give rise to Δ-wave-configured QRS complexes during sinus rhythm that disappear during the usual orthodromic type of AV tachycardia with a depolarization wavefront utilizing the specific conduction system as its antegrade limb and the accessory pathway as its retrograde limb (Wolff-Parkinson-White syndrome). In a minority of patients, antidromic (wide-QRS) tachycardia with reversed wavefront propagation is observed. Concealed accessory connections permanently block antegrade conduction and are functionally silent during sinus rhythm, but they maintain orthodromic tachycardia by their retrograde conduction property. In patients with Wolff-Parkinson-White (WPW) syndrome, the anomalous connection may facilitate rapid conduction of atrial fibrillation (AF) to the ventricles and thus present a life-threatening hazard.

For decades, the therapeutic options offered to these patients have consisted of lifelong antiarrhythmic medication or—if this proved ineffective, was not tolerated, or was deemed unacceptable—surgical intervention. Surgery for the WPW syndrome, aided by intraoperative electrophysiology, has been refined to the extent that it is presently associated with a high rate of success and low morbidity and mortality rates. Nevertheless, a curative therapeutic modality that circumvents surgery is more than welcome, particularly because the vast majority of patients suffering from tachyarrhythmias mediated by an accessory connection are free of organic heart disease.

180

Several large studies published recently have now established the ablation of an accessory fiber using catheter-induced radiofrequency current as the first line of treatment in specialized centers for adult and pediatric patients. The reported success rates usually exceed 90%, serious complications such as cardiac tamponade secondary to myocardial perforation and coronary artery spasm with or without myocardial infarction are extremely rare, and the incidence of procedure-related deaths is well below 0.5%; surgical dissection of accessory AV connections has been rendered all but obsolete (Table 12.1).

The outcome of an attempt at catheter ablation is critically dependent on the precision of accessory pathway localization, because radiofrequency current induces lesions confined to several millimeters in width as well as in depth. Accessory pathway localization is performed by catheter mapping techniques under biplane fluoroscopic guidance. Conventionally, the anatomic site of an accessory connection is approximated by the site of earliest ventricular activation during sinus rhythm or atrial pacing and/or by the site of earliest atrial activation during tachycardia or ventricular pacing. Improved catheter technology has enabled the direct bipolar recording of accessory pathway activation, and this has subsequently become the preferred mode of localizing an accessory fiber in some institutions. Catheters with an orthogonal electrode configuration are primarily useful to search for left-sided accessory pathway activation potentials within the coronary sinus, but it has recently been shown that catheters with a longitudinal electrode configuration and a distal 2-mm interelectrode distance may be successfully used to detect accessory pathway (Fig. 12.1) activation at all locations inside the heart.

Although standard-production electrode catheters were initially used for ablation purposes, new catheter designs have significantly contributed to the increased acceptance of the catheter ablation procedure. These catheters, 5- to 7-French in diameter, usually have a deflectable tip to ease maneuverability along the AV anuli, and the tip electrode is prolonged to 3 or 4 mm. Compared with the standard 2-mm tip-electrode catheters, current breakdowns caused by a sudden impedance rise due to the formation of blood coagulum are encountered less frequently with the large-tip catheters, and more electrical power (in the 25–40-W range) can be applied. It has been shown that blood coagulation occurs if the electrode-tissue

Table 12.1
Success Rates and Complications in Catheter Ablation of Accessory Pathways Performed at the University of Hamburg by the End of September 1993

Site of AP[a]	Success Rates (%)	Complications
Right free wall	90	0/77
Left free wall	97	5/388
Posteroseptal	93	3/162
Midseptal	100	1/24
Anteroseptal	95	2/39

[a]AP, accessory pathway.

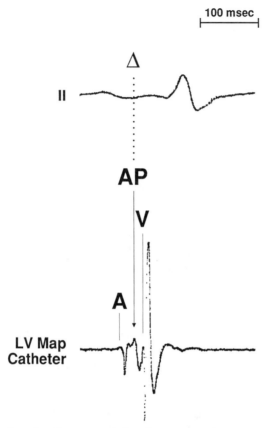

Figure 12.1. Recording during sinus rhythm of accessory pathway activation (AP) coinciding with the onset of the Δ wave and preceding local ventricular activation (V) in a patient with a left free wall accessory pathway. The mapping/ablation catheter is located at the ventricular aspect of the mitral valve anulus. A, local atrial activation potential.

interface temperature exceeds 100°C, and thermistor-controlled electrode catheters have since become available to avoid this phenomenon.

Because an accessory fiber has both an atrial and a ventricular insertion, an ablation attempt may be directed at either site. Programmed stimulation studies have revealed that the vulnerable link along the axis atrium-accessory pathway-ventricle is the atrium-accessory pathway interface in the majority of right-sided pathways, whereas left-sided pathways most often block conduction at the accessory pathway-ventricle interface. Consequently, a (femoral or jugular) venous approach appears to be the logical choice to ablate accessory connections located on the right free wall and along the septum. Septal accessory pathways require particular attention, as they may bridge the AV groove in close vicinity to the conduction system. However, anteroseptal fibers (located anterosuperiorly to the bundle of His) as well as midseptal fibers (located between the bundle of His and the coronary-sinus ostium) can be differentiated from the structures of normal conduction and be safely ablated from an atrial catheter position.

Accessory fibers traversing the pyramidal posteroseptal space from the postero-medial aspect of either atrium to insert into the posterior ventricular septum (usu-ally referred to as posteroseptal pathways) may be ablated using a variety of approaches depending on the actual course of the fiber. Using a femoral venous access, possible ablation sites identified by precise catheter mapping are the immediate vicinity of the coronary-sinus ostium, the proximal coronary sinus, and the middle cardiac vein draining into it. An arterial approach using the retrograde introduction of the ablation catheter into the left ventricle may also be attempted for posteroseptal accessory connections.

The insertion of a catheter into the left ventricle to probe for an accessory path-way was introduced in 1986; it was later established as the standard approach to ablate the ventricular insertion of left free wall accessory pathways. Recently, transseptal puncture to access the atrial insertion of such pathways has been advo-cated as an equally efficacious alternative. With increasing investigator experience, localization and ablation of manifest accessory pathways (i.e., in patients with WPW syndrome) may be attempted during sinus rhythm using a single catheter and foregoing all pacing and mapping catheters. This technique yielded good results for left free wall accessory pathways, with a significantly reduced overall session duration and fluoroscopy time compared with patients investigated with multiple catheters; it appears particularly suited to a pediatric patient population.

Although highly effective, radiofrequency current ablation of accessory path-ways is associated with a varying number of unsuccessful pulses preceding the final, successful pulse. Early studies aimed at identifying the predictors of a suc-cessful pulse have been reported. Local electrogram stability and a number of local parameters were found to be associated with a higher probability of success. Among them were the recording of a presumed accessory pathway activation potential, the timing of local atrial relative to local ventricular activation (AV inter-val), as well as the timing of local ventricular activation relative to the onset of the QRS complex (ΔV interval) for manifest accessory pathways; and the recording of a presumed accessory pathway activation potential, the timing of local ventricular relative to local atrial activation (V-A interval), as well as the presence of retro-grade continuous electrical activity for concealed accessory pathways. A major lim-itation of these reports is that the accessory pathway was regarded as a uniform entity, and a purely statistical analysis was applied to local electrogram parameters to predict the outcome of a radiofrequency current application. Different approaches that take into account a number of important variables likely to influ-ence the outcome of any single pulse, such as the anatomy of the AV groove, the geometry and location of the accessory pathway, and the orientation of the catheter electrodes with respect to the presumed course of the accessory pathway, have not been reported yet.

Left free wall accessory pathways represent a uniform enough set of fibers for such a systematic approach to be performed. Analysis of local electrograms recorded at the subannular aspect of the mitral valve annulus and of the relative outcome observed in response to radiofrequency application shows that the vast majority of these fibers, whether located anteriorly, laterally, or posteriorly, appear to have a rather circumscript ventricular insertion and a partially subendocardial course, and that they bridge the mitral annulus at sites that permit close contact with the ablating catheter. Ablation of these pathways at their ventricular insertion can be expected with a few pulses, provided that the pathway is precisely located via electrogram criteria. Exceptions are most likely represented by pathways with an epicardial course or a wide ventricular insertion, and by pathways embedded in an "adverse" anatomy of the AV groove that may prevent close enough contact with the ablating catheter. In our experience, consistent inability to record a ΔV interval less than 10 msec is likely to point at a more epicardial ventricular insertion of the accessory pathway; ablation at its atrial insertion may be more easily obtained in such cases. Repeated occurrence of transient block despite catheter manipulation for an "optimal" ablation site in the same area indicates a branched ventricular insertion (or a subepicardial course), and ablation using the ventricular approach may be achieved through a cumulative energy effect. A local atrium to ventricle amplitude ratio of less than 0.1 invariably indicates poor contact of the ablating catheter with the mitral annulus, regardless of the values of all other electrogram parameters.

In contrast to the rapid ventriculoatrial conduction facilitated by most accessory fibers during orthodromic AV tachycardia, some concealed anomalous connections may exhibit slow and decremental conduction properties analogous to those of the AV node. They frequently give rise to the permanent form of junctional reciprocating tachycardia (PJRT) with inverted P waves in leads II, III, aVF, and V3–V6 and an R-P interval longer than the P-R interval. Once diagnosed and differentiated from the atypical form of atrioventricular node reentrant tachycardia (AVNRT), PJRT lends itself to abolition by catheter ablation with preservation of AV nodal conduction. The accessory fiber is generally confined to the posteroseptal space, but a recent preliminary study reported additional sites for the anomalous connection in PJRT along the posterior to lateral region of the mitral valve ring. Differentiation of the accessory pathway site with a subsequent decision on the optimal ablation approach may be achieved by analyzing the P-wave polarity in leads I and V1: posteroseptal accessory connections consistently show a biphasic retrograde P wave in lead I, which by contrast is negative in patients with a left free wall (posterolateral) accessory connection. Additionally, lead V1 allows differentiation of posteroseptal accessory pathways into right-sided ones (retrograde P negative in V1) and left-sided ones (retrograde P positive in V1).

Catheter ablation procedures have recently also shed light into the ongoing debate about the anatomic course and the electrophysiologic properties of the so-called Mahaim fibers. Conventionally believed to arise in the AV node and to insert in the bundle branches and ventricular myocardium (nodofascicular/nodoventricular fiber), these anomalous connections give rise to antidromic (preexcited) reentrant tachycardia utilizing the Mahaim fiber in antegrade and the specific conduction system in retrograde direction. Preliminary reports have now provided strong evidence supporting the notion that the majority of clinically encountered Mahaim fibers, although indeed inserting in the vicinity of the right bundle branch, arise in the free wall aspect of the tricuspid valve ring and should therefore be considered atrioventricular. They exhibit antegrade-only decremental conduction properties, and the optimal target site for catheter ablation appears to be the endocardial breakthrough of the fiber beneath the tricuspid anulus.

Catheter ablation of an accessory AV fiber is indicated in all symptomatic patients, to avoid potentially fatal arrhythmia-related sequelae. It should be performed only in specialized centers by investigators with extensive experience in the electrophysiologic investigation of patients with this cardiac abnormality. In the asymptomatic patient, the decision to proceed with catheter ablation should be carefully weighed and probably advocated if an occupational hazard (e.g., airline pilot, athlete) is present.

AV Nodal Reentry Tachycardia

Radiofrequency current catheter ablation has not only led to new interest and insight into the pathophysiology of AVNRT, but also offers a new method to treat patients with this arrhythmia. In fact, the results of radiofrequency ablation have led to a dramatic change in therapy of AVNRT from a palliative approach with drugs to a curative approach. Two different techniques have been successfully used. The so-called anterior approach is used to modify or ablate fast pathway conduction. This technique is very similar to that used for complete interruption of AV nodal conduction in patients with AF. After recording His bundle activity, the ablation catheter is withdrawn anterosuperiorly to record a large atrial potential with no or only a minimal His bundle potential. Radiofrequency energy is titrated at this site starting at 10 W (up to 30 W) until junctional ectopic beats are recorded. To avoid high-degree AV nodal block, radiofrequency current application must be terminated as soon as no retrograde P wave can be recorded during junctional beats.

The results and complication rates for this technique are summarized in Table 12.2. The success rate is between 82–100%, with a risk of producing complete heart block of between 10–25%. In experienced hands, the success rate should be close to 100% and careful titration of energy may avoid a high incidence of third-degree AV block; but with the anterior approach to the fast pathway, the risk of total AV block still exists.

As an alternative, the "posterior" approach is aimed at modifying or ablating slow pathway conduction. It may be guided either by electrophysiologic landmarks or by purely anatomic criteria as judged from different radiographic views. The electrophysiologic approach introduced by Jackman et al. is based on the recording of a slow pathway activation potential. Believed to represent the atrial insertion of the slow AV nodal pathway, this potential is observed in the posteroseptal right atrium as a sharp bipolar deflection succeeding or preceding atrial activation during antegrade or retrograde slow pathway conduction, respectively. It can be recorded in the anterior, posterior, and inferior vicinity of the coronary sinus

Table 12.2
Success Rates and Complications in Catheter Ablation of A-VNRT[a]

	Success Rates (%)		Complications	
	FP	SP	FP	SP
Lee et al. (1991)	82		3/39	
Jazayeri et al. (1992)	100	97	4/19	0/35
Wu et al. (1992)	100	100	0/10	0/16
Jackman et al. (1992)		98		1/80
Haissaguerre et al. (1992)		100		0/64
Kay et al. (1992)	100	88	1/4	0/34

*a*FP, fast pathway; SP, slow pathway.

ostium, and sometimes even within the coronary sinus itself. Radiofrequency current is delivered at sites where such a potential is present.

Because the electrocardiographic characteristics of the slow pathway potential (morphology as well as timing with respect to the local atrial and ventricular potentials) and its presence or absence after radiofrequency current application are very different depending on the ablation center, the true nature of the potential is still under debate. Jackman et al. gave evidence by pacing techniques that the potential may indeed represent activity from the atrial insertion of the slow pathway. Because pacing techniques have not always been performed in subsequent publications by other authors, perhaps such potentials presented in those studies may represent a different type of electrical activity. The recording of such a potential may or may not be associated with successful slow pathway modification, and different origins of the potential cannot be excluded. In some instances, it may even represent activation from a dead-end pathway within the AV node. Indeed, we now know that such pathways exist in the anterior as well as the posterior AV node in the rabbit heart.

Different techniques have been reported for the "anatomic" posterior approach to slow pathway ablation/modification. In two studies, catheters placed at the bundle of His and inside the coronary sinus served as reference points marking the anterior and posterior border, respectively, of the triangle of Koch. Radiofrequency current was then applied at the tricuspid anulus, regardless of any pathway activation recordings, with the ablation catheter in a posteroseptal position. When current delivery at this site failed to modify or ablate slow pathway conduction, the catheter was gradually moved anteriorly along the tricuspid anulus toward the midseptal area, and current was applied at each successive site until AVNRT was no longer inducible. Other authors reported successful block of the slow pathway at its entrance to the Koch triangle by placing successive lesions between the tricuspid anulus and the coronary sinus ostium, moving the catheter from inferior (amplitude of ventricular activation exceeds that of atrial activation) to superior (amplitude of atrial activation exceeds that of ventricular activation).

Table 12.2 summarizes the results of the posterior approach. Regardless of the technique used—slow pathway potential recording or "anatomical"—the results are impressive. The success rate varies between 88–100%, with only a minimal incidence of inadvertent complete heart block (>1%). The risk of inducing third-degree AV block may be somewhat higher in inexperienced hands, but it will still be significantly lower than for the anterior approach, as long as the ablation catheter is kept in the posterior septal area, i.e., in the vicinity of the coronary sinus ostium. Catheter displacement toward the midseptal area may be associated with a higher incidence of total AV block.

Except for complete heart block, other complications in ablation of AVNRT are extremely rare. They consist mainly of complications due to catheter placement rather than to radiofrequency current application. However, it should not be forgotten that the induction of total AV block is a serious complication that should be avoided by all means, particularly in young patients. We therefore recommend using only the posterior approach. This approach may also be associated with the occurrence of junctional ectopic beats during radiofrequency current application. Current delivery must be interrupted immediately if loss of the retrograde P wave occurs, as this indicates conduction block in the fast pathway and, consequently, a catheter position dangerously close to the AV node. One should also be aware of the fact that total AV block may occur even if radiofrequency current is applied to the posterior region.

In patients with AVNRT in whom a sustained tachycardia can be induced during the ablation session, the endpoint of the study should be the inability to induce a sustained arrhythmia, even if single AV nodal echo beats remain inducible. There are patients in whom sustained AVNRT cannot be induced in the electrophysiology laboratory. Yet in these same patients, AVNRT is the suspected mechanism of the clinical tachycardia, based on surface ECG criteria, duality of AV nodal conduction curves, or single AV nodal echoes. In these cases the presence of a junctional ectopic arrhythmia during radiofrequency current application is our endpoint. The incidence of recurrences (>10% after 1 year) in this group is no different from those who have an inducible sustained tachycardia at the beginning of the study. Undoubtedly, the recurrence of AVNRT during follow-up necessitating a repeat attempt at catheter ablation is preferable to the inadvertent induction of total AV block, which requires permanent pacemaker implantation.

In general, radiofrequency current application to block either fast or slow pathway conduction has become the treatment of choice for patients with symptomatic AVNRT. It has almost totally replaced drug treatment in these patients. However, despite the euphoria regarding this revolutionary treatment, one should not forget that the follow-up in these patients is still limited to a few years. Thus, the long-term effects of such a procedure on AV nodal conduction is not yet known. Whether patients undergoing this technique will have a greater incidence of high-degree AV nodal block in later years compared with a normal population needs to be assessed.

Atrial Flutter

DIRECT CURRENT ABLATION

By delivering one to two direct current shocks in the "low posterior right atrial septal area," early investigators successfully treated patients with symptomatic and drug-refractory type I atrial flutter or at least achieved pharmacologic control. It is noteworthy that this technique offered an alternative therapeutic approach to AV node-His bundle ablation. However, because direct current shocks immediately restore sinus rhythm and its electric and barotraumatic effects cannot be precisely localized, the question has remained as to where exactly the critical site for ablation of atrial flutter is located.

RADIOFREQUENCY CURRENT ABLATION

Recent studies have provided evidence that discrete lesions produced by radiofrequency current in a relatively small area of endocardium can terminate and prevent recurrence of atrial flutter. This may be accomplished by current application either at the isthmus between the tricuspid annulus and the inferior vena cava, and/or at the isthmus between the tricuspid annulus and the coronary sinus os, provided that an exact entrainment pace map can be obtained from these areas. At successful sites, the recording of low-amplitude, fragmented, or double-spiked activation potentials preceding the P-wave onset by 20–50 msec suggests that a critical portion of the reentrant circuit is anatomically and electrophysiologically defined, which may account for the consistent morphology and rate of atrial flutter among all patients. However, the predictive value of these parameters for a successful radiofrequency pulse outcome is limited, as proved by the possibility of recording them at unsuccessful sites as well.

According to preliminary results based on rather small series and short follow-up periods, a successful outcome by radiofrequency current ablation technique in atrial flutter is achieved in a lower percentage of patients (60–75%) and by way of a higher median number of current applications as compared with accessory pathway-mediated tachycardias and AV nodal reentrant tachycardia. These findings suggest a fairly extended critical area of slow conduction and support a complex model of reentrant circuit sustaining atrial flutter. In this setting, cumulative energy applied at close sites within the critical area is likely to play an important role in favoring a successful outcome by this procedure; by inducing structural changes in the atrial substrate, previous pulses might also modify the morphology of the local activation potential, thus reducing its predictive value for a single pulse.

After the successful termination of atrial flutter by radiofrequency current ablation, late recurrences have been reported in 16–25% of cases over a follow-up period of 4–12 months. Furthermore, AF can be frequently recorded during extended follow-up. At present it is not clear whether its occurrence is a procedure-related late event or whether it reflects the natural progression of an atrial disease. Answering a number of still unsolved questions is likely to improve the clinical impact of radiofrequency current ablation in patients with atrial flutter. First, if a critical area of slow conduction exists in the atrial flutter reentrant circuit, and if it can be localized in the same or similar location among patients, its extent has not yet been precisely defined. It is also reasonable to assume that such an area might vary slightly from patient to patient, which render precise mapping difficult and subsequent pulse applications not effective enough in large series.

Second, more than one single critical area might be present in the reentrant circuit, thus favoring early or late recurrence after apparently successful applications. Third, radiofrequency current-induced lesions might create the conditions for a nearby area to assume the role of slow conduction in the reentrant circuit after ablation of the first such area. Finally, late pathophysiologic modification induced by electrocoagulation might result in a "new" substrate that itself could favor the recurrence of slow conduction in the same area, although through a different electrophysiologic conduction pattern.

In light of the complex mechanisms involved in the pathophysiology of atrial flutter, development of catheter mapping and ablation techniques appears to be a critical requisite before radiofrequency current ablation can have an impact comparable to that reported in the treatment of other reentrant tachycardias.

Atrial Fibrillation

DIRECT CURRENT ABLATION

Since the introduction of direct-current shock therapy in clinical practice from 1981, AV node-His bundle ablation has proved an effective palliative treatment in patients with drug-resistant AF. Patients with no or minimal heart disease are likely to benefit more than those with significant organic heart disease, but an improved quality of life, as defined by an improved stress capacity and the ability to return to work, is observed in the majority of cases. Relevant in-hospital complications have been documented after shock delivery, including postshock ventricular tachyarrhythmias, myocardial perforation, and pericardial effusion. In patients with organic heart disease, a 1.5% incidence of sudden death occurring 3 days to 6 months after direct current ablation has been reported.

RADIOFREQUENCY CURRENT ABLATION

Initial experimental and clinical studies have documented that incomplete AV nodal block could be induced by using radiofrequency energy. Modulation of antegrade conduction, as defined by a 50% increase of the baseline A-H interval, or a prolongation of Wenckebach cycle length exceeding 400 msec, could be obtained in 37% of cases. Although the clinical efficacy of this approach was maintained in only 13% of all patients during follow-up, these data provide evidence that AV nodal modulation may represent an alternative approach to ablation in selected patients with drug-refractory atrial tachyarrhythmias. The success rate of total AV nodal ablation, which is presently approximately 90% with a right-sided approach, can be further improved by a complementary left-sided approach performed during the same session. With the aim of modifying the antegrade conduction properties, attempts have been performed to deliver radiofrequency current to the anterosuperior anatomic input to the AV node in a large series of patients.

Atrial Tachycardia

Similar to atrial flutter, precise localization of an arrhythmogenic focus in atrial tachycardias requires a three-dimensional map and, unlike accessory AV pathways, lacks the support of reliable electrogram markers. However, because of the small extension of the focus, atrial tachycardias appear more suitable to definitive cure by radiofrequency current ablation than does atrial flutter.

Preliminary data on small patient groups confirm that radiofrequency current ablation can effectively eliminate atrial tachycardias in 80–100% of cases. At ablation sites, local atrial activation during tachycardia may precede the onset of P wave by up to 60 msec; in one series, a clear distinction was found in this interval between ectopic atrial tachycardia (0 to –50 msec) and reentrant atrial tachycardia, as defined by its easy inducibility and termination during programmed electrical stimulation (–70—120 msec). In addition to earliest local atrial activation, mechanical block of tachycardia induced during catheter manipulation and rapid termination within less than 10 seconds of the beginning of radiofrequency application are good predictors of definitive abolition of these arrhythmias. Local atrial activation potentials do not appear to show any unique morphology at successful sites.

During atrial mapping, coronary sinus recording does not appear to be a reliable substitute for direct atrial mapping if the ectopic atrial tachycardia involves a site other than the right atrial appendage. In such cases, direct atrial recording can be achieved through a catheter advanced in the left atrium via a patent foramen ovale or a transseptal puncture.

No procedure-related complications have been reported so far, although application of radiofrequency current in close proximity to the sinus node, as required in sinus node tachycardia, can be associated with transient depression of sinus node function. In case of recurrence during follow-up, as observed in 10–20% of cases, repeated attempts can be safely performed in a subsequent session.

In patients with ventricular dysfunction, elimination of atrial tachycardia leads to immediate relief of symptoms, followed by progressive improvement of ventricular function, which usually normalizes over weeks to months. Because of the promising results observed in preliminary series and the unsatisfying control of cardiac rhythm by antiarrhythmic drugs, radiofrequency current ablation may became the therapy of choice in atrial tachycardia.

VENTRICULAR TACHYCARDIA

Clinical Role of Catheter Ablation for Ventricular Tachycardia

The availability of radiofrequency energy sources together with use of newer steerable catheters have greatly altered our therapeutic approach to the management of patients with ventricular tachycardia. Use of ablative procedures has proven exceedingly safe and effective for patients with ventricular tachycardia without cardiac disease. These include patients with tachycardia emanating from the right ventricular outflow tract as well as those with left septal tachycardia.

In patients with myocardial ventricular tachycardia, either due to coronary artery or myocardial disease, catheter ablation is reserved for patients with sustained, virtually incessant ventricular tachycardia of one morphology, particularly those patients who fail drug therapy and are not considered optimal candidates for surgical ablation of the ventricular tachycardia focus. Optimal candidates for surgery include those patients with well-preserved left ventricular function, those with single ventricular foci located in the anteroapical area, and patients who require revascularization or valve repair. Patients with virtual incessant ventricular tachycardia are not candidates for defibrillator therapy because they would be exposed to repeated shocks.

Our experience increasingly demonstrates that patients with myocardial ventricular tachycardia, particularly those with a single focus who prove refractory to drug therapy, can be considered for catheter ablative therapy. The use of radiofrequency energy has significantly diminished the risk and hence allows for repeated attempts at ablative therapy. Recent advances in ablative techniques have mandated that the clinician integrate use of these techniques in the management of patients with ventricular tachycardia. Future advances will in large measure depend on development of multiple electrode array catheters, allowing for simultaneous recordings from multiple endocardial sites. In addition, development of newer energy sources allowing for a wider zone of myocardial ablation may be required for the successful cure of patients with myocardial ventricular tachycardia due to coronary artery disease or cardiomyopathic processes.

Myocardial Ventricular Tachycardia in Coronary Artery Disease

The most frequent cause of sustained ventricular tachycardia is that associated with coronary artery disease. Both canine experimental observations as well as clinical reports support the presence of intramyocardial reentry as the basis for this arrhythmia. Initial attempts to locate the ventricular tachycardia focus at cardiac catheterization involved positioning of the catheter during ventricular tachycardia in order to find the earliest endocardial potential relative to the surface complexes.

At present, newer mapping techniques have been introduced to better locate the ventricular tachycardia focus. One technique involves pace mapping, as described below. In addition, entrainment mapping has been found to be effective. This technique may be used in two ways. First, an area remote from the tachycardia is paced, and the tachycardia is entrained to the paced cycle length. With termination of pacing, the putative early site again appears prior to inscription of the surface QRS. Another technique, introduced by Morady et al., involves pacing directly from the putative ventricular tachycardia site. Successful pacing from this area will show a long interval from stimulus to surface QRS, with a QRS complex identical to that during ventricular tachycardia. This technique, designated concealed entrainment, is explained by direct pacing from within the critical slow zone of the ventricular tachycardia circuit. The impulse is conducted orthodromically with an obligate delay owing to slowed conduction within the circuit itself. Others have emphasized the importance of finding middiastolic potentials during ventricular tachycardia. These potentials are thought to emanate from the tachycardia circuit. Once the putative critical slow conduction zone of the reentrant circuit is identified, radiofrequency energy is applied to desiccate this focus. It should be emphasized that mapping techniques are crucial to successful identification of the ventricular tachycardia site. Activation mapping (finding the earliest endocardial potential relative to the surface ECG during ventricular tachycardia) identifies the presumed exit site of the ventricular tachycardia. Because in clinical situations multiple electrode mapping is not available, one is never certain whether the true earliest site has been recorded. Pace mapping that reliably mimics the spontaneous ventricular tachycardia morphology is another technique for identifying the ventricular tachycardia exit site. Unfortunately, the dense scarring associated with infarction ventricular tachycardia may make the infarct zone unexcitable or may produce similar maps from areas several centimeters from the true site of origin. In contrast, identification of middiastolic potentials (during ventricular tachycardia) or use of concealed entrainment serves to identify the critical zone of slow conduction. Which of these techniques is preferable for proper identification of the critical site for successful ablation remains unclear.

Prior reports using high-energy direct current shocks for catheter ablation have been reviewed. For the most part, only limited reports are available concerning use of radiofrequency energy for patients with ventricular tachycardia. It is clear that because radiofrequency lesions can be repeatedly applied with greater safety, the efficacy of this approach might exceed that reported for direct current ablation. One of the largest series of patients with ventricular tachycardia due to coronary artery disease treated with radiofrequency ablation included 15 highly selected patients with ventricular tachycardia. These patients had a total of 20 ventricular tachycardia forms. Patients proved resistant to at least two antiarrhythmic agents, and the mean ventricular tachycardia cycle length was 438 ±82 msec. They described successful ablation in 11 of 15 (75%) of the patients, with a mean follow-up of 9.1 ±3.3 months. The successfully treated patients were maintained on antiarrhythmic agents. Interestingly, these authors used a variety of mapping techniques. They either targeted the exit site of ventricular tachycardia (i.e., endocardial activation mapping or pace mapping) or the critical slow zone of the ventricular tachycardia circuit (i.e., middiastolic potentials or concealed entrainment). It is difficult to draw definitive conclusions from this small and selected patient group, because patients had to be hemodynamically stable in order to allow for the extensive mapping required. Moreover, less than 10% of the patients seen at this center for sustained ventricular arrhythmias proved to be suitable candidates for ablation.

Although the available experience using radiofrequency ablation for selected patients with ventricular tachycardia appears promising, the results are clearly not as effective as those described for surgical ablation of ventricular tachycardia in patients with coronary artery disease. A variety of reasons might explain the disparity of results. First, the volume of tissue excised at surgery (40–60 mm^2) far exceeds that which is destroyed by ablative procedures (i.e., 2–4 mm^2). Experimental as well as clinical observations suggest that the ventricular tachycardia circuit may be quite large. In addition, the ventricular tachycardia circuit often involves intramyocardial as well as epicardial regions and is not exclusively confined to the subendocardial regions.

Nevertheless, the available data suggest that radiofrequency ablation may be fruitfully used in patients with frequent or incessant ventricular tachycardia, inasmuch as these patients may not be suitable candidates for defibrillator therapy. Successful ablation of the dominant ventricular tachycardia focus may, therefore, significantly simplify the medical regimen. In addition, it is reassuring that, to date, no significant complications have been reported for catheter ablation of patients with ventricular tachycardia associated with coronary artery disease.

Bundle Branch Reentry Tachycardia

Bundle branch reentrant tachycardia is a form of ventricular tachycardia involving the specialized intraventricular conduction system. The mechanism usually involves antegrade conduction over the right bundle branch with retrograde conduction over the left bundle. The converse may be rarely observed. Bundle branch reentrant tachycardia occurs almost exclusively in patients with either severe myocardial disease or in those with significant disease of the specialized intraventricular conduction system. The incidence of bundle branch reentrant tachycardia appears to be higher in patients with idiopathic cardiomyopathy compared to those with ischemic heart disease.

The salient electrophysiologic features include induction of a tachycardia with left bundle branch block contour with an H-V interval ≤ the H-V during sinus rhythm. In addition, variation in the H-H interval that precedes variation in the ventricular cycle length excludes ventricular tachycardia of myocardial origin. Registration of the right bundle branch potential is of paramount importance, because this structure is an obligate portion of the tachycardia circuit. During bundle branch reentrant tachycardia, the interval from the right bundle deflection to the onset of ventricular activation shortens. This finding effectively excludes a supraventricular mechanism.

A steerable electrode catheter with a 4-mm distal electrode tip is advanced to the usual His bundle position. The catheter is then advanced over the summit of the right ventricular septum to record a right bundle branch potential. Once located, radiofrequency energy of 40 W is applied for 60 seconds to destroy the right bundle branch. This technique is usually readily successful because the main right bundle branch is draped superficially over the right side of the septum. In our experience, we have found that isolated destruction of the right bundle branch does not necessarily require permanent pacemaker insertion. The most important caveat in terms of appropriate management of these patients is exclusion of the presence of concomitant myocardial ventricular tachycardia, which in our experience occurs in approximately 30% of patients with bundle branch reentrant tachycardia.

Right Ventricular Outflow Tract Ventricular Tachycardia

A group of patients without known heart disease but who are afflicted with ventricular tachycardia emanating from the right ventricular outflow tract has been well described. In these patients, the tachycardia is often exercise- or isopro-terenol-induced and shows a left bundle branch block and inferior axis pattern on surface ECG recordings. These tachycardias may be interrupted by either carotid sinus massage or infusions of adenosine and are thought to be caused by abnormal automaticity or afterdepolarizations. The technique we use for ablation of these tachycardias involves placement of the ablation catheter into the pulmonary artery and gentle withdrawal of the catheter in order to map all margins of the right ven-tricular outflow tract. Activation mapping is of limited help because the earliest endocardial site is only 30–40 msec earlier than the surface recordings. The most reliable mapping technique appears to be use of the paced map, with 100% con-cordance between paced and spontaneous ventricular tachycardia for all 12-leads. Once this area is identified, radiofrequency energy is applied, as described earlier, to destroy the focus.

In the largest experience to date using radiofrequency ablation for ablation of ventricular tachycardia arising from the right ventricular outflow tract. The authors demonstrated a very high success rate (90%) in ablation of tachycardia located in this region without significant complications. These results are supported by our own experience showing a comparable success rate in 20 consecutive patients stud-ied. The most serious side effect observed in our experience was development of tamponade due to perforation of the right ventricular outflow tract. This complica-tion required emergency thoracotomy for closure of the wound.

Idiopathic Left Septal Ventricular Tachycardia

Another type of ventricular tachycardia seen in patients without apparent car-diac disease arises from the posteroinferior aspect of the left septum. These tachy-cardias show a characteristic right bundle branch block and superior axis morphology. They appear to be reentrant in origin in that they can be readily pro-voked and terminated by standard pacing procedures. The unusual features of this tachycardia include the ability to induce the tachycardia from the atrium (in marked distinction from myocardial ventricular tachycardia in patients with coro-nary artery disease). In addition, these tachycardias are often sensitive to infusions of verapamil.

Patients with this form of tachycardia may be treated with either a retrograde aortic approach or with a transseptal approach. The rationale is to carefully explore the inferoposterior portion of the left side of the ventricular septum. This often requires looping the catheter against the lateral wall of the left ventricle and directing its tip toward the septum. The tachycardia is induced using standard pac-ing techniques with or without isoproterenol, and endocardial mapping is used to identify the earliest endocardial activation site. Once the latter is found, the tech-nique of pace mapping, as described previously, is used to identify the ventricular tachycardia exit site. Ablative lesions using radiofrequency energy are applied to destroy the reentrant circuit.

We have successfully ablated left septal ventricular tachycardia foci in six of seven consecutive patients. As with patients with right ventricular outflow tract ventricular tachycardia, the importance of pace mapping is emphasized for proper location of the ventricular tachycardia focus. In only one of the seven was the focus located in the anterior septal region. The cause of failure in one patient is not evident, but she is presently controlled with high-dose verapamil therapy. The only complication observed in our series was the development of aortic insufficiency in one patient due to repeated manipulation of the catheter across the aortic valve. The aortic insufficiency was mild (by echocardiographic assessment), and no specific therapy was required.

SUGGESTED READING

Calkins H, Sousa J, Rosenheck S, et al. Diagnosis and cure of the Wolff-Parkinson-White syndrome or paroxysmal supraventricular tachycardias during a single electrophysiologic test. N Engl J Med 1991;324:1612–1618.

Evans GT, Scheinman MM, Zipes DP, et al. The Percutaneous Cardiac Mapping and Ablation Registry: final summary of results. PACE 1988;11:1621–1626.

Feld GK, Fleck RP, Chen PS, et al. Radiofrequency catheter ablation for the treatment of human type-I atrial flutter. Identification of a critical zone in the reentrant circuit by endocardial mapping technique. Circulation 1992;86:1233–1240.

Jackman WM, Beckman KJ, McClelland JH, et al. Treatment of supraventricular tachycardia due to atrioventricular nodal reentry by radiofrequency catheter ablation of slow-pathway conduction. N Engl J Med 1992;327:313–318.

Jackman WM, Wang X, Friday KJ, et al. Catheter ablation of accessory atrioventricular pathways (Wolff-Parkinson-White syndrome) by radiofrequency current. N Engl J Med 1991;324:1605–1611.

Kay GN, Chong F, Epstein AE, Dailey SM, Plumb VJ. Radiofrequency ablation of primary atrial tachycardias. J Am Coll Cardiol 1993; 21:901–909.

Klein LS, Shih HT, Hackett FK, Zipes DP, Miles WM. Radiofrequency catheter ablation of ventricular tachycardia in patients without structural heart disease. Circulation 1992; 85: 1666–1674.

Lee MA, Morady F, Kadish A, et al. Catheter modification of the atrioventricular junction with radiofrequency energy for control of atrioventricular nodal reentry tachycardia. Circulation 1991;83:827–835.

Lesh MD, Van Hare GF, Scheinman MM, Ports TA, Epstein LA. Comparison of the retrograde and transseptal methods for ablation of left free wall accessory pathways. J Am Coll Cardiol 1993;22:542–549.

Tchou P, Jazayeri M, Denker S, Dongas J, Caceres J, Akhtar M. Transcatheter electrical ablation of the right bundle branch: a method of treating macroreentrant ventricular tachycardia attributed to bundle branch reentry. Circulation 1988;78:246–257.

13 Implantable Cardioverter-Defibrillator: Indications and Outcomes

INDICATIONS

In an attempt to guide physicians in selecting patients for implantable cardioverter-defibrillator (ICD) therapy, two separate consensus groups have published similar guidelines. One of these was organized by the American College of Cardiology (ACC) and the American Heart Association (AHA), and the other by the North American Society of Pacing and Electrophysiology (NASPE). The wording of the indications by the different committees was slightly different, but the substance was similar. In each case the indications were divided into three categories:

1. Class I: ICD is indicated by general consensus;
2. Class II: ICD is an option but there is no consensus; and
3. Class III: ICD therapy is generally not justified.

Class I Indications

1. A patient with ventricular tachycardia (VT) or ventricular fibrillation (VF) in whom electrophysiologic testing or Holter monitoring cannot be used to predict efficacy of therapy. This indication is intended to include the patient who is noninducible at electrophysiologic study (EPS).
2. A patient with recurrent VT or VF despite drug therapy as guided by EPS testing or Holter monitoring. This indication includes the patient who failed an antiarrhythmic drug that was predicted effective by EPS or Holter monitoring.
3. A patient with spontaneous VT or VF in whom drugs are not tolerated. This indication includes patients with an adverse drug effect or poor compliance.
4. A patient with VT or VF who remains persistently inducible. There are no qualifications in terms of the number of drug trials, the rate of the VT on drugs, or hemodynamic stability during VT.

Class II Indications

1. A patient with syncope of uncertain cause and with sustained VT or VF induced at EPS in whom drugs are not tolerated, ineffective, or not taken.

Class III Contraindications

1. A patient with sustained VT or VF due to acute myocardial ischemia, acute myocardial infarction (MI), or metabolic/toxic etiologies that are reversible.
2. A patient with recurrent syncope of uncertain cause who is not inducible to any ventricular arrhythmia.

196

3. A patient with incessant VT or VF that cannot be controlled with antiar-rhythmic drugs such that device firing might be frequent.
4. A patient with VF secondary to Wolff-Parkinson-White syndrome.
5. A patient with medical, surgical, or psychiatric contraindications.

It is noteworthy that these clinical indications and contraindications are within the guidelines set by the FDA in 1985. These guidelines are flexible and grant the practicing physician a certain amount of latitude in selecting suitable candidates for device therapy. They allow for placement of the ICD as a means of secondary prevention, as in the case of the survivor of cardiac arrest secondary to VT/VF.

Not included within the indications are various clinical criteria that would ordi-narily be addressed by the implanting physician. First, there is nothing within the guidelines that specifically require the patients to undergo coronary angiography in order to assess the potential need for revascularization. Implicit within the guidelines is that the malignant rhythm is not secondary to an acute myocardial ischemic event. Second, the best prognostic factor in selecting patients at high risk for sudden cardiac death (SCD) is left ventricular ejection fraction (LVEF). The LVEF in conjunction with electrophysiologic testing allows for the selection of patients who are less likely to benefit from pharmacologic therapy.

The group of patients with reduced LVEF who have no history of a serious arrhythmia but in whom an arrhythmia is induced by electrophysiologic testing is not mentioned within the guidelines. This is of particular importance for patients with nonischemic dilated congestive cardiomyopathy with diminished LVEF, because it is well recognized that up to 50% of these patients eventually succumb to SCD, despite what appears to be effective antiarrhythmic drug therapy by EPS. Third, the guidelines were drawn up before the general availability of third-gen-eration ICDs for use in patients with hemodynamically stable VT that is pace-ter-minable. As devices become available with new functions, indications may need to be revised, expanded, or altered to allow more appropriate utilization.

Nevertheless, the relatively broad nature of the indications have made possible several prospective primary prevention studies. There are three major clinical tri-als that are currently exploring this expanded role for the ICD. They are called Coronary Artery Bypass Grafting-Patch (CABG-Patch), the Multicenter Automatic Defibrillator Implantation Trial (MADIT), and the Multicenter Unsustained Tachycardia Trial (MUSTT). These trials have many similar features. All three are large, multicenter, and have a randomized, prospective design. All three enroll patients who are at high risk of suffering VT/VF as defined by having known coronary artery disease, a low EF (<40% at least, although criteria differ), and some marker of electrical instability (either a positive signal averaged ECG and/or inducibility at EPS). Patients eligible for the CABG-Patch trial must be candidates for elective aortocoronary bypass surgery, have an EF <36%, and a pos-itive signal averaged ECG. The MADIT Trial eligibility criteria are somewhat more complex. Patients are eligible for randomization if they have coronary artery disease, an EF <36%, and have asymptomatic nonsustained VT on monitor.

Patients at EPS who are inducible into sustained VT and not suppressed with intravenous procainamide are then randomized either to "traditional" therapy (as defined by the investigator) or to an ICD implant; since 1993, ICDs with nonthoracotomy lead systems have been used in the trial. The MUSTT eligibility criteria are similar to the MADIT criteria. Patients must have coronary artery disease, an EF <40%, and be asymptomatic or minimally symptomatic due to nonsustained VT. Patients are randomized based on their inducibility at EPS. The three study protocols vary, and a proportion of each study population will be randomized to ICD therapy. All three trials have total cardiac mortality as an endpoint and SCD as a secondary endpoint. Each trial will evaluate the role, if any, of the ICD in reducing sudden and total cardiac mortality in the patient groups studied. Both CABG-Patch and MUSTT are funded by the National Heart, Lung, and Blood Institute. The results of these trials will not be available until at least 1996. The impact of these trials on clinical care will be enormous if benefit is derived from the ICD in (patients such as those enrolled in) the Multicenter Automatic Defibrillator Intervention Trial (MADIT), Multicenter Unsustained Tachycardia Trial (MUSTT), CABG Patch Trial, Dilated Cardiomyopathy Trial (CAT), and Defibrillator Implantation as Bridge to Later Transplantation (DEFIBRILAT). It is likely that future ICD implantation guidelines will take into account the results of these studies as well as the technologic advances in devices.

The indications for ICD therapy may also change as the technology is applied to atrial arrhythmias. There is a burgeoning experimental experience in atrial fibrillation (AF), for example, with the hope of ultimately developing a stand-alone atrial defibrillator. Several technological issues will need to be considered before this can be deemed practical for clinical investigation. Patient discomfort must be minimized, and there must be no chance of provoking a malignant ventricular arrhythmia or heart block with an intraatrial shock. This is an especially important consideration given the non-life-threatening nature of almost all cases of AF and the potential for frequent rhythm reversions. Development of unique lead systems for energy delivery is a critical feature of this research effort.

CLINICAL OUTCOME

Despite attempts through community education and public policy, proportionately few patients are successfully resuscitated from SCD without at least some major morbidity. Survivors of cardiac arrest typically have diminished LVEF and in most cases there is coronary artery disease or a dilated cardiomyopathy. These patients have a very high risk of recurrent cardiac arrest with resultant death if left untreated. Also, given the extent of the underlying cardiac disease and LV dysfunction and the frequent presence of comorbid illnesses, such as hypertension and diabetes mellitus, it is apparent that they are also at increased risk of nonarrhythmic cardiac death as well as noncardiac death.

The success of the ICD in diminishing SCD has been reported in numerous nonrandomized reports. Coupled with the potentially deleterious effects of antiarrhythmic drugs and the relative novelty of ablative therapy—with its limited success and applicability—ICD therapy has been touted as the treatment of choice for patients at risk for SCD. Recently, however, critics of ICD therapy have noted the absence of prospective, randomized, multicenter trials documenting the safety and efficacy of nonpharmacologic over pharmacologic therapy. These critics argue that the previously reported studies may have overestimated the overall clinical efficacy of the ICD. The current debate within the cardiology community is whether such a clinical trial is indeed necessary to better assess the presumed mortality reduction among those receiving a device compared to the outcome in those receiving drugs.

Conversely, there are those who believe that because the ICD has so dramatically decreased SCD in cardiac arrest survivors, randomizing patients to an alternate form of therapy would be unethical and not justifiable simply to gain a scientific perspective. Furthermore, the technology of the devices is progressing so rapidly that the results of a randomized trial may not be applicable to future implantation techniques or devices. For example, one would expect lower morbidity and mortality for nonthoracotomy ICD implantation to improve as better lead systems and generators become available. To fully appreciate the impact on total mortality of antiarrhythmic drugs versus implantable devices, the National Heart, Lung, and Blood Institute has commenced a prospective, randomized, controlled study called AVID (Antiarrhythmic Drugs versus Implantable Devices) that will randomly assign survivors of cardiac arrest to implantation of a nonthoracotomy ICD or to therapy with drugs (amiodarone or sotalol).

In assessing the clinical outcome of ICD recipients, it is essential to include operative risk as well as the results of long-term therapy, including all causes of death. The remaining portion of this section addresses these issues.

Operative Morbidity and Mortality

Despite technological advances and evolving surgical techniques, implantation of the ICD carries with it operative risk. Operative mortality with a thoracotomy approach is approximately 3%, compared with 1% with a nonthoracotomy implant. The decrease in risk with nonthoracotomy lead systems has been one factor supporting the position of those currently advocating the use of the ICD in prospective studies of high-risk patients who have not had an arrhythmic event and for those patients who have an unacceptable surgical risk with thoracotomy. Eventually, the use of smaller devices placed in the pectoral region will most likely further improve outcome and reduce implant risk.

Several factors are known to contribute to operative risk: surgical approach (thoracotomy more than nonthoracotomy), advanced age, concomitant cardiac surgery, comorbid illness, poor LVEF, and class IV NYHA status. In one study, the operative mortality was 0% in patients with a LVEF of >30% and 5.1% in those with an LVEF of <30%. In another, there was a 42% operative mortality in patients with class IV heart failure, pointing out that, as in many other clinical situations, functional status may be a much more important risk variable than the measured ejection fraction.

The most serious postoperative complication is ICD system infection, which occurs in 1–5% of implants. It typically presents insidiously within the first 1–2 months postoperatively but, when discovered, demands immediate attention. There is typically ICD pocket swelling, erythema, and tenderness without associated fever, leukocytosis, or bacteremia. Subcutaneous tracking via the leads is common and may lead to sepsis and distant organ seeding. Total ICD system explanation is usually required to eradicate the infection.

Other postoperative complications associated with the thoracotomy approach to implantation are pericarditis (commonly subclinical), mild atelectasis, and paroxysmal AF. Other uncommon complications include deep vein thrombosis, lead migration or dislodgement, or pneumonia. Rare complications include cardiac tamponade, cerebrovascular accident, and MI.

Another serious complication in postthoracotomy patients is exacerbation of ventricular arrhythmias. This occurs quite frequently, typically within 2 weeks of surgery, and accounts for over 40% of the postoperative deaths. The postoperative arrhythmias of 46 patients who had epicardial lead ICD or nonthoracotomy lead ICD implant are depicted in Figure 13.1. A likely mechanism for VT/VF in this setting is the pericarditis associated with epicardial patch placement. Unfortunately, some of these deaths occurred in patients whose devices had been deactivated in the immediate postoperative period to avoid inappropriate and/or frequent device discharges secondary to AF or nonsustained VT. The incidence of arrhythmia aggravation has decreased substantially with the increased use of transvenous lead systems.

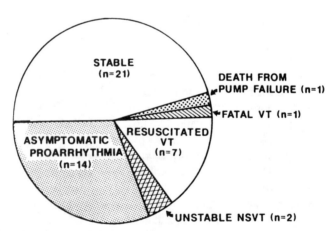

Figure 13.1. Clinical course of 46 patients who underwent implantation of an ICD without concomitant surgery. Forty-three had epicardial leads placed and three had a nonthoracotomy system. Asymptomatic proarrhythmia is defined as a 7-fold increase in ventricular ectopy in asymptomatic stable patients. NSVT, nonsustained VT. (From Kim SG, Fisher JD, Furman S, et al. Exacerbation of ventricular arrhythmias during the postoperative period after implantation of an automatic defibrillator. J Am Coll Cardiol 1992;18:1200–1206.)

Clinical Efficacy

Clinical studies have proven conclusively that the ICD is capable of terminating VT/VF. This has been the case with VT/VF induced during initial implantations, pulse generator replacements, or in the electrophysiology (EP) laboratory, and with electrocardiographically documented spontaneous arrhythmia. This finding probably reflects the remarkable stability of the defibrillation threshold when measured in several different clinical situations.

To best demonstrate the efficacy of the ICD in the absence of a randomized study, a variety of methods for presenting survival data have emerged. In the earliest studies of clinical outcome, ICD recipients were compared with historical controls from the same or different institutions. Mirowski first utilized this type of analysis to demonstrate a 52% reduction in overall mortality. The principal limitations in these studies include disparities in baseline characteristics, including cardiac substrate, left ventricular function, coronary anatomy, and concomitant therapy.

Some studies have reported the long-term outcome of patient populations with respect to SCD and overall mortality (Table 13.1). These are not controlled, prospective, randomized groups, however. The patients in these studies were at high risk in that they had diminished LVEF, survived a cardiac arrest, and may have had inducible but not suppressed VT/VF. The unifying feature of these studies is that they all demonstrated a low SCD incidence in patients with the ICD. Some investigators have chosen to examine the issue of outcome as a function of the severity of underlying heart disease. A commonly used and easily measured marker is left ventricular ejection fraction. When patients receiving an ICD are stratified by LVEF, patients with better function tend to have a more favorable outcome.

Another method of assessing ICD efficacy entails utilization of an "appropriate discharge" as a surrogate endpoint, with the supposition that the discharge represents an episode of SCD that was aborted. Appropriate discharges typically are defined as those occurring with premonitory presyncope, syncope, or during sleep, if an electrocardiogram (ECG) is not recorded at the time. This allows for comparison of the actual observed mortality with that of the appropriate discharge, aborted SCD, or expected mortality. Several studies have evaluated the incidence of shock occurrence and their relationship to actual mortality. In one study, the actual versus expected incidence of survival at 1, 2, and 3 years was 97%, 90%, and 85% versus 59%, 39%, and 31%, respectively. Studies such as this suggest a tremendous survival advantage for ICD recipients. A notable limitation is the inability to definitively equate an appropriate discharge with SCD, because the discharge may have been spurious, prompted by hemodynamically stable VT, a self-terminating nonsustained VT, or even supraventricular tachycardia. Moreover, it is not certain that even if the shock were appropriate, the arrhythmia would have resulted in death. Lastly, the implantation of the ICD and the subsequent increase in arrhythmia could have resulted in an arrhythmia that might not have occurred without the ICD. Many investigatores have called into question the reliability of shock analysis as a surrogate for outcome. They point out that the occurrence of any kind of shock does not necessarily correlate with an increased

Table 13.1
Clinical Outcome of ICD Patients

Study	Patients	Mean Follow-up (years)	Mean EF (%)	SCD (%)	Cardiac Death (%)	Total Death (%)
Veltri et al., 1992	403	2.5	35	4	23	30
Winkle et al., 1989	270	?	34	2.6	11	15
Grimm et al., 1993	241	2.1	31	7	21	30
Axtell et al., 1991	200	2.3	36	3	8.5	17
Powell et al., 1993	150	2.0	35	3	13	19
Fogoros et al., 1990	119	1.8	?	2.5	11	12
Palatianos et al., 1991	111	2.8	33	2.7	15	18

mortality risk. Advanced devices now have stored memory for data logging and bipolar electrograms during events, which will enable better interpretation of clinical events.

Yet another means by which clinical efficacy has been reported is via retrospective case control study. Utilizing this approach, 60 patients treated with an ICD and 120 patients treated with best drug, which in many cases was amiodarone, were compared. The patients were matched via five variables known to be predictive of outcome: age, LVEF, presenting arrhythmia, underlying heart disease, and drug therapy. This study demonstrated not only a clear reduction in SCD but also a significant reduction in overall mortality in ICD recipients. At 3 years, the total mortality was 51% in case controls versus 35% in ICD recipients, P<.01. The strength of the case control method in this study was the selection of important variables for matching. The key weakness is the potential that other variables could have biased ICD therapy to a healthier population, which would account for the differences in overall outcome. This is not unexpected in ICD clinical use because surgical risk is predicated on the same factors that influence mortality risk.

Results of two studies reporting on concurrent unmatched, nonrandomized groups of patients who accepted versus those who declined ICD therapy have yielded disparate results. One of these reported that the survival of patients declining ICD therapy was significantly lower compared with patients who accepted therapy. These results held for SCD, cardiac death, and all-cause death when compared with patients who had accepted ICD implantation during an 8-year cumulative experience at one institution. After a mean follow-up of 2 years, 65% of patients discharged without an ICD were dead, with approximately 50% succumbing to SCD. The other study, however, reporting on a smaller population followed over a shorter period of time, found no significant difference in survival at 18 months (84% with and 78% without ICD).

In 1987, the first prospective, multicenter, randomized controlled study in survivors of cardiac arrest documented to be secondary to ventricular tachyarrhythmias was initiated (Cardiac Arrest Study of Hamburg). This study seeks to compare the incidence of SCD, cardiac, and total mortality among four treatment groups: propafenone, metoprolol, amiodarone, and ICD. The study's primary endpoints include total mortality and cardiac arrest rates in ICD and drug-treated patients. Enrollment continues in this important study and the final results should be available soon. A preliminary report suggested an increased mortality with propafenone, but no significant treatment advantage for device therapy versus the other drug therapies.

Cost Effectiveness and Quality of Life

The cost effectiveness of device therapy has been explored in several ways. In an early study, Medicare information from 1984, including hospital expenses and the cost of rehospitalization, was analyzed. The net cost was $17,100 per life-year saved in a high-risk patient population, with a predicted further reduction to $7,400 per life-year saved with the advent of devices that had greater longevity, and programmability, and that could be implanted without thoracotomy. Another analysis considered the issue of early implantation versus sequencing the implant after unsuccessful drug therapy, and concluded that there could be a considerable cost savings if the ICD was implanted earlier, in addition to a substantial savings in hospital days. In addition, these savings could be extended with the availability of nonthoracotomy systems. Another study compared the costs of the ICD with amiodarone and conventional antiarrhythmic therapy. It found an increased life expectancy with the ICD but with a higher associated cost. However, the study concluded that the $13,800–$29,200 cost per year of life saved was reasonable and comparable to other medical interventions, especially if ICD therapy was found to be associated with a better quality of life. Additional savings can probably be generated by using a nonthoracotomy lead system, although some of those gains might be eroded by a prolonged length of stay. It is important to emphasize that, as consistent as these data are, they are not completely reliable because these issues have never been examined in a large prospective, randomized study. AVID has been designed to include a cost assessment that should help in determining the relative value of drug versus device therapy of patients with malignant ventricular arrhythmia. These analyses will need to assess not only the costs of the initial hospitalization, but also the cost of subsequent hospitalization, medications, and adverse outcomes from device or drug therapy.

Another major issue in considering the ICD as primary therapy for patients with VT/VF is quality of life. Although a few reports have painted an optimistic picture of patients who receive a device, most authorities believe that many of these patients are susceptible to psychological trauma. One study found a high level of anxiety and anger in patients who received devices, although this was reduced after the first 6 months, perhaps because of diminishing shock rates over time. Others have found that the ICD had no significant impact on patients' psyches because all patients with life-threatening arrhythmias were anxious and depressed with any therapy. Some of this may come as a result of severe limitations in activities that are frequently imposed on these patients, such as restrictions on operating an automobile. Severe sleep disturbances have been reported in patients with devices, giving rise to dream shocks that caused considerable psychological upheaval in some. These problems are very important because they can significantly affect such important life-style issues as return to work and productivity. Whether modern ICD therapy, especially with nonthoracotomy lead systems, will have a positive impact on quality of life is unknown. This question will also be studied in AVID, which will consider quality of life within the context of the patient's overall medical and cardiac condition.

FIRST-GENERATION ICDS

The first-generation device, the automatic implantable defibrillator (AID), was first implanted in February 1980, after years of development in the animal laboratory by its inventors Michel Mirowski and Morton Mower. It sensed arrhythmias using a transcardiac (superior vena caval spring electrode to left ventricular apical epicardial patch) modified bipolar electrocardiographic signal. It weighed 250 g, delivered shocks of 25 and 30 J, and had a total discharge capability of 100 shocks.

This first device employed a relatively crude density algorithm called the probability detection function (PDF) for arrhythmia sensing. It had no cardioverting capability. The PDF, which is a histogram of the time spent by the ventricular electrogram signal on the isoelectric line, was good at detecting VF but not VT. Despite these limitations in arrhythmia sensing, the initial clinical results with the AID device were very positive. Of the first 52 patients receiving the AID between 1980 and 1982, 33% received successful defibrillating shocks. There was an actual 1-year SCD mortality of 8.5% and all cause mortality of 22.9%. The expected (i.e., calculated by assuming those patients who received a shock would have died without an AID) 1-year SCD rate was 48%. Although these statistical assumptions have been challenged, the remarkable clinical efficacy of the AID device was apparent from the outset. Subsequent iterations of the first-generation ICD added improvements such as bipolar endocardial or epicardial electrode rate counting and VT cardioverting capabilities. The devices could also be ordered from the manufacturer with customized rate cut-offs above or below the nominal, fixed value of approximately 150–155 bpm. However, the devices remained large in size and nonprogrammable, despite being remarkably effective for rapidly terminating ventricular tachyarrhythmias.

SECOND-GENERATION ICDS

The second-generation devices offered limited programmability. The detection rate for VT could be programmed between 110–200 beats/minute. A delay between onset of sensing a tachycardia and obligate charging of the ICD capacitors to deliver a committed shock could also be programmed from 2.5–10 seconds. This extended delay is a useful feature in patients having runs of asymptomatic nonsustained VT to reduce the number of unnecessary shocks. For patients with a low defibrillation threshold energy, the ICD could also have its first sequential shock energy output programmed to lower values than the usual maximum 30 J value; this results in faster delivery of therapy due to an abbreviated capacitor charge time and increased ICD longevity due to reduced battery drain. However, second-generation devices were still capable of only delivering shocks to terminate arrhythmias, lacked bradycardia pacing capability, and stored little information about device function or charging history for use in clinical follow-up. Retrievable data in these devices included only the number of shocks, capacitor charge time, and shock electrode impedance.

THIRD-GENERATION ICDS

Improvements in Tachycardia Detection

Refer to Table 13.2 for a review of the characteristics of third-generation devices.

Table 13.2
Characteristics of Third-Generation Devices

	Ventritex Cadence V110	Medtronic Jewel 7219D	CPI PRxIII	Teletronics 4211	Intermedics ResQ 101-01
Weight (grams)	198	132	179	270	240
Tachycardia detection					
Rate	Yes	Yes	Yes	Yes	Yes
Duration	Yes	Yes	Yes	Yes	Yes
Antitachycardia pacing					
Fixed	Yes	Yes	Yes	Yes	Yes
Adaptive	Yes	Yes	Yes	Yes	Yes
Scan	Yes	Yes	Yes	Yes	Yes
Autodecremental	Yes	Yes	Yes	Yes	Yes
Tiered therapy	Yes	Yes	Yes	Yes	Yes
Detection algorithms	RT, SO, EHR	RT, SO, RS	RT, SO, RS, EHR	RT, SO	RT, SO, RS, EHR
Shocking energy (stored) (joules)	0.1–42 J	0.2–34 J	0.1–37 J	0.1–30 J	0.2–40 J
Waveform	Bi	Bi	Bi	Bi	Bi
Committed	No	No	No	No	Yes
Bradycardia pacing	Yes	Yes	Yes	Yes	Yes
Holter					
Total episodes	Yes	Yes	Yes	Yes	Yes
Last R-R intervals	No	Yes	Yes	Yes	No
EGM					
Real-time	Yes	Yes	Yes	Yes	Yes
Stored	Yes	Yes	Yes	Yes	No
Noninvasive EPS	Yes	Yes	Yes	Yes	Yes
Life span (nonshocking)	5	5?	4–5?	5+	2+

*Bi, biphasic; EGM, electrogram; EHR, extended high rate detection; EPS, electrophysiology study; RS, rate stability; RT, rate; SO, sudden onset.

SUDDEN ONSET

This feature monitors the cardiac cycle length to detect the sudden onset of a high ventricular rate. VT begins abruptly and usually achieves a relatively stable and short cycle length within 2 seconds of onset. Sinus tachycardia develops more gradually. The sudden onset detection criterion may preclude misdiagnosing sinus tachycardias as relatively slow VTs. Caution must be taken when using this detection algorithm to increase the specificity of arrhythmia detection when confronted with VTs that tend to occur during periods of sinus tachycardia and that have rates that are not much faster than the immediately preceding sinus tachycardia.

Third-generation devices use similar algorithms for detecting sudden onset, although the terminology differs. For example, the Medtronic PCD maintains a running average of the cycle length of the four current R-R intervals and compares it to the running average of the cycle length of the four previous R-R intervals. If the value of the current four R-R intervals' average cycle length is less than a programmed percentage (e.g., 80%) of the previous four R-R intervals' cycle length, the sudden onset criterion is fulfilled (Medtronic, technical manual). In a clinical study of 37 PCD patients, an onset algorithm of 87% permitted detection of all clinical VT episodes; however, premature ventricular contractions (PVCs) in association with sinus acceleration were occasionally falsely detected. Any SVT (such as AV nodal reentry or paroxysmal AF) that has an abrupt onset can also be misdiagnosed as VT.

RATE STABILITY

VT usually has fairly stable R-R intervals compared with AF; as an exception, slow VTs can have more marked cycle length variability early after onset, but they then usually stabilize in rate in about 30 beats. The rate or cycle length stability criterion attempts to enhance specificity of VT detection when tachycardia occurs at mean rates similar to those of paroxysmal or chronic AF in a patient prone to both arrhythmias. The algorithm measures each R-R interval and determines whether it differs from a running average of previous R-R intervals by more than a programmed value; this programmable interval value is measured in milliseconds and can vary between 6–120 msec, depending on the particular ICD.

In the PCD clinical trial, there was no report of nondetection of a clinical VT in patients in whom this feature was used (Medtronic PCD PMA submission). In a subsequent clinical report, the interval stability criteria were evaluated in 42 patients. Using a stability value of 40 msec, the device appropriately treated 399 VT episodes. More importantly, 10 patients had either fixed or paroxysmal AF that was appropriately identified, and VT therapy was not delivered.

SUSTAINED RATE DURATION

Some VTs might not meet the sudden onset or rate stability criteria because they occur during a sinus tachycardia that has a similar rate or because of overly stringent detection criteria. The sustained rate duration feature allows the clinician to program a fixed time period after which device therapy will automatically be delivered if primary detection criteria (such as high rate plus sudden onset) were not met and the tachycardia persists. The value is programmable from 10 seconds to 60 minutes in the CPI PRxIII and from 10 seconds to 5 minutes in the Ventritex Cadence V110. The feature is not available in the Medtronic PCD. Nearly all third-generation devices confirm that the tachycardia is still present before delivering ATP or a shock. In essence, these devices are noncommitted.

Improvements in Tachycardia Termination

A variety of pacing schemes to terminate VT have been studied, and each may have a role in terminating reentrant VT. The most useful algorithms offer both decremental burst pacing and ramp pacing, usually with adaptive coupling intervals. The adaptive method determines the pacing cycle length as a percentage of the basic VT cycle length. This method allows for variability in spontaneous VT cycle length and is superior to fixed cycle length burst pacing. Decremental burst pacing introduces each successive pacing train at a shorter initial coupling interval and paced cycle length than the preceding train; ramp pacing shortens each successive cycle length within the pacing train by a fixed amount measured either in absolute msec time intervals or as a percentage of the VT cycle length.

Both pace-termination algorithms have equal efficacy when tested on a large group of patients (although one method may be superior to the other when tested in an individual patient). Other modes are described but are much less useful clinically.

Antitachycardia pacing (ATP) can terminate most episodes of spontaneous VT and VTs induced in the EP laboratory. At least 75% of VT episodes can be pace-terminated at least some of the time, although up to a 43% incidence of acceleration of VT rate can occur on occasion when attempting to apply ATP to repeated episodes of VT. ATP is more successful when treating slower VTs. VT episodes can also be treated with low-energy cardioversion (LEC) (0.75–2.0 J). One early clinical study employed a transvenous lead and a truncated exponential shock of 0.025–2.0 J. Successful cardioversion of 47 episodes of VT was observed in five of seven patients tested. Shocks of energy less than 0.5 J were well tolerated by the nonsedated patient. By substituting painless ATP or LEC for high energy (< 5J) shocks, patient acceptance of the ICD is improved.

It is difficult to predict which tachycardia will be successfully pace-terminated other than by rate criteria. It is important to test proposed antitachycardia programs in the EP laboratory after ICD implant, whenever the patient's antiarrhythmic drug treatment has been charged, or when the patient's structural heart disease has changed—e.g., new MI. The latter two situations in particular can cause profound and unpredictable alterations in the rate of VT, defibrillation threshold, and other parameters.

Improvements in Lead Systems

During the 1980s, the epicardial lead system employing two- or three-patch electrodes was the standard configuration. Three-patch systems were used primarily in patients who had marginal DFTs with a two-patch system. With the FDA approvals in 1993–1994 of nonthoracotomy ICD lead systems, however, epicardial electrodes have been virtually abandoned in favor of nonthoracotomy leads for all new ICD implants.

Nonthoracotomy ICD lead systems are also still continuing to undergo rapid development. There are many similarities but some important differences between the FDA-approved lead systems that are manufactured by CPI and Medtronic. The CPI Endotak C 0070 series is a single tripolar lead that can be used in conjunction with a subcutaneous patch or a recently approved Endotak SQ Array. It is 100 cm in length and uses a Teflon-coated drawn brazed strand (DBS) cable-coated in silicon rubber (CPI Technical Manual). The lead body is 9.6 F and requires a 14F introducer to place via either subclavian vein (although the left is preferable for optimizing the defibrillating voltage gradient). The shocking electrodes consist of a proximal (or right atrial) spring electrode with surface area of 617 mm^2, and a distal (or right ventricular) spring electrode with surface area of 379 mm^2. The distance between the tip and proximal spring electrodes can be selected as 15 cm (Model 0073) or 18 cm (Model 0075). The porous, passive fixation tip electrode has a 9-mm^2 surface area and provides integrated bipolar rate sensing/pacing with the distal spring electrode. The distal tip and spring electrodes are separated by 6 mm. The transvenous lead may provide effective defibrillation when used alone in up to 60–70% of patients but may be used with a subcutaneous patch (Model 0063) electrode when defibrillation threshold requirements mandate it. This electrode is constructed of silicone-coated titanium and has a surface area of 28 cm^2; it is very similar to a standard epicardial patch (see Third Generation ICD Comparisons below). Recently, the Endotak SQ Array electrode was approved as an alternative to the patch that may produce less chronic discomfort at the subcutaneous implant site in the left lateral/posterolateral chest wall. This lead consists of three electrically common multifilar coil elements with a total surface area of 3900 mm^2 joined by a silicone-insulated cable at a molded silicone yoke. Each element is 20 cm in length and the entire lead length from element tip to terminal connector pin is 70 cm.

The Medtronic Transvene lead system is also a two- or three-electrode lead system (Medtronic Technical Manual); unlike the CPI Endotak lead system, all shocking electrodes are housed in separate leads and the rate-sensing/pacing electrodes are separate dedicated bipolar electrodes with an active fixation screw. The right ventricular lead (Model 6936) is 110 cm long and insulated with polyurethane; the lead can be passed through an 11F introducer. The right ventricular shock electrode surface area is 426 mm^2. The Model 6936 lead contains a distal tip electrode that requires active fixation in the endocardium with the helical screw serving as part of the active cathode for bipolar pacing/sensing with a proximal anodal ring electrode. The right ventricular shock electrode lead is used in concert with a second lead (Model #6933) that is usually placed in the left innominate vein. It is also 110 cm in length, has a shocking coil surface area of 90 mm^2, and has no active fixation mechanism. The third component of the system is a subcutaneous patch (Model 6939). It has a conduction surface area of 660 mm^2 and is similar to the epicardial patch system.

Shock Waveforms

All first- and second-generation defibrillators as well as several now-obsolete third-generation ICDs deliver a truncated monophasic shock waveform with a fixed tilt of 60%. This waveform yielded adequate defibrillation thresholds in approximately 95% of patients receiving a standard bipolar epicardial system and 72–88% of patients receiving nonthoracotomy systems.

Virtually all current third-generation ICDs offer a biphasic shock waveform to improve defibrillation efficacy (Fig. 13.2). The shock can be delivered in a bipolar fashion or simultaneously in a tripolar electrode system between two common electrodes serving as cathode with a single anode (or vice-versa). A biphasic shock waveform's polarity is reversed partway through the time course of the shock's delivery along the same pathway.

Basic clinical data have consistently shown that biphasic shocks are more efficient than monophasic shocks for defibrillation. In a comparison of monophasic and biphasic shock waveforms in 22 patients undergoing epicardial lead system

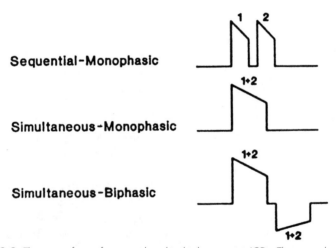

Figure 13.2. The types of waveforms employed in third-generation ICDs. The monophasic waveform has been used in all second-generation devices. The sequential waveform differs from a monophasic waveform in that at the end of pulse I a separate monophasic pulse is delivered across a second independent pathway. In a three-electrode system, the right ventricular cathode might deliver a pulse first to the right atrial electrode and second to the subcutaneous patch. A biphasic waveform differs from a monophasic waveform in that at the end of phase I of the biphasic waveform, the defibrillation and shock polarity are reversed. Delivery is then continued along the same pathway but in the opposite direction. Defibrillation thresholds using biphasic waveforms are lower than with either monophasic or sequential waveforms. (From Saksena S., An A, Mehra R, et al. Prospective comparison of biphasic and monophasic shocks for implantable cardioverter-defibrillators using endocardial leads. Am J Cardiol 1992;70:304–310.)

implantation, the mean DFT for the monophasic pulse was 8.5 J, compared with 6.3 J for the biphasic pulse. In two recent series using the Endotak lead and a biphasic pulse, the DFTs were less than 20 J in 32 consecutive patients.

There are several theories why biphasic shocks are so effective. Some investigators believe that the biphasic pulse may facilitate depolarization of more myocardium than a monophasic pulse. Others think the polarity reversal during the second phase of the shocks causes less postshock myocardial dysfunction. Finally, some researchers argue that the biphasic pulse prolongs refractoriness and protects ventricular cells from defibrillation wave fronts at the cellular level.

Telemetry Functions

Second-generation ICDs only stored data about battery and capacitor function and had limited information about device discharges. Enormous progress has been made in this area. The third-generation ICDs provide information about time and date-stamped numbers and types of events, arrhythmia R-R intervals, therapies delivered, and therapy success or failure at terminating the arrhythmia episodes. Data retrieved by interrogating the ICD are printed in tabular form. Three FDA-approved ICDs, the Ventritex Cadence V-110, the Medtronic Jewel PCD 7219D, and the CPI PRxIII 1720/1725 can store electrograms up to 150 seconds long, including pre-therapy rhythm, detection, and therapy delivery. This information can be of great help in diagnosing the cause of shocks as well as troubleshooting for lead problems as a cause of spurious shocks. Other valuable stored information in third-generation devices includes information about electrode status (shock and pacing lead impedances and pacing threshold), and battery life (indicating the need for generator replacement).

Generator Design

Key to the development of the third-generation ICDs is the concept of a hierarchial approach to ventricular arrhythmia treatment. This concept treats slower VTs first with painless therapy (ATP), and then moves on to more aggressive cardioversion and defibrillation. Faster and more hemodynamically destabilizing VT and VF would still receive prompt high-energy cardioversion and defibrillation therapy as well as those VTs created by rate acceleration after unsuccessful attempts at delivering ATP and/or LEC shocks for "slow" VT. To carry out such therapy, a device must be extremely flexible and easy to program, have reliable tachycardia detection criteria, and have the capacity to easily test and validate therapies through noninvasive programmed stimulation.

At the core of this concept are the twin goals of patient comfort and safety. Patient comfort is maximized by attempts at using ATP before cardioversion or defibrillation. Patient safety is assured by limiting the duration of potentially ineffective therapy (ATP) and moving quickly toward established, more aggressive, and effective therapy (defibrillation).

The current devices allow many complex modifications of this simple scheme. Multiple tachycardia zones can be defined by rate (e.g., 150–175, 176–200, and >200 beats/minute) with different first therapies in each zone (e.g., ATP zone 1, low-energy cardioversion zone 2, and defibrillation zone 3). In each zone, therapy moves from a less aggressive therapy to the "gold standard" of defibrillation. Programming these zones of VT/VF detection and therapy, and making sure each zone is successful in achieving arrhythmia detection and termination, requires careful attention and may demand extended programming time in the EP laboratory.

SPECIFIC THIRD-GENERATION DEVICES

Ventritex Cadence

The Ventritex Cadence is the prototypical third-generation ICD, and its features are outlined in Table 13.2. Most of the patients in the clinical trial experience had underlying coronary artery disease, just as in second-generation device trials. Although most patients had sustained VT, only a minority of patients had a cardiac arrest; almost one-half presented with palpitations and sustained VT. This latter population represents an extension of the previous ICD patient populations, a large percentage of whom were cardiac arrest survivors.

Device implantation was originally carried out with a standard epicardial patch-patch configuration. In one early series, there were eight postoperative deaths and an operative mortality of 2.5%. This device was the first to widely apply a biphasic waveform that was used in 99% of the implantations. The resulting DFT was a low 11.7 J (407 V). There were no patients in whom an ICD could not be implanted because of high DFTs. In late 1994, however, the FDA granted approval to implant the Cadence ICD with CPI Endotak nonthoracotomy leads; similar approval to "mix-and-match" the Cadence with the Medtronic Transvene leads is also expected soon.

Follow-up data showed this device to be remarkably effective. In the follow-up period, there were three SCDs and 15 non-SCDs; thus, the 1-year SCD-free survival was 99%, and the 1-year survival from all cardiac causes was 95%. These data are as good or better than the survival data shown for second-generation devices. Comparable all-cause survival data are expected because the ejection fraction of the entire group averaged 32%, which is similar to the second-generation ICD series.

During clinical follow-up, 238 of 338 patients (70%) had ECG documented episodes of VT or VF and were treated with either ATP, cardioversion, or defibrillation. Cardioversion was programmed as the initial therapy in 580 of these episodes: it was successful as the initial therapy in 90%, and additional shocks were needed in 10%. In 13,425 episodes of spontaneous VT, ATP was programmed as first therapy. It was successful in 93.5% of attempts, unsuccessful in only 4.8% (thus requiring a shock), and responsible for acceleration in only 1.7% (also requiring a shock). The most popular programmed pacing algorithm was adaptive burst pacing, with the adaptive percentage programmed between 80–85% of the tachycardia cycle length. Of the other ATP enhancements, scanning was programmed "on" in 82% of the episodes and decremental ramp pacing programmed "on" in 23% of the episodes.

There was no difference in survival between patients receiving ATP and those not receiving ATP. This laid to rest some earlier concerns that ATP might add to mortality because it delayed delivery of high energy shock therapy. False or spurious shocks continued to be a clinical problem and were experienced by 38% of the patients during the trial, as documented by stored electrograms. This figure is similar to that noted with second-generation devices.

There were a number of lead-related problems that plagued the trials using epicardial electrodes. A total of 12% of patients had a variety of difficulties, including problems with the lead adapter (between another manufacturer's leads and the generator header) and migration or fracture of endocardial leads. The current Cadence ICD has obviated these problems by offering three versions of ICD with different headers. There were seven premature generator failures caused by component failure. The stored electrograms are extremely helpful clinically in understanding what rhythm prompted therapy. SVT can usually be distinguished from VT by electrogram morphology and R-R intervals. Based on this analysis, changes in antiarrhythmic drug therapy or device programming can be made. The ease of detection of lead fracture is especially useful.

Generator life is predicted to be 4–5 years. There have been very few premature device failures. Backup bradycardia VVI pacing has functioned well and was used clinically in approximately 10% of patients in the trial. Ventritex is just entering a transvenous lead system into clinical trials.

Medtronic Jewel PCD 7219D

The third-generation Medtronic Jewel PCD 7219D received FDA approval in 1995 and is a remarkable improvement over the previous third-generation ICD known as the Model 7217 PCD. Its features are summarized in Table 13.2. Most of the patients in the clinical trials of both devices (77%) had coronary disease and the presenting rhythm was VT in 55% and SCD in 45%. The mean ejection fraction was 34%. The most striking improvements in the Jewel 7219D over its 7217 predecessor are its incorporation of a biphasic shock waveform, improved diagnostics including stored electrograms, noncommitted first-shock therapy in the VF zone, simplified implant support device and "user-friendly" programmer (Model 9790), and remarkably small size. With a volume of 83 cc and a mass of 132 g, the Jewel 7219D is presently the smallest FDA-approved ICD and is suitable for infraclavicular implant in either a prepectoral or subpectoral location in carefully selected patients. In the most recent database of the Jewel 7219D with Transvene lead (compared with the still investigational 7219C "Active Can" Jewel), the mean DFT was 13.5 J. There were four perioperative deaths (within 30 days postimplant) yielding an operative mortality of 2.6%. The primary implant success rate (achieving a defibrillation threshold of 24 J or less) was 89%.

The 3-month cumulative survival for SCD was 100%, and the all-cause survival was 97%, which is comparable to second-generation ICD survival data. During the trial a total of 13 patients (9%) had spontaneous VT. Of those patients, the majority had ATP programmed on as the first therapy, and this was successful in terminating over 90% of the tachycardias. The remainder were programmed with cardioversion as the primary therapy. When cardioversion was used as a first therapy, it was successful over 90% of the time.

The memory function stores up to 255 detected VT, fast VT (FVT), and VF episodes and the successes or failures of each therapy. To help sort out the approp-riateness of therapy, the last 5 VT, FVT, or VF episodes provide interval markers for up to 30 intervals predetection and 20 intervals after the start of last therapy, in addition to detection interval stability and onset values at the time of the episode. A choice of five 2.5 second episodes of predetection electrogram or one episode with 5 seconds of predetection electrogram and 5 seconds of postdetection electrogram is available.

CPI Ventak PRxIII 1720/1725

The CPI Ventak PRxIII received FDA approval in May 1995, and its features are summarized in Table 13.2. The majority of patients (75%) had coronary artery disease, and 62% presented with monomorphic VT and 30% with VT/VF. The mean ejection fraction was 32%.

The device was implanted primarily using the Endotak lead system, with a perioperative mortality of 1–2%. The 1-year survival from SCD was 98.5%, and survival from all causes was 93%. Again, SCD survival was excellent, as with the Cadence and PCD trials.

Nearly 50% of patients were programmed to a multizone configuration. There was a total of 2733 episodes of spontaneous ventricular arrhythmia. ATP therapy was successful as first therapy over 90% of the time, with an acceleration incidence of 8.5%. ATP was most successful at heart rates between 131–160 beats/minute (94%) but was only slightly less effective at rates between 191–220 beats/minute (85%). As with the Cadence and Jewel ICDs, the Ventak PRxIII provides a markedly expanded array of diagnostic information, more stored electrogram time (150 seconds) than any other device available, biphasic shock output, and a very efficient programming system.

Telectronics Guardian 4211

The ongoing clinical trial of the Telectronics third-generation device, called the Guardian ATP, Model 4211, had enrolled more than 400 patients worldwide by May 1994. Its features are summarized in Table 13.2. Most patients had either coronary artery disease (71%) or cardiomyopathy (28%). The majority of patients presented with VT (72%) and a smaller percentage with VF (13%). The mean ejection fraction was 33%. The following results include over 155 patients receiving the 4211 ICD with the still-investigational Telectronics Enguard PFX nonthoracotomy lead system.

There were 10 operative deaths, for an operative mortality of 1.8%. During follow-up, 1-year freedom from SCD was 100%. The mean defibrillation threshold ranged from as low as 7.4 J for the 4211 patch configuration to 11 J for the 4211 Enguard PFX system. A primary implant success rate of 98.7% was achieved using the 4211 Enguard PFX system, although in 22% of the implants, a dual pathway shock electrode configuration incorporating a subcutaneous patch was necessary. As with the other ICDs, the 4211 ICD yielded a high primary ATP conversion success rate of 92.1%, with only a 1.8% acceleration rate. Although the 4211 ICD is a large device (mass 270 g, volume 184 cc), it has demonstrated remarkable battery longevity with current data supporting a projected longevity 6 years, based on 100% pacing and monthly shock frequency.

Intermedics RES-Q 101-01 System

The Intermedics clinical trial of its third-generation device began in March 1992 and culminated in recent FDA approval. During the initial period of the trial, there were oversensing and device header design problems that suspended the trial for a time and delayed full-scale patient enrollment. As of May 1994, 429 patients had been enrolled in the clinical trial encompassing both a conformal epicardial patch electrode system, a nonthoracotomy lead system using a 10-cm right ventricular endocardial coil and subcutaneous patch electrode, and a 5-cm RV endocardial coil with a 5-cm superior vena cava coil. The performance of the RES Q ICD appears comparable to the aforementioned ICDs. The 1-year total survival is 91% and SCD survival 98.3%. The device is physically large (mass 240 g, volume 150 cc) but is capable of delivering up to 10 sequential biphasic shocks at maximum 700 V output (or nearly 40 J). It has limited ability to provide details of therapy delivery histories and lacks stored electrogram capability.

NONTHORACOTOMY LEAD SYSTEMS

The other area of innovation in ICD therapy is the development of reliable nonthoracotomy lead systems. Currently there are two FDA-approved lead systems.

CPI Endotak

The original CPI Endotak clinical trial combined a second-generation device (Ventak 1550, 1555, 1600) with the CPI Endotak series 0600 lead system (see Improvements in Lead Systems above). A total of 536 patients were evaluated and Endotak implantation was attempted between September 1990 and February 1992 at 35 investigational centers. Most of these patients had coronary disease (76%) and presented with either VT (51%) or VF (37%). Of these, 403 (75%) met protocol and had a device implanted. A number of clinical variables were analyzed to predict successful DFT criteria; those predicting a failure to achieve adequate DFTs at implantation included low ejection fraction, prior use of amiodarone, male gender, and greater body surface area.

A variety of potential lead arrays were tested at implantation, including lead-only (employing a unidirectional pulse) and lead-patch configuration (employing both unidirectional and bidirectional pulses). DFTs of less than 25 J (monophasic) were required for a system to be implanted. There were five perioperative deaths (1.2% operative mortality at 30 days), six SCDs during follow-up, and freedom from SCD was 97.2% at 1 year.

A chief concern regarding a transvenous lead system is its ability to sense VF reliably after implant. The instances of nonsensing with the Endotak were very few. At operation testing, there was one sensing problem in 566 inductions. At pre-discharge testing, there were 12 instances of nonsensing in 713 inductions (0.84%). Two of these were examples of subsequent failed detection after an initial unsuccessful shock. In all of these cases, the problem was either corrected or the device was explanted. Criticisms had been raised that use of an integrated shock/sensing electrode system might predispose to VF undersensing after a failed first shock. This was considered to be caused by the proximity of the RV coil (jointly serving as both a shock electrode and anode for sensing/pacing) to the tip cathode serving as a dedicated sensing/pacing electrode. The recently FDA-approved Endotak C 0070 series lead appears to have addressed this concern by promoting greater physical separation between the two electrodes.

Arrhythmia conversion testing at 6 weeks after discharge was also successful. There were 613 arrhythmia inductions and 33 (5%) required external cardioversion. Four of these patients went on to receive a transthoracic system and two a new Endotak system. Careful testing of the lead system is mandatory before hospital discharge and perhaps also at 6 weeks, especially because a significant rise in the defibrillation threshold of up to 5 J may occur.

During the follow-up period, 42% of patients received shocks. Approximately 20% of the shocks seemed to be "appropriate." There were six SCDs, and all seemed the result of failure of the ICD to defibrillate adequately. There were 168 examples of successful conversion after unsuccessful first-shock therapy. There were three cases of lead dislodgement, and only one occurred after the 6-week test. The overall survival and total device conversions were similar to the Ventak 1600 (epicardial patch system) data. The current practice of combining a biphasic shock output with the Endotak lead system appears to provide even greater defibrillation efficacy and a higher implant success rate with use of only the transvenous electrode, i.e., subcutaneous patch not needed.

Medtronic Transvene

The Medtronic Transvene clinical trial was conducted concurrently with investigation of the now-obsolete Medtronic third-generation monophasic shock output PCD (7217B). There were 757 patients who received the device in 78 centers between October 1989 and October 1990. Of these centers, 43 were international and 35 were in the United States. Coronary artery disease was present in 74%; sustained VT was present in 50%, and SCD in 38%. The mean ejection fraction (EF) was 36%.

The criterion for implant was three of four episodes of VF converted with 18 J or less. Device implantation was attempted in 854 patients and was successful in 88%. Of the 757 patients who received the PCD, 543 (71.8%) met the implant criteria. However, 737 of the 757 had at least a 10-J safety margin. Operative mortality was 0.7%. The important differences between patients meeting and not meeting the criteria include a higher incidence of male gender, a higher incidence of SCD, and a higher incidence of amiodarone usage. The mean DFT for all systems was 14.8 J. The most frequently used lead systems were right ventricle-superior vena cava-subcutaneous (RV-SVC-SQ) (65%), RV-Coronary Sinus-SQ (30%), and RV-CS-SVC (5%).

There were three SCDs and 18 cardiac deaths during follow-up. Freedom from SCD was 99.8% at 1 year. There was a 6.6% incidence of lead-related problems, including chronic lead dislodgement (4.4%), right ventricular perforation (0.7%), subclavian thrombosis (0.1%), subcutaneous patch crinkling (0.9%), or RV lead fracture (0.5%). The incidence of either loss of capture or sense-related problems was 0.9%. Most recently, the development of a Model #6936 Transvene lead implanted in the right ventricle with a Jewel PCD 7219C biphasic "Active Can" ICD in the left infraclavicular region serving as the second shock electrode is yielding primary implant success rates of 96% and mean defibrillation thresholds of 11.4 J.

Both the Endotak and Transvene data demonstrate that:

1. Implantation of a nonthoracotomy lead system can be accomplished in 70–80% of patients using a monophasic waveform ICD and potentially in over 90% of patients when a biphasic waveform device is used. With biphasic devices, the potential is also very high for implanting a pure transvenous lead system that obviates need for a subcutaneous patch electrode that causes chronic discomfort at its implant site.
2. Perioperative mortality is lower when a nonthoracotomy lead system is used compared with an epicardial electrode system (1% nonthoracotomy vs. 2.2% epicardial system).
3. Long-term survival is excellent and freedom from SCD is comparable to the older epicardial lead systems.
4. Complications resulting from the epicardial lead itself are low. Long-term sensing problems were not seen with either lead system. Early dislodgement was noted in 4.4% of cases in the Transvene series. The dislodgement rate was <1% in the Endotak series. This complication appears to decline as experience with the lead grows.

SUGGESTED READING

Bardy GH, Ivey TD, Allen MD, et al. A prospective randomized evaluation of biphasic versus monophasic waveform pulses on defibrillation efficacy in humans. J Am Coll Cardiol 1989; 14:728–733.

Dreifus LS, Fisch L, Griffin JC, Gillette PC, Mason JW, Parsonnet V. Guidelines for implantation of cardiac pacemakers and antitachyarrhythmia devices: a report of the American College of Cardiology/American Heart Association

Task Force on Assessment of Diagnostic and Therapeutic Cardiovascular Procedures. J Am Coll Cardiol 1991;18:1–13.

Furman S, Kim SG. The present status of implantable cardioverter defibrillator therapy. J Cardiovasc Electrophysiol 1992;3:602–625.

Kelly PA, Cannom DS, Garan H, et al. The automatic implantable cardioverter-defibrillator: efficacy, complications, and survival in patients with malignant ventricular arrhythmias. J Am Coll Cardiol 1988;11:1278–1286.

Keren R, Aarons D, Veltri EP. Anxiety and depression in patients with life-threatening ventricular arrhythmias: impact of the implantable cardioverter-defibrillator. PACE 1991;14:181–187.

Kim SG, Fisher JD, Furman S, et al. Benefits of implantable defibrillators are overestimated by sudden death rate and better represented by the total arrhythmic death rate. J Am Coll Cardiol 1991;17:1587–1592.

Lehmann MH, Saksena S. Implantable cardioverter defibrillator in cardiovascular practice: report of the Policy Conference of the North American Society of Pacing and Electrophysiology. NASPE Policy Conference Committee. PACE 1991;14:969–979.

O'Donoghue S, Platia EV, Brooks-Robinson S, Mispireta L. Automatic implantable cardioverter-defibrillator: is early implantation cost-effective? J Am Coll Cardiol 1990;16:1258–1263.

Winkle RA, Mead RH, Ruder MA, et al. Ten-year experience with implantable defibrillators. Circulation 1991;84(suppl I):II–426.

14 Normal Sinus Rhythm and Its Variants (Sinus Arrhythmia, Sinus Tachycardia, Sinus Bradycardia), Sinus Node Reentry, and Sinus Node Dysfunction

NORMAL SINUS RHYTHM

Sinus rhythm is the dominant rhythm in the normal heart. Normal sinus rhythm (NSR) is defined by a physiologically normal atrial rate (60–100 beats/minute while awake and sedentary) and a P-wave vector on the electrocardiogram (ECG) indicating a high lateral right atrial origin (upright in leads I, II, III, AVL, and AVF). Sinus rhythm usually results from impulse initiation by spontaneously depolarizing P cells, within the sinoatrial (SA) node, and conduction of the impulse through the node and out to the atrium. Under certain circumstances, however, as demonstrated during electrical mapping intraoperatively under general anesthesia, impulse initiation may shift to areas around but outside of the histologically defined, spindle-shaped SA node. Although all P-cell regions within the SA node have properties of automaticity, usually one group is dominant, i.e., has the most rapid firing rate at any instant and serves as the cardiac pacemaker, while the other P-cell regions remain latent as they are reset by or interfered with by impulses generated by the dominant focus. Whether the dominant focus is a single cell or nest of cells with the most rapid rate of depolarization, or whether it really is several groups of cells electronically linked remains uncertain.

In infants and children, sinus rates are age related. Sinus rates in children are higher than in adults and decline through childhood. However, the age-related decline in resting rate does not continue through adulthood. Although intrinsic SA node function does decrease during the adult years, it is balanced by a progressive decrease in parasympathetic influence and α_1-receptor sensitivity.

In NSR, impulse initiation in the dominant pacemaker region is followed by impulse conduction through the node and the perinodal region out to the atrium. Thus, the sinus node possesses both automatic and conductive properties. Under physiologic conditions, automaticity and conduction are enhanced by sympathetic input and depressed by parasympathetic input and are subject to a continually shifting balance between the autonomic limbs. Normal SA node function is also modulated by several additional factors, including adrenal catecholamines, thyroxin, temperature, pH, and electrolyte status. When parasympathetic (vagal) influence is blocked pharmacologically with atropine or by transplantation (denervation), sinus rate increases, sometimes by more than 50%. However, it will not exceed 120 beats/minute in normals. With total pharmacologic autonomic denervation using both atropine and propranolol, the intrinsic sinus rate in normals is usually higher than before such blockade, but generally less than 100 beats/minute, and can be predicted by the formula, intrinsic heart rate (IHR) = 118.1 −(0.57 × age). Thus, at rest, parasympathetic influence usually predominates, while with physiologic stress, such as exercise, vagal withdrawal and adrenergic stimulation combine to increase sinus rates.

Sinus Arrhythmia

During NSR, the cyclical changes in sinus rate that are synchronized to breathing and autonomically mediated are called sinus arrhythmia (Fig. 14.1). Respiratory phasic changes in cardiac parasympathetic nerve traffic result in alterations in P-cell automaticity, conduction velocity within and around the SA node, and shifts in the region of the dominant pacemaker. These factors, which have been confirmed by observations made on directly recorded sinus node electrograms in humans, result in the cyclical changes in sinus rate as determined by atrial cycle lengths (P-wave-to-P-wave intervals). Sinus arrhythmia is most pronounced in the young and decreases as parasympathetic influence on the SA node decreases with age. Exercise (vagal withdrawal), parasympathetic blockade (atropine), or denervation (transplantation) will abolish sinus arrhythmia. When marked, sinus arrhythmia can be difficult to distinguish from sinus pauses or atrial ectopy and can be sensed as palpitations in occasional patients. Treatment consists of reassurance.

The range of variation in sinus cycle length (SCL) (normalized by dividing by the average SCL) and the maximal change in SCL between any two consecutive cycles is greater in patients with sinus node dysfunction than in normals. This probably relates to periods of bradycardia or pathologic pauses in such patients. Conversely, a decrease in the cycle-to-cycle variation (typically referred to as heart rate variability) during moderate to prolonged periods of monitoring can also reflect pathophysiology. Decreased heart rate variability, for example, which probably reflects decreased absolute or relative parasympathetic nerve traffic and increased sympathetic influence, has been associated with adverse prognosis following myocardial infarction.

Vagal activity is also a dominant factor in the circadian variation in sinus rate that occurs with the daily sleep-wake cycle. Enhanced vagal activity in normals during sleep can result in sinus rates less than 40 beats/minutes, pauses greater than 1.5 seconds, and both SA and A-V nodal Wenckebach patterns. (Commonly, circadian variation is attenuated in the presence of sinus node disease.)

Sinus Tachycardia

Electrocardiographically defined sinus rates greater than 100 beats/minute are called sinus tachycardia (Fig. 14.1). Sinus tachycardia may be physiologic, pathologic, or pharmacologic. Vagal withdrawal, enhanced catecholamines, thyrotoxicosis, fever, and pharmacologic stimulants can all enhance sinus node automaticity and thereby increase the sinus rate. During exercise, the sinus rate should increase

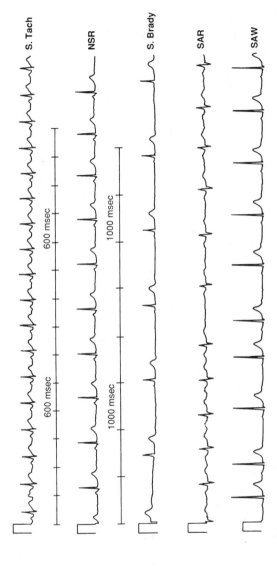

Figure 14.1. Electrocardiographic rhythms strips. Rhythm strips (*top to bottom*) demonstrate sinus tachycardia (*S. Tach*) (P-P intervals less than <600 msec), normal sinus rhythm (*NSR*) (P-P intervals between 600–1000 msec), and sinus brady-cardia (*S. Brady*) (P-P intervals >1000 msec). Also displayed is sinus arrhythmia (*SAR*) and sinoatrial Wenckebach (*SAW*).

progressively in normal individuals proportionately to the isotonic load until an age-related maximum is achieved. This upper rate, which is approximately 220 beats/minutes minus age, is an effect mediated by vagal withdrawal, adrenergic stimulation, and possibly by mechanical effects of decreased atrial stretch and altered sinus node artery pulse pressure. The rate limit of approximately 200 beats/minute in young adults is probably not incidental. Rather, it likely relates to SA node refractory, excitability, and conductive properties. In normals, the duration of sinus node depolarization, as determined by sinus node electrography, is 100–150 msec. However, because time dependence exists in the SA node, recovery of excitability outlasts the voltage excursion of sinus node action potentials by more than 100 msec; because intranodal conduction velocity is exceedingly slow, normally less than 0.05 meters/sec, an intercycle time frame less than 300 msec (heart rate greater than 200 beats/minute) would be difficult to achieve.

The blunting of maximal sinus rate with age is normal; however, a greater degree of blunting of maximal achievable sinus rate with disease is not and is termed chronotropic incompetence. Chronotropic incompetence may result in symptoms of exertional fatigue or dyspnea. Many drugs and diseases can directly or via autonomic interaction (see later discussion) alter sinus rate. Additionally, conditioning by isotonic (aerobic) exercise will reduce resting heart rate through augmented peripheral muscle efficiency and therefore adequacy of a lower resting cardiac output as well as by enhancing vagal tone and reducing sympathetic neural inputs. Physical conditioning typically results in slow sinus rates at rest (less than 60 beats/minute). Rates of 50–60 beats/minute awake or less than 40 beats/minute with sleep in normals would be expected. Conditioning does not reduce the maximal achievable sinus rate with exercise, however; rather, it prolongs the amount of aerobic exercise time prior to obtaining one's maximal rate and reduces the cardiac output and sinus rate required for any submaximal level of activity.

Sinus tachycardia may be pathologic under several circumstances. Pathologic sinus tachycardia is recognized when sinus tachycardia is inappropriate for the level of activity. Most commonly, pathologic sinus tachycardia is mediated by increased levels of sympathetic nerve traffic or circulating catecholamines, thyrotoxicosis, or the ingestion of agents with sympathomimetic or direct stimulating effects. These compounds include caffeine or cocaine. Each of the aforementioned circumstances reflects enhanced automaticity. Typically, other signs of catecholamine, thyroxin, or stimulant excess are also present, such as tremor, sweating, increased cardiac output, esthesia, chest discomfort, among others. The so-called hyperkinetic heart syndrome probably reflects such pathophysiology. Removal of the offending agent and/or β-blocker administration will usually ameliorate the symptom. Also, sinus tachycardia, which is usually transient and probably due to altered parasympathetic input, has been reported following radiofrequency ablation in the AV nodal region. Occasionally, persistent sinus tachycardia is pathologic and idiopathic. Perhaps paradoxically, pathologic sinus tachycardia can also result from disordered sinoatrial (SA) conduction. As in the

AV node, regions of impaired conduction can serve as a substrate for reentry, and reentry in the SA nodal region can mimic paroxysmal sinus tachycardia.

Sinus Bradycardia

When sinus rhythm is present at a rate less than 60 beats/minute, this is called sinus bradycardia (Fig. 14.1). Sinus bradycardia, like sinus tachycardia, may be physiologic, pathologic, or pharmacologic. Sinus bradycardia is a physiologic response to conditioning and a normal response to periods of increased parasympathetic tone. Enhanced parasympathetic tone itself may be physiologic, as during sleep, or pathologic. The latter may be triggered by gastrointestinal, genitourinary, pharyngeal, or other disorders involving tissues that are richly innervated by the vagus, or may represent an enhanced sensitivity to or disproportionate increase in or response to vagal traffic triggered by normal reflexes, such as baroreceptor stimulation. Vagally induced sinus bradycardia may be responsive to atropine, but need be treated only if symptomatic. Atropine doses less than 0.5 mg may cause a paradoxical increase in vagal-induced bradycardia. These effects are mediated by central nervous system (CNS) effects and should be avoided. Physiologic sinus bradycardia should be distinguished from the pathologic type because of differences in treatment and prognosis. Findings that might indicate physiologic sinus bradycardia are a correlation of the bradycardia with physiologic increases in vagal tone, such as sleep, micturition, nausea and vomiting, or sinus bradycardia in a well-conditioned individual, e.g., one who participates regularly in aerobic exercise. Also, physiologic sinus bradycardia should be reversible with atropine because the efferent mechanism involves vagotonia. Sinus bradycardia under other circumstances, particularly in the setting of coexisting pathological disorders involving the myocardium, coronary flow, or components of the conduction system distal to the sinus node, should suggest a pathologic rather than a physiologic mechanism, as should sinus bradycardia in the setting of cardioactive drugs or CNS disorders. Pathologic and/or symptomatic sinus bradycardia are part of the constellation of sinus node disorders collectively known as sick sinus syndrome (SSS) and is discussed later in this chapter.

SINUS NODE REENTRY

In many ways, the SA node is functionally similar to the AV node. Resting potentials less negative than those of Purkinje tissue or working myocardial cells, "slow channel"-dependent action potentials, and a structurally complex node all promote slow rates of intranodal and perinodal conduction. Similarly, and relatedly, both nodes demonstrate decremental conduction (decreasing conduction velocity in association with premature stimuli of increasing prematurity during relative refractoriness), inequalities in bidirectional conduction, and occasionally "dual pathway" properties. As in the AV node, the presence of decremental conduction with premature stimulation (some regions may slow, some may block) and the existence of more than one "functional" pathway for conduction within the SA nodal region provide the potential conditions to support reentry: slow conduction and unidirectional block.

Sinus node reentry has been demonstrated and mapped in atrial preparations, and reentry in the sinus node region has been confirmed in humans. In clinical practice, paroxysmal supraventricular tachycardia (PSVT) due to sinus node reentry is infrequent (Fig. 14.2). In the experience of Wellens, only 10% of patients who undergo clinical electrophysiologic study for tachycardias have sinus node reentry. Others, however, have reported slightly higher frequencies. Current techniques do not allow us to tell in vivo how much of the reentrant pathway is within the node versus in the perinodal tissue. In general, the cycle length of PSVT due to sinus node reentry is generally longer (the rate is slower) than with other PSVTs. Rates of 110–150 beats/minute, often with some cycle-to-cycle variation, are most common. Thus, symptoms, such as palpitations or dizziness, are less frequent and severe than with other more rapid PSVTs. Additionally, at least when studied in the clinical electrophysiology laboratory, sinus node reentry typically is self-terminating in 1–6 beats and is sustained only infrequently.

Sinus node reentry can be presumed when several ECG and intracardiac atrial electrogram criteria are fulfilled. These include (a) when the sinus node return cycle length following an atrial premature depolarization (APD) is shorter than what would occur with an interpolated APD; (b) when visible (and not buried in the preceding QRST complex), the echo beat P-wave vector in multiple ECG leads and its atrial activation sequence are the same as in sinus rhythm, and the RP′/P′R ratio is greater than 1; (c) for single echoes, when the postecho sinus return cycle exceeds the basic sinus cycle length; and (d) when neither A-H pro-

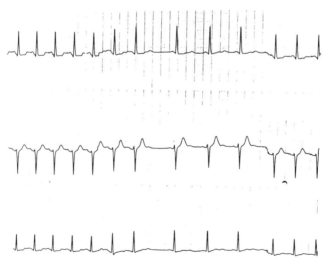

Figure 14.2. Example of sinus node reentry. Note the abrupt onset and offset of the arrhythmia, the same P-R interval, and the P waves, which are identical in sinus rhythm and during the tachycardia.

longation nor AV conduction is prerequisite to inducing or supporting the reentrant beat(s). When sustained, sinus node reentrant tachycardia usually responds to the same drugs that suppress AV nodal reentry (e.g., digitalis, β-blockers, verapamil, diltiazem, or class I or III antiarrhythmics) and usually can be terminated by "vagal maneuvers," and antitachycardia-pacing algorithms. Additionally, radiofrequency ablation may be attempted as a cure, guided by careful sinus node identification, though. Still, injury to the sinus node is a risk, so the procedure should be used only in resistant cases.

SINUS NODE DYSFUNCTION (SICK SINUS SYNDROME)

Sinus node dysfunction (SND) exists when nonphysiologic alterations in sinus rhythm are present. SND encompasses both disordered SA node automaticity and SA conduction. The recognition of SND (or sick sinus syndrome, a term popularized by Ferrer) is electrocardiographic. Symptoms are frequent, but are not necessarily present. The recognition of SND is important with regard to the mechanism of symptoms, the treatment of symptoms, the initiation of cardioactive pharmaceuticals, and prognosis.

Recognition

Electrocardiographically, SND is recognized by the appearance of any or all of the following developments: inappropriate sinus bradycardia, sinus pauses (representing impaired automaticity or SA exit block), or alternating periods of sinus bradyarrhythmias and nonsinus tachyarrhythmias. This may present as a bradycardia followed by an escape tachyarrhythmia (the bradycardia-tachycardia syndrome [Fig. 14.3]) or as a tachyarrhythmia that after termination is followed by a long offset pause (the tachycardia-bradycardia syndrome [Fig. 14.4].

Most commonly the tachyarrhythmia is paroxysmal atrial fibrillation (AF) or flutter. Because dysfunction of other segments of the cardiac conduction system, particularly the AV junction, frequently coexists with SND, several additional ECG findings should suggest the possibility of concomitant SND. These include AF or flutter with a slow ventricular rate in the absence of drugs, other AV nodal conduction disorders, APDs with prolonged post-APD pauses, and AF in the absence of any demonstrable associated cardiac disorder or known extracardiac cause (lone AF). Lone AF can represent a default or escape rhythm in the setting of persistent sinus nodal arrest or exit block. The latter is important to recognize because both direct current or pharmacologically mediated cardioversion may result in asystole or marked bradyarrhythmias rather than NSR under these circumstances. Automaticity of AV junctional and ventricular pacemakers is also often depressed in SND, so that escape rhythms are slower than expected. Lastly, as suggested earlier, sinus "bradycardia" may be relative, rather than absolute, presenting as NSR with chronotropic incompetence.

During sinus rhythm, pathologic sinus pauses may result from SA arrest and/or exit block. Sinus arrest, a disorder of automaticity, is recognized as pauses that are

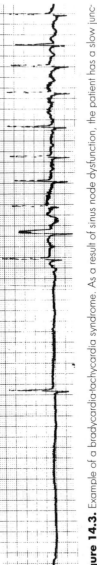

Figure 14.3. Example of a bradycardia-tachycardia syndrome. As a result of sinus node dysfunction, the patient has a slow junctional rhythm at a rate of approximately 20 beats/minute, resulting in the occurrence of AF.

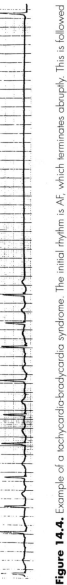

Figure 14.4. Example of a tachycardia-bradycardia syndrome. The initial rhythm is AF, which terminates abruptly. This is followed by a 6.3-second pause and a junctional beat.

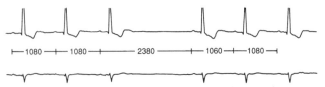

Figure 14.5. An ECG rhythm strip illustrating a sinus pause. Use the interval measurements to determine whether it is due to S-A exit block or S-A arrest.

out of proportion to sinus arrhythmia and that are not multiples of the basic underlying cycle length (Fig. 14.5). This contrasts with sinus node exit block, a disorder of conduction that exists when an impulse generated within the SA node fails to conduct out to the atrium or does so slowly. First-degree sinus node exit block can be identified by intracardiac electrophysiologic studies (see later discussion) but cannot be recognized on the routine electrocardiogram, as sinus node depolarization is not visible on it. Although sinus node depolarization may be visible on appropriately obtained signal-averaged electrocardiograms (ECGs), we have found that any degree of sinus arrhythmia precludes accurate measurements. First-degree sinus node exit block, a prolongation of sinoatrial SA conduction time, is analogous to the prolonged P-R interval seen when AV nodal conduction is slow. Also analogous to AV nodal conduction is type I and type II second-degree sinus node exit block. Type I sinus node exit block is recognized by Wenckebach periodically of P-P intervals (a progressive shortening of consecutive P-P intervals until one abruptly lengthens), similar to the R-R interval periodicity in AV Wenckebach (Fig. 14.1). Type II second-degree sinus node exit block is recognized by an abrupt P-P interval lengthening to a value that is a multiple of (e.g., twice, three times, four times) the basic sinus cycle length. Third-degree SA nodal exit block, as well as cessation of automaticity, both of which are rare, would cause atrial standstill in the absence of an escape rhythm.

Prevalence

Because sinus bradyarrhythmias are often asymptomatic and may be physiologic rather than dysfunctional, it is impossible to determine the frequency of SND within any population. In screening studies, such as cardiovascular detection programs, the incidence has been reported to be under 0.2%. However, the absence of routine prolonged ambulatory monitoring in most such programs ought to underestimate the true incidence. In contrast, if one does not distinguish between pathologic and physiologic sinus bradyarrhythmias, the incidence is substantial. For example, in a University of Illinois study of 50 normal young men and women, 24% of men and 8% of women had rates less than 40 beats/minute with sleep. (The average, maximum, and minimum waking and sleeping heart rates were also greater in women than in men.) Other studies reveal that sinus pauses in excess of 2 seconds can occur in apparently normal subjects and in up to 37% of trained athletes. Pauses in excess of 3 seconds, however, are rare in normals, frequently correlate with symptoms, and should provoke clinical assessment.

Significance

The recognition of sinus node dysfunction is important in several respects. First and foremost is its relationship to symptoms. If sinus rates are sufficiently slow or pauses are sufficiently long so as to impair cerebral or peripheral blood flow, symptoms will ensue. The extent of bradycardia or length of pause that results in symptoms, however, varies among individuals because stroke volume, peripheral resistance, and local vascular patency also contribute to the extent of regional blood flow at any heart rate. Chronotropic incompetence often leads to exertional fatigue or dyspnea. Symptoms associated with undue resting bradycardia most commonly are fatigue, dizziness, or minor personality changes. Symptoms most commonly associated with undue pauses are dizziness, syncope, or manifestations of escape rhythms. Importantly, all of these symptoms are nonspecific; that is, many processes can produce identical symptoms, and thus, no symptom is specific for SND. Accordingly, the treatment of symptomatic SND requires documentation of the association between the dysrhythmia and the symptom or the reasonable exclusion of alternate explanations for the symptom. Rarely, marked sinus bradycardia will cause dyspnea or worsened angina that reflect the associated increase in ventricular filling and diastolic pressure.

The recognition of SND is also important in relation to implications for concomitant therapy. An asymptomatic bradycardia may become symptomatic if worsened by the administration of an agent that is depressive to the sinus node (Table 14.1). Many of these agents, such as digitalis, the β-blockers, verapamil, diltiazem, and the class I and III antiarrhythmics are used in the treatment of paroxysmal supraventricular tachyarrhythmias. In patients with the bradycardia-tachycardia syndrome, however, reduction of or control of the tachycardia may occur at the expense of worsening of the bradycardia. Digitalis is the least likely of these agents to do this in SND patients, in our experience. A β-blocker with intrin-

Table 14.1
Cardioactive Drugs That May Induce or Worsen Sinus Node Dysfunction

β-Blockers
Calcium channel blockers (e.g., verapamil, diltiazem)
Sympatholytic antihypertensives (e.g., α-methyldopa, clonidine, guanabenz, reserpine)
Cimetidine
Lithium
Phenothiazines (rarely)
Antihistamines
Antidepressants
Antiarrhythmic agents
    May cause SND in normals: amiodarone
    Frequently worsens *mild* SND: flecainide
    Infrequently worsens *mild* SND: digitalis, quinidine, procainamide, disopyramide, moricizine[a]
    Rarely worsens *mild* SND: lidocaine, phenytoin, mexiletine, tocainide
Opioid blockers

[a]Note: the anticholinergic properties of disopyramide may reduce the risk of SND.

sic sympathomimetic activity, such as pindolol, may also be tolerated in some patients. Frequently, pacemaker implantation is pursued to support antiarrhythmic therapy in patients with asymptomatic SND.

SND is also important to recognize because of the potential for embolism. The bradycardia-tachycardia syndrome has had a sufficiently high incidence of associated systemic emboli to warrant the use of anticoagulants. Similarly, right atrial thrombi have been documented when underlying atrial disorders coexist with SND.

Lastly, some data suggest that SND may have an adverse effect on survival. However, when SND is idiopathic and unassociated with apparent underlying structural heart disease or more distal conduction system dysfunction, mortality may not be increased, though symptoms may develop or worsen with time. If AF becomes persistent as a default rhythm in SND, the prognosis of AF itself becomes a factor.

Diagnostic Evaluation

Generally, therapy for SND is required only for symptom relief or to support concomitant drug therapy, as noted previously. However, the relationship between the dysrhythmia and symptoms should be established as clearly as possible, because many of the common symptoms are nonspecific. In addition, they may be unrelated to SND. Periods of sinus bradycardia or pauses are frequent in normal individuals, particularly nocturnally (with sleep) or with other periods of high vagal tone, as was noted earlier. Because symptoms are typically brief and/or intermittent, they are rarely present during routine ECGs. More often, prolonged ambulatory ECG recordings and/or transtelephonic event recordings are needed to capture a symptomatic episode. The documentation of symptoms simultaneously with a bradydysrhythmia is a strong enough piece of evidence to declare a relationship between the two and to pursue therapy. In the case of suspected chronotropic incompetence, an exercise ECG may similarly be diagnostic. In patients with the hypersensitive carotid sinus syndrome, appropriate symptoms (such as symptoms in association with shaving, head turning, buttoning a collar, tying a tie) coupled with a hypersensitive response on physical examination, can establish a diagnosis. The hypersensitive response on physical examination is represented by a pause in excess of 3 seconds in response to moderate unilateral massage of 5 seconds.

Noninvasive techniques, however, are often inadequate because of the transient nature of symptoms. In an early study using Holter recordings in patients with known SND, the sensitivity was only 60–75%. In a study of 44 symptomatic patients, a diagnosis was achieved in only 48%, despite an average duration of almost 6 days of continuous recordings. Similarly, chronotropic incompetence may vary (perhaps with autonomic tone); thus, exercise test reproducibility is limited, and a normal response may not exclude SND.

When ambulatory electrocardiographic surveillance fails to capture a symptomatic episode or fails to reveal a bradycardia severe enough in itself to warrant therapy (a rate less than 30 beats/minute or pauses greater than 3 seconds), electrophysiologic techniques may be used.

Electrophysiologic (EP) studies are designed to be diagnostic, i.e., to demonstrate the severity of SND and, if possible, to provoke the clinical symptoms. EP studies can also be used to provide prognostic information. Additionally, when performed serially, EP studies can provide information about the efficacy, safety, or intolerance of proposed medications for concurrent disorders. For example, serial EP studies (predrug and postdrug administration) can be used to tell whether a drug may worsen a bradycardia or a posttachycardic pause if it fails to prevent the paroxysmal tachycardia itself. Acute drug studies using intravenous (i.v.) or oral agents are highly predictive of long-term effects in patients with SND. Sinus node pauses after overdrive pacing in the EP laboratory closely approximate pauses following spontaneous tachyarrhythmias, both before and after drug administration.

The target of EP evaluation of the SA node is an assessment of automaticity, conduction, occasionally refractoriness, and possible associated tachyarrhythmias and conduction defects. Because a detailed review of sinus node EP testing is beyond the scope of this chapter, only an overview will be presented here.

There is no technique that purely assesses automaticity. However, the heart rate response after atropine and the behavior of sinus rhythm after overdrive atrial pacing come the closest. In normal individuals, incremental dosing of atropine will produce progressively more rapid sinus rates until all vagal influence is abolished. In our experience, at this point the sinus rate will plateau around 110–120 beats/minute. In patients with intrinsic SND, this peak rate will be lower. A sinus rate that does not exceed 90 beats/minute after atropine is indicative of intrinsic SND. However, those with autonomically mediated extrinsic SND will appear normal by this test. Also, if the baseline bradycardia were due to SA exit block, e.g., 2:1, and the atropine were to reverse the conduction defect, the sinus rate would also improve, though not simply from enhanced automaticity.

Overdrive pacing is probably the most commonly used single test to screen for SND in the EP laboratory. It is based on observations made in the tortoise heart over a century ago, which revealed that cardiac pacemakers can be suppressed by overdrive stimulation and will take a finite and reproducible time to recover their normal automatic firing rate after such overdrive suppression. In clinical practice, this technique uses trains of atrial pacing (usually 30–60 seconds), at several cycle lengths shorter than the spontaneous sinus cycle length to suppress the sinus node. Following termination of pacing, the interval until the recovery of the first sinus beat is measured (Fig. 14.6). (Occasionally the interval to the complete return of the prepacing sinus rate is also assessed.) Cycle lengths of 400, 500, 600, 700, 800, 900, 1000 msec, and so on are used. This technique assumes that the paced impulses conduct into the sinus node and continuously reset and suppress the pacemaker focus. After termination of pacing, the speed of recovery of a sinus impulse is taken as an index of sinus node function—reflecting in large part automaticity. In theory, the more disordered the automatic properties of the SA node, the more severely it will be suppressed by overdrive, the slower it will recover, and the longer will be the postpacing pause. However, the impulse, once formed, must conduct out of the node, and prolonged postpacing pauses have also been docu-

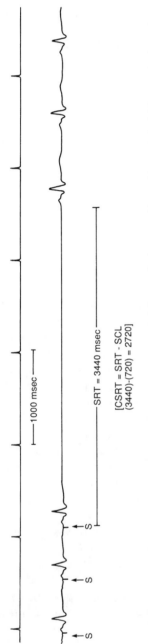

Figure 14.6. A lead II rhythm strip showing the sinus recovery time (*SRT*) following the last paced beats (*S*, stimulus) of 30 seconds of overdrive pacing. Calculation of the corrected SRT is demonstrated (see text for discussion).

mented to occasionally reflect postpacing exit delay or exit block for one or more impulses.

To facilitate interpatient comparisons, the following guidelines may be helpful. Because the absolute value of the postpacing pause would not be expected to be the same in patients with different native sinus rates, the longest pause is usually normalized or "corrected," most often by subtracting the prepacing sinus cycle length. A corrected sinus node recovery time (CSRT) obtained in this way is less than 525 msec in normals. (The absolute value taken in normals varies a little among laboratories.) In truth, however, overdrive pacing is more complex than just an assessment of suppression of automaticity. Rapid atrial pacing reflexively initiates vagal activation, which depresses both AV nodal and SA nodal conduction. The increase in A-H intervals and eventual development of AV nodal Wenckebach patterns with incremental atrial pacing is a commonly recognized manifestation of the former. Atriosinus entrance block can also occur with incremental atrial pacing, in which case all atrial paced impulses may not penetrate the sinus node. The same would be true if perinodal or intranodal conduction were impaired by disease. For this reason, multiple pacing rates must be used to determine the maximal obtainable sinus recovery time and, in the setting of disease or substantial vagotonia, the maximally recorded sinus recovery time may appear normal, despite dysfunction. That is, if impaired conduction sufficiently limits sinus nodal penetration by the paced impulses, the node will not be suppressed, and recovery intervals will not be prolonged. Such "falsely shortened" sinus node recovery times (SRTs) reduce the sensitivity of sinus recovery time assessment to the range of 55–75%.

Fortunately, in most such circumstances, the longest recovery time is noted at a fairly long-paced cycle length rather than at a rapid pacing rate, especially if the reproducibility of postpacing pauses is assessed at each paced cycle length tested and the average of those obtained at each cycle length is considered. Other evidence of SND obtained from postpacing observations is secondary pauses, that is, cycles after the first with cycle lengths longer than the first. These secondary pauses are not seen in normals, but their utility in symptom assessment is uncertain.

When the postpacing pause is sufficiently long so as to induce the patient's clinical symptoms, then both the diagnosis and mechanism of symptoms are clearly established, and therapy goals will be clear. When the postpacing pauses are sufficiently long to establish sinus node dysfunction, but the link to symptom remains undocumented, the interpretation must be handled like the interpretation of notable but asymptomatic sinus bradycardia on ambulatory monitoring. Therapy is usually pursued when alternative explanations for the symptoms have been excluded. Although CSRT values greater than 525 msec are abnormal, there is no single value that, if exceeded, always correlates with symptoms.

Because determination of the CSRT is not in itself highly sensitive for SND, though a prolonged CSRT has high specificity, additional EP tests have been developed. These focus on SA nodal properties other than automaticity. Most frequently, these have involved an assessment of SA conduction. One clue to disordered SA conduction has already been mentioned—namely, the instance when the longest SRTs occur at the slowest pacing rates. However, SA conduction can also be assessed without the stress of overdrive pacing and its inherent increase in vagal tone.

The earliest methods to determine the time it takes an impulse to conduct from the dominant pacemaker region of the sinus node out to the atrium, the sinoatrial conduction time (SACT), were all indirect. That is, they used observations made during atrial premature stimulation or during short trains of slow atrial pacing to calculate the SACT. These two stimulation approaches both assume that, following a beat that retrogradely captures the SA node in the absence of overdrive suppression, the return sinus cycle as measured on the atrial electrogram will encompass the conduction time from the atrial paced beat into the SA node, the sinus cycle length following reset of the pacemaker focus by the atrial beat, and the conduction time of this next sinus beat out of the node.

If the sinus cycle length of this recovery beat within the node is the same as the average SCL, the atrial cycle will equal the SCL plus the SACT into and out of the node. Thus, 1/2 of the difference between the post-APD atrial cycle length and the average SCL will approximate the average unidirectional SACT. Using such approaches, the average SACT is generally less than 120–130 msec and has been found to be abnormal in some patients with normal CSRTs. SACT values longer than 130 msec represent first-degree SA exit block. In this regard, the SACT calculation has been of diagnostic and prognostic value. Occasionally, patterns of 2:1 or more advanced SA block are precipitated by the atrial premature stimuli or slow atrial pacing and can replicate spontaneous long pauses or symptoms. In such cases, the SACT testing helps identify the need for therapy. Hence, the interpretation and utility parallels that of the CSRT.

More recently, a direct technique to determine SACT has been utilized. Sinus node electrograms can be recorded using appropriate catheter placement and filters and by directly visualizing the depolarization of the sinus node as well as atrial activation on such sinus node electrograms (SNE), the SACT can be directly measured (Fig. 14.7).

It should be stated that the recognition of abnormal SA conduction can be useful not only as a direct determinant of SND or as a factor in falsely short SRTs, but also in to improve the sensitivity of CSRT testing. It has been demonstrated that when SA entrance block has limited overdrive suppression and hence has falsely shortened the SRT, repetition of the overdrive pacing runs following the administration of atropine (to prevent or alleviate vagally induced depression of SA conduction) may reveal the inherent defect in automaticity and produce long and diagnostic pauses. This should be performed when CSRTs are normal, but the longest ones occur at a long-paced cycle length or when the SACT is prolonged.

For diagnostic purposes, when the aforementioned constellation of EP tests is used to confirm SND in the absence of clear noninvasive documentation, the sensitivity is variable. Individual reports for CSRT or SACT have ranged from 18–75%, with an increase generally reported when the tests are used in combina-

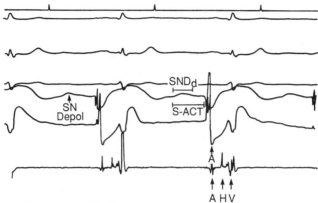

Figure 14.7. A human sinus node electrogram (SNE). From top to bottom are shown: 1000-msec time pips; ECG leads I, AVF, V1; the human sinus node electrogram; a high right atrial electrogram 1 cm proximal to the SNE; and the His bundle electrogram (where atrial (A), His bundle (H), and ventricular (V) depolarization is indicated). On the SNE, the sinus node depolarization (SN Depol), the denoted measurement of the sinoatrial conduction time (S-ACT), and the duration of the sinus node depolarization (SNDd) are depicted. See text for discussion.

tion. The specificity probably approximates 90%. In patients with syncope of uncertain etiology, the combination of EP tests is more likely to document SND than is a 24-hour Holter monitor recording.

For prognostic purposes, abnormal EP test results are also useful. There is a significant incidence (60%) of symptom development during follow-up in patients with asymptomatic sinus bradycardia who have a prolonged CSRT. Conversely, patients with asymptomatic sinus bradycardia but a normal CSRT have a less than 30% incidence of subsequent symptom development. For patients who are already symptomatic, pacemaker implantation in patients with prolonged CSRT will be associated with resolution of symptoms more than 90% of the time.

In addition to determining the SACT and examining observations made during overdrive atrial pacing, an assessment of the duration of sinus node refractory periods has been suggested as having clinical utility. Its role remains uncertain and underexamined, however, and it is not widely used. More recently, we have shown that the duration of the sinus node depolarization on sinus node electrograms (Fig. 14.7) is prolonged in patients with modest or severe SND and thus has direct clinical utility. The duration of the sinus node depolarization is prolonged when the P cells' action potentials are prolonged, automaticity is impaired, or intrasinus or perisinus impulse conduction is slow. As such, it correlates closely with the findings of an abnormal CSRT or SACT. Noting the duration of sinus node refractory periods is probably no more sensitive as an identifier of SND than is an abnormal CSRT or SACT. Nevertheless, it may be quicker to determine in some patients and is not subject to the "pseudonormalization" seen with the CSRT when entrance block is present.

One additional test to expose SND is the use of i.v. adenosine (150 μg/kg). An increase in SCL of greater than 675 msec following adenosine has similar sensitivity (69%) and specificity (100%) to that of a prolonged CSRT. However, further experience with this protocol will need to be gathered before its widespread use can be justified. Additionally, as with the CSRT itself, a modestly high false-negative rate (36%) may limit its utility.

Therapy

The therapy of SND is generally based upon symptoms. In general, a bradycardia or a pause of sinus origin that is asymptomatic requires no therapy. Exceptions to this rule, however, occur when one must add an agent for the treatment of a concomitant disorder, such as a tachyarrhythmia or hypertension, and that agent has a likelihood of worsening the SND significantly (Table 14.1). Prophylactic treatment of the SND is then justifiable. When the degree of the bradycardia or the length of the pause is so severe that any further worsening is likely to produce symptoms or place the patient at risk for having an unstable escape rhythm, another exception exists. Acceptable indications for pacemaker implantation in this respect, for example, are rates in the 30s or pauses in excess of 3 seconds.

Specific corrective therapy is possible only when a reversible cause has been established. For example, sinus bradycardia due to myxedema will resolve with the treatment of the hypothyroidism. Similarly, the hypersensitive carotid sinus syndrome may resolve with carotid sinus denervation. However, in most circumstances, therapy must be aimed at symptom prevention, independent of cause. When the pathophysiologic mechanism is parasympathetic excess, belladonna alkaloids, such as atropine and its congeners, may be tried either prophylactically or therapeutically. However, most patients with SND are older and either have intrinsic SA node dysfunction or do not tolerate the anticholinergic side effects, such as constipation, sicca, visual blurring, prostatism, lethargy, or confusion. Such patients may also have a discrete contraindication to these agents, such as glaucoma, sluggish bowel, angina, prostatic hypertrophy, or obstructive pulmonary disease. Thus, anticholinergics are generally used as emergency i.v. therapy, in younger patients, or for short-term treatment.

Occasionally, agents that produce sympathetic activation in response to drug-induced vasodilatation (such as hydralazine) or β-blockers with intrinsic sympathomimetic activity may help reduce or prevent sinus bradycardia. There have been no reported studies linking the efficacy of such agents to the mechanism of the bradycardia. However, it is likely that patients with intrinsic sinus node dysfunction are less responsive. For the overwhelming majority of patients with SND, pacemaker implantation is the therapy of choice. Underlying disease pathophysiology, ventricular compliance characteristics, the status of associated conduction defects and arrhythmias, and the status of ventriculoatrial (VA) conduction are important considerations in selecting pacemaker node(s) and site(s).

Pacemaker therapy in SND is directed at symptoms, not at longevity. The progression of effectively treated SND is determined by the associated heart disease (e.g., left ventricular dysfunction, myocardial ischemia, valvular disorder), and longevity is usually not prolonged in SND by pacemaker insertion. Quality of life, however, may be notably enhanced when pacemaker insertion is directed at symptom relief and the symptoms have been adequately correlated with SND.

In the presence of associated AV conduction defects (which are common and usually AV nodal in origin), pacing must be ventricular or dual chamber. In its absence, atrial pacing may suffice, particularly when AV nodal conduction is normal at detailed EP testing. When the disorder being treated presents as occasional pauses, an AAI or a VVI pacer to prevent such pauses may be all that is needed initially. There are patients, however, who develop persistent bradycardia with time and begin to pace most or all of the time. This possibility as well as the status of VA conduction should be considered prior to pacer implantation vis-à-vis potential pacing modes and lead site(s) that should be available. In the presence of frequent or persistent sinus bradycardia, whether initial or later in the course, attention to the hemodynamics of pacing is required, and dual chamber devices will often be found necessary.

In the presence of chronotropic incompetence (which should be considered prior to pacer implant), a rate-responsive unit such as a VVIR or DDDR is optimal, and will be needed for full symptom relief. AAIR devices are occasionally useful but are less predictably effective if AV conduction becomes impaired over time. In the presence of atrial tachycardias such as paroxysmal AF, DDI(R) or VVI(R) features may be necessary. The specific mode(s) will depend upon the type of tachycardia, status of AV and VA conduction, and chronotropic competence. Because AF is a common sequelae of SND long term, this possibility should be considered prior to pacemaker implantation. Lastly, in the bradycardia-tachycardia patients, atrial pacing at a rate in the mid- to upper normal range (e.g., 80–85 beats/minute) with an AAI or a dual chamber device will often reduce and occasionally eliminate the paroxysmal fibrillating periods. Clearly, the numerous issues described in this chapter must be considered when implanting a pacemaker for SND. Thus, before the implantation is performed, the decision as to type and features of the device to be implanted should be reviewed with or by a physician knowledgeable in current pacemaker methodology.

SUGGESTED READING

Bigger JT Jr, Reiffel JA. Sick sinus syndrome. Ann Rev Med 1979;30:91–118.

Fujimura O, Yee R, Klein GJ, Sharma AD, Boahene KA. The diagnostic sensitivity of electrophysiologic testing in patients with syncope caused by transient bradycardia. N Engl J Med 1989;321:1703–1707.

Kerr CR, Strauss HC. The measurement of sinus node refractoriness in man. Circulation 1984;68:1231–1237.

Reiffel JA. Electrophysiologic evaluation of sinus node function. Cardiol Clin 1986;4:401–416.

Reiffel JA, Bigger JT Jr. Current status of direct recordings of the sinus node electrogram in man. PACE 1983;6:1143–1150.

Reiffel JA, Bigger JT Jr. The relationship between sinoatrial conduction time and sinus cycle length revisted. J Electrophysiol 1987;1:290–299.

15 Atrial Tachycardia

ATRIAL PREMATURE DEPOLARIZATIONS, JUNCTIONAL PREMATURE
DEPOLARIZATIONS, MULTIFOCAL ATRIAL TACHYCARDIA, AND ATRIAL
TACHYCARDIA

Atrial Premature Depolarizations

PREVALENCE AND SIGNIFICANCE

Atrial premature depolarization (APDs) occur commonly in both the young and
the elderly with or without significant heart disease. They should therefore not be
considered an abnormal finding. The prevalence of APDs is highly dependent on
the technique used to evaluate the population. The frequency and prevalence of
APDs appear to increase with age. Variability with regard to APDs is similar to that
reported for ventricular premature depolarizations. As with ventricular premature
depolarizations, there may also be a circadian variation in the frequency of APDs,
but there is significant interpatient variation. Cardiac conditions associated with
APDs are mitral valve prolapse, myocardial infarction (MI), especially with left
ventricular dysfunction, hypertrophic cardiomyopathy, mitral stenosis, mitral
regurgitation and any cause for congestive heart failure (CHF). Other medical
conditions, such as acute and chronic pulmonary disease, chronic renal failure,
and neurologic disorders, have also been associated with an increased frequency
of APDs. Smoking, alcohol, and coffee are considered potential precipitants of
APDs. Smoking and alcohol intake are known to increase sympathetic tone, which
may affect the frequency of APDs.

ELECTROCARDIOGRAM MANIFESTATION AND DIAGNOSIS

APDs may have a variety of manifestations on the electrocardiogram (ECG)
(Figs. 15.1–15.4). The diagnosis of an APD is made when a P wave with a morphology different from the morphology of the sinus P wave is noted earlier than
the anticipated sinus P wave. The APD may be associated with a normally conducted QRS complex and normal or short P-R interval, a normal QRS complex
with a prolonged P-R interval, a conducted but aberrant QRS complex, or it may
not be conducted.

Early APDs may also impinge upon the refractory period of the His-Purkinje
conduction system and lead to variable degrees of aberrant conduction (Fig. 15.2).
In general, right bundle branch block aberrancy is more common than left bundle
branch block aberrancy because of the longer refractory period of the right bundle branch.

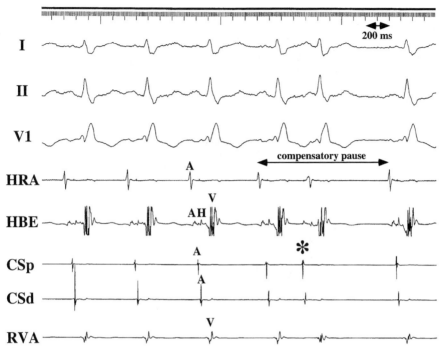

Figure 15.1. Simultaneous surface electrocardiographic recordings from leads I, II, and V1 as well as intracardiac recordings from the high right atrium (*HRA*), His bundle electrogram (*HBE*), proximal (*CSp*) and distal (*CSd*) coronary sinus, and right ventricular apex (*RVA*). An APD is noted (*asterisk*, second to last beat in the tracing). For the sinus beats, earliest activation occurs in the high right atrium, followed by the His bundle electrogram and coronary sinus. For the APD, earliest atrial activation occurs in the coronary sinus electrogram. With the APD, there is conduction delay in the AV node reflected by an increase in the A-H interval from 50 msec at baseline to 65 msec with the APD. In addition, though not typical for APDs, there is a fully compensatory pause.

Finally, the site of origin of an APD can also affect its conduction through the atrioventricular (AV) node. An APD originating in the low right atrium near the AV node may result in a short P-R interval (<120 msec) and may even be mistaken for a junctional premature depolarization. The AV nodal conduction time, and the P-R interval, may also differ, depending on the input pathway to the AV node.

A nonconducted APD (Fig. 15.3) may give the false appearance of a sinus pause, and a nonconducted APD may be obscured by the T wave. Evaluation of multiple leads may be required to detect the APD, as it may cause a discernible deflection in only a limited number of ECG leads and may be manifest only as a deformity of the normal T wave.

An APD that occurs relatively late in the cardiac cycle may not reach the sinus node and will therefore not reset the sinus node (zone of collision or interference). In this case, a fully compensatory pause may be noted. More commonly, an APD will depolarize the sinus node and reset it (zone of reset). A postextrasystolic pause

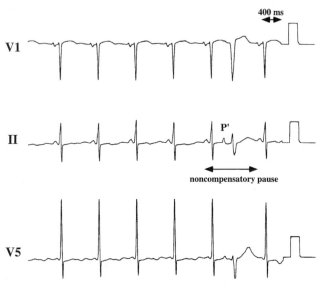

Figure 15.2. Simultaneous electrocardiographic recordings from leads V1, II, and V5 demonstrating an atrial premature depolarization (*P'*) conducted with a long P-R interval and aberrant ventricular conduction. In this case, there is a noncompensatory pause, which is typical for an APD.

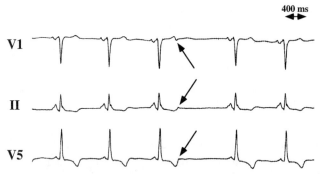

Figure 15.3. Simultaneous electrocardiographic recordings from leads V1, II, and V5 demonstrating an APD (*arrows*). In lead V1, the APD causes a clear deformity in the T wave. In lead II, the APD causes a small but noticeable deformity in the T wave. In lead V5, the APD is almost completely obscured by the T wave.

that is not fully compensatory is frequently observed. APDs may transiently depress sinus node function, thereby causing a post-APD interval that is longer than the previously noted sinus cycle length; this explains the presence of a post-extrasystolic pause that is not fully compensatory.

A very early APD may find the sinus node refractory, giving rise to an interpolated APD (zone of interpolation) or sinus echoes (zone of sinus echoes). These types of responses are the least common.

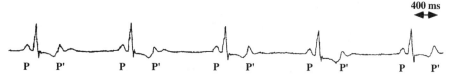

Figure 15.4. Holter recording from a patient with atrial bigeminy leading to an effective ventricular rate of 38 beats/minute. P, normal P wave; P′, nonconducted atrial premature depolarization. (Courtesy of James Rosenthal, M.D.)

ELECTROPHYSIOLOGY

There are no indications for performing electrophysiologic studies in patients with APDs. Findings related to APDs include an activation sequence that is different from the sinus activation sequence (Fig. 15.1). Functional bundle branch block may be associated with a prolongation of the H-V interval. Typically, nonconducted APDs demonstrate block at the level of the AV node.

ASSOCIATED SYMPTOMS

Most subjects with APDs are asymptomatic. However, APDs may lead to symptoms of palpitations or the sensation of skipped beats. Sensation of skipped beats may be due to nonconducted APDs or ineffective contraction because of poor filling of the left ventricle during the premature beat. Atrial bigeminy with nonconducted APDs may lead to ventricular rates approaching 40 beats/minute, possibly leading to symptoms related to the bradyarrhythmia (Fig. 15.4). APDs may precipitate a sustained supraventricular tachyarrhythmia.

PHYSICAL EXAMINATION

Palpation of the peripheral pulse will demonstrate either premature pulse waves or pauses related to APDs. Early APDs may lead to cannon A waves on the jugular venous pulsations. This may be particularly helpful in differentiating early nonconducted APDs from sinus pauses. Auscultation of the heart may detect early heart sounds or pauses. APDs may lead to changes in a variety of cardiac murmurs (such as those due to mitral valve prolapse) because of the reduction in diastolic filling time.

THERAPY

In the asymptomatic individual, no therapy is required for APDs. For patients with symptomatic APDs, reassurance of the benign nature of APDs and discontinuing potential precipitating habits such as smoking, coffee intake, alcohol intake, and stress, may alleviate the symptoms. Otherwise, initial therapy should include a β-blocker, if there is no contraindication. β-Blockers have been successful in controlling both the symptoms related to APDs and their frequency.

Digoxin, calcium channel blockers, and type Ib antiarrhythmic agents have not been clearly shown to have benefit in patients with symptomatic APDs. Type Ia, type Ic, and type III antiarrhythmic agents may be used to diminish the frequency of APDs in the patient who is symptomatic. Treatment with these agents must be balanced with the risk for proarrhythmia associated with these agents.

JUNCTIONAL PREMATURE DEPOLARIZATIONS

PREVALENCE AND SIGNIFICANCE

Junctional premature depolarizations (JPDs) occur less commonly than both atrial and ventricular premature depolarizations. The prevalence of JPDs has not been well studied. JPDs may occur in subjects with normal hearts or those with structural heart disease, young or old. The etiology is the same as for APDs.

ECG MANIFESTATION AND DIAGNOSIS

JPDs may have a variety of manifestations on the surface ECG (Fig. 15.5). Most frequently, JPDs are detected when there is a premature beat with a normal QRS complex and (a) a P wave with a P-R interval (<90 msec) that is too short to be considered to be conducted through the AV node; (b) no P wave (in which case it may be buried within the QRS complex or there may be no retrograde atrial activation (Fig. 15.6); or (c) a P wave that occurs at the terminal portion of the QRS complex. The location of the P wave relative to the QRS complex provides no definitive information regarding the site of origin within the AV junction, but is simply a manifestation of the relative anterograde and retrograde conduction velocities. JPDs frequently conduct anterograde with bundle branch block. In this case, they may be indistinguishable from premature ventricular depolarizations on the ECG. JPDs may conduct retrograde to the atrium and demonstrate conduction block to the ventricles. When this occurs, they appear like APDs and are indistinguishable from nonconducted APDs on the surface ECG. Thus, JPDs may resemble either APDs or ventricular premature depolarizations.

Finally, JPDs may fail to conduct both antegrade to the ventricles and retrograde to the atria, in which case they are concealed junctional premature depolarizations (Fig. 15.7). This may have no effect on the surface ECG or may be manifest on the surface ECG as either sudden prolongation of the P-R interval for a single beat or Mobitz I (Wenckebach) or Mobitz II second-degree AV block. Concealed junctional bigeminy may give rise to 2:1 AV block. The definitive differentiation between concealed JPDs leading to the appearance of Mobitz II second-degree AV block versus actual Mobitz II second-degree AV block is virtually impossible on the surface ECG, but nevertheless remains an important distinction. The P wave morphology of JPDs is generally related to the retrograde acti-

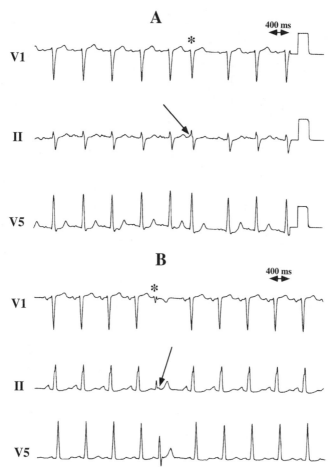

Figure 15.5. Simultaneous electrocardiographic recordings from leads V1, II, and V5 demonstrating a JPD (*asterisk*). In both *A* and *B*, the arrow marks the sinus P wave, which occurs just prior to the JPD in *A* and just after the JPD in *B*. In *A*, the QRS configuration for the junctional premature depolarization is identical to that of the sinus beats. In *B*, the junctional premature depolarization demonstrates a different QRS configuration.

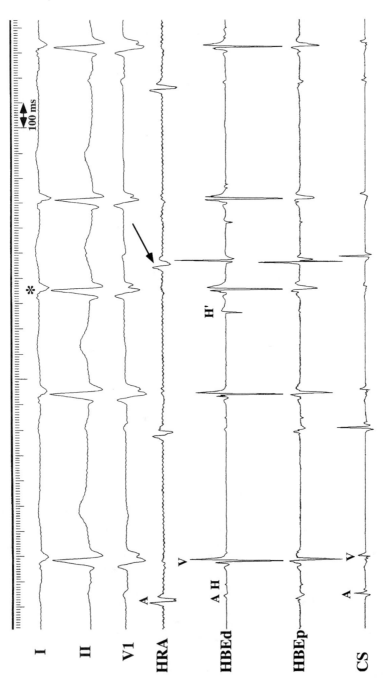

Figure 15.6. Simultaneous surface electrocardiographic recordings from leads I, II, and V1 as well as intracardiac recordings from the high right atrium (*HRA*), distal (*HBEd*) and proximal (*HBEp*) His bundle electrogram, and coronary sinus (*CS*). An interpolated junctional premature depolarization (*asterisk, H'*) is noted. The sinus beat following the junctional premature depolarization conducts through the AV node with a prolonged A-H interval.

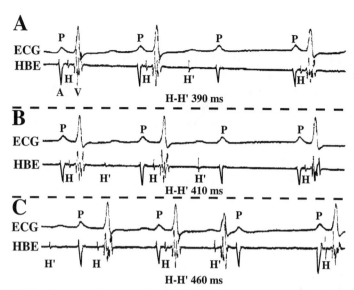

Figure 15.7. Simultaneous surface ECG and intracardiac His bundle electrograms (*HBE*) in a patient with JPDs. *H'* indicates a JPD. **A.** A JPD occurs at a coupling interval of 390 msec and demonstrates both anterograde and retrograde conduction block; thus, there is no activity on the ECG corresponding to the JPD. However, the following P wave fails to conduct to the ventricles. The electrocardiographic appearance is that of Mobitz II second-degree AV block, while the intracardiac recordings demonstrate that AV block is due to a concealed JPD. **B.** There are two JPDs in this tracing. The first one results in prolongation of the following P-R interval. Another JPD occurs following this conducted P wave and produces block of the next P wave. In this case, the electrocardiographic appearance is that of Mobitz I second-degree AV block (Wenckebach); however, intracardiac recordings demonstrate that this pattern is due to two concealed JPDs. **C.** There are again two JPDs. The first JPD produces sudden prolongation of the following P-R interval. The second JPD at a coupling interval of 460 msec successfully conducts to the ventricles. The following sinus P wave is therefore not conducted. (Adapted from Rosen K, Rahimtoola S, Gunnar R. Pseudo A-V block secondary to premature nonpropagated His bundle depolarizations. Documentation by His bundle electrocardiography. Circulation 1970;42:367–373.)

vation of the atria via the AV node. Thus, the P wave is generally inverted in ECG leads II, III, and aVF, upright in aVR, flat or biphasic in lead I, and usually upright in V1.

ELECTROPHYSIOLOGY

Junctional premature depolarizations generally do not require invasive electrophysiologic investigation unless there is a question of infra-His conduction disease, as in the patient with possible Mobitz II second-degree AV block. However, JPDs do occur occasionally during routine electrophysiology studies. If there is anterograde conduction, the H-V interval will be either the same as baseline or prolonged (ruling out a ventricular origin of the premature beat). If there is retrograde activation of the atria, atrial activation will occur following the His bundle activation. The H-A conduction time may be variable, depending on the site.

ASSOCIATED SYMPTOMS

Most subjects with JPDs are asymptomatic. However, JPDs may lead to symptoms of palpitations or the sensation of skipped beats. The sensation of skipped beats may occur because of concealed JPDs or ineffective contraction due to poor filling of the left ventricle during the premature beat. Concealed JPDs that lead to second-degree AV block may be associated with symptoms of lightheadedness or near syncope, particularly if they occur in a bigeminal pattern.

PHYSICAL EXAMINATION

Palpation of the peripheral pulse will demonstrate either a premature pulse wave or pauses related to JPDs. Auscultation of the heart may detect these changes as well.

THERAPY

In the asymptomatic individual, no therapy is required for JPDs. Therapeutic options may include β-blockers or calcium channel blockers. Digoxin probably will not control symptomatic JPDs. Type Ia antiarrhythmic agents may be tried in some cases. For patients refractory to these options, type Ic or type III antiarrhythmic agents may be offered. Patients with concealed JPDs giving rise to pseudo-AV block and symptomatic bradycardia should be treated with agents that will suppress the JPDs rather than with pacemaker implantation.

MULTIFOCAL ATRIAL TACHYCARDIA

PREVALENCE AND SIGNIFICANCE

Multifocal atrial tachycardia (MAT) has been noted in 0.05–0.38% of ECGs interpreted in hospitals. It is most commonly noted in an elderly population with a mean age in the upper 60s and 70s. The incidence of MAT in an outpatient setting has not been adequately studied, probably as a result of its association with acute illnesses.

Common illnesses found in patients with MAT include chronic obstructive pulmonary disease either with or without an acute exacerbation, pneumonia, nonpulmonary infections, CHF, postoperative state, diabetes mellitus, coronary artery disease, lung carcinoma, and pulmonary embolus. In patients admitted for acute respiratory decompensation of their underlying chronic obstructive pulmonary disease, the incidence of MAT has been reported between 6–17%. The finding of MAT is significant, as many studies have shown that these patients have a very high in-hospital mortality ranging from 25–56%. Death is not directly caused by the arrhythmia, but by the severity of the underlying disease. While MAT has a particularly strong association with advanced pulmonary disease, it has been noted in other settings, such as acute MI, electrolyte imbalance (particularly hypokalemia and hypomagnesemia), and mitral stenosis.

ETIOLOGY

Many factors contribute to the precipitation of MAT. The most common clinical precipitant is hypoxia due to an acute pulmonary or a cardiac problem. Other conditions associated with increased sympathetic tone, such as acute MI, sepsis, and the postoperative state, are also common precipitants of MAT. Electrolyte abnormalities, particularly hypokalemia and hypomagnesemia, may play a role in precipitating MAT.

ECG MANIFESTATION AND DIAGNOSIS

The diagnosis of MAT is made on the ECG when an atrial tachycardia (rate more than 120 beats/minute) is noted with at least three different P wave morphologies and with different P-P, P-R, and R-R intervals (Fig. 15.8). There must be an isoelectric interval between P waves. When the atrial rate is slower and associated with three different P wave morphologies, a diagnosis of wandering atrial pacemaker is more appropriate (Fig. 15.9). Because of the varying intervals in MAT, the ventricular response may be irregularly irregular and may be confused with coarse atrial fibrillation (AF). This distinction becomes more difficult because of the strong association of AF with MAT. AF or flutter may be noted prior to or following MAT in approximately half the cases. It may be important to examine multiple ECG leads to confirm the diagnosis. Some degree of AV block is commonly noted during MAT. Typical ventricular rates during MAT range from 100–170 beats/minute.

ELECTROPHYSIOLOGY

There are no indications for performing electrophysiologic studies in patients with MAT. Typically, this arrhythmia cannot be induced or terminated in the electrophysiology laboratory. Electrophysiologic recordings during MAT would be expected to show an atrial tachycardia with varying pathways of atrial activation.

ASSOCIATED SYMPTOMS

Subjects with MAT predominantly have complaints related to their underlying disorder, such as shortness of breath related to an exacerbation of chronic obstructive pulmonary disease or CHF. Patients may also have complaints related to the arrhythmia such as palpitations, lightheadedness, and chest pain. Given the

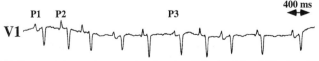

Figure 15.8. Electrocardiographic recording from lead V1 of multifocal AT. Note the multiple P wave morphologies (P1–P3). In addition, there are multiple P-R intervals as well as irregular R-R intervals.

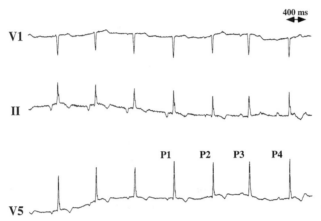

Figure 15.9. Simultaneous electrocardiographic recordings from leads V1, II, and V5. The tracing demonstrates a wandering atrial pacemaker. Four P wave morphologies can be identified (P1–P4). Because the rate is approximately 80 beats/minute, the diagnosis is wandering atrial pacemaker rather than multifocal AT.

advanced age and significant incidence of cardiac disease in these patients, they may not tolerate the rapid rates associated with MAT.

PHYSICAL EXAMINATION

Physical examination is notable for an irregular and perhaps irregularly irregular pulse, often leading to the incorrect diagnosis of AF. The presence of A waves on the jugular venous pulse may aid in the differentiation of MAT from AF. The predominant findings on physical examination are usually related to the underlying precipitating illness.

THERAPY

Therapy for MAT should be directed at correcting the underlying abnormalities, which include poor oxygenation and electrolyte abnormalities. Occasionally, patients will require adjunctive therapy for control of the tachycardia. A variety of treatment strategies have been attempted. Cardioversion is ineffective for MAT. Digoxin, and type I antiarrhythmic agents have also generally been ineffective for treatment of MAT. β-Blockers and verapamil have both been described to be effective for treatment of MAT by either restoring sinus rhythm or slowing the rate.

β-blockers do appear to be more efficacious in patients with MAT, but extreme caution must be exercised with the use of these agents in patients with obstructive pulmonary disease, as many of these patients cannot tolerate β-blockers. Magnesium therapy has also been shown to be effective in treating MAT, even in patients with normal serum magnesium levels. For those patients with pulmonary problems being treated with agents such as aminophylline or theophylline, which may be responsible for precipitating or exacerbating MAT, these agents should be discontinued, and alternative therapy should be considered.

ATRIAL TACHYCARDIA

PREVALENCE AND SIGNIFICANCE

Short bursts of atrial tachycardia (AT) occur occasionally on Holter monitoring in 2–6% of normal young subjects. In the healthy, active, elderly population, short bursts of AT have been noted in 1–13% of subjects, with most episodes lasting less than five beats. In patients with mitral valve prolapse, the incidence of AT has been reported to be between 3–29%, with a mean prevalence of approximately 20%. The rates of these tachycardias are generally slower than for other types of supraventricular tachycardia, with mean reported rates of approximately 115 beats/minute. AT has been noted in the setting of acute MI, present in 4–19% of patients.

Although an increased mortality has been reported in patients with AT versus those without, this is related to the severity of the underlying infarction. Short bursts of AT lasting up to 8 seconds have been noted in 40% of patients with mitral stenosis. In hospitalized patients with chronic obstructive pulmonary disease, AT may be noted in 20% of patients. In general, this variety of AT represents a benign arrhythmia, much like the presence of APDs.

Paroxysmal, sustained ATs account for approximately 10–15% of all cases of paroxysmal supraventricular tachycardia referred for electrophysiologic evaluation. Patients with AT are more likely to have organic heart disease than patients with other types of paroxysmal supraventricular tachycardia. The incidence of concomitant heart disease has been reported to vary from 33–100% and includes coronary artery disease, valvular disease, congenital heart disease, and other cardiomyopathies. This type of AT has been reported in all age groups, ranging from infants to the elderly.

Incessant AT is a much rarer entity than paroxysmal AT (PAT). This tachycardia is present more than half of the day. The exact prevalence of this disorder is difficult to gauge because of its low incidence. Most reports have been in children, though this arrhythmia has been documented in adults. The incessant nature of these tachycardias may lead to tachycardia-related cardiomyopathies, which may improve dramatically when the tachycardia is controlled.

PAT with block has been noted in 0.25–0.40% of ECGs. PAT with block has been classically associated with digitalis toxicity. The differentiation of this disorder from other varieties of atrial or sinus tachycardias may be difficult. Because of the presence of AV block, the nonconducted P wave may be obscured by either the QRS complex or T wave. Carotid sinus pressure or intravenous (i.v.) administration of adenosine may be used to increase the degree of AV block, allowing better visualization of the P waves. Similarly, esophageal lead recordings may be used to document the presence of AT with block. For the rare patients with digitalis-induced PAT with block at rates greater than 220 beat/minute, differentiation from atrial flutter is essential. Patients with AT will have isoelectric intervals between P waves. In addition, discontinuation of digoxin or potassium repletion will slow the tachycardia and then cause digitalis-induced AT to terminate.

Administration of digitalis will increase the rate of digitalis-induced PAT. In patients with PAT, discontinuation of digitalis does not always result in control of the arrhythmia. While digitalis toxicity should be suspected in a patient with PAT with block who is receiving digitalis, it is important to recognize that the AT may be a primary rhythm disorder requiring therapy. In the absence of digitalis toxicity, this tachycardia should be approached and treated as a paroxysmal, sustained AT. As in patients with MAT, there is a high in-hospital mortality associated with PAT with block, probably because of the severity of the underlying heart disease. The reported mortality has ranged from 20–60%. However, the mortality rates associated with this arrhythmia are likely to be significantly lower when the presence of digitalis toxicity is recognized, allowing for institution of appropriate therapy.

ETIOLOGY

Short bursts of AT may occur in the setting of a variety of precipitating factors. Myocardial ischemia or infarction, alcohol ingestion, hypoxia, theophylline toxicity, and electrolyte abnormalities (i.e., hypokalemia) may predispose to the short bursts of AT. Sustained, reentrant ATs may be found in patients with previous atrial surgery, such as those who have undergone procedures for correction of congenital heart disease. It may also be noted in a variety of other structural heart diseases.

The etiology of automatic ectopic ATs is unclear. Frequently, there is an associated cardiomyopathy, but it is unknown whether this is primary or secondary to the tachycardia. The high incidence of structural heart disease in patients with AT compared with the incidence of other types of paroxysmal supraventricular tachycardia suggests that structural or functional abnormalities of the atria might predispose to AT.

Finally, PAT with block occasionally results from digitalis toxicity. These patients usually have structural heart disease, providing the rationale for digitalis therapy. Hypokalemia and hypoxia may accentuate the toxic effects of digitalis. Pulmonary disease is also frequently noted in these patients.

ECG MANIFESTATION AND DIAGNOSIS

The electrocardiographic manifestations of AT are variable. The P wave in AT may be located preceding the QRS complex (Fig. 15.10)—long RP tachycardia—during the QRS complex, or following the QRS complex. Thus, the P-R interval may be variable, depending on the AV nodal conduction characteristics as well as atrial location of the abnormal focus. Because the ventricles are not a critical component of the tachycardia in AT, variable degrees of AV block may be noted as well.

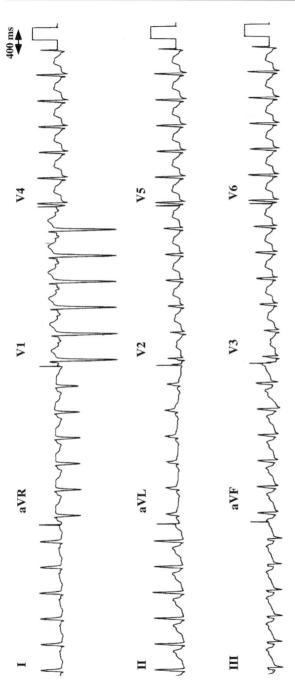

Figure 15.10. 12-lead ECG of AT. This is a long RP tachycardia. Examination of the 12-lead ECG reveals no information regarding the mechanism of the AT.

AV block may be useful in establishing the diagnosis in that AV block noted during tachycardia rules out the possibility of AV reentrant tachycardia and makes the diagnosis of AV nodal reentrant tachycardia less likely. The P wave morphology on the surface electrocardiogram is not a reliable indicator of the site of origin of the tachycardia.

The electrocardiographic diagnosis of AT may be difficult to make, especially if the P wave is hidden in the QRS complex. Diagnosis may also be difficult if the P wave occurs in the ST segment. However, even in long RP tachycardias, other diagnoses, such as atypical AV nodal reentrant tachycardia (fast-slow variety) or AV reentrant tachycardia utilizing a slowly conducting accessory pathway, need to be considered. The permanent form of junctional reciprocating tachycardia may appear identical to an incessant AT on the ECG. In patients with automatic ectopic AT, the tachycardia rate may vary throughout the day with alterations in autonomic tone. In PAT with block, AV block may be exhibited in a 2:1 or Wenckebach fashion (Fig. 15.11).

ELECTROPHYSIOLOGY

Electrophysiologic studies are not indicated or useful in patients with short bursts of AT or in patients with PAT due to digitalis toxicity. However, in patients with other types of paroxysmal or incessant ATs, electrophysiologic studies are frequently indicated to evaluate the mechanism of tachycardia and to aid in therapy. AT due to abnormal automaticity may be difficult to induce during electrophysiologic studies. They are most often noted spontaneously or following infusion of isoproterenol.

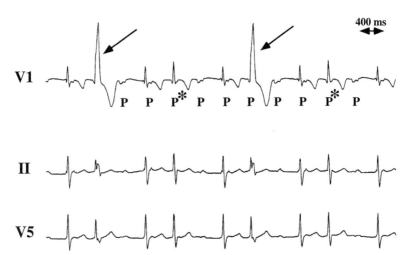

Figure 15.11. Simultaneous electrocardiographic recordings from leads V1, II, and V5 demonstrating an AT with type I, second-degree AV block (Wenckebach). The P waves are labeled. The blocked P waves are marked with an asterisk. The wide complex beats (arrows) may reflect aberrant conduction or premature ventricular depolarizations.

ASSOCIATED SYMPTOMS

Patients with short bursts of AT are mostly asymptomatic. However, they may develop palpitations. Patients with sustained ATs may have symptoms of palpitations, chest pain, near syncope, syncope, fatigue, shortness of breath, or exercise intolerance. In addition, patients with incessant tachycardia may develop CHF due to tachycardia-related myopathy. Patients with PAT with block due to digitalis toxicity may have other signs of digitalis toxicity. Because of the AV block, the ventricular response is rarely greater than 120 beats/minute. Thus, symptoms related to the tachycardia may be minimal.

PHYSICAL EXAMINATION

Physical examination may be useful in identifying potential underlying structural heart disease. It may also be important in detecting patients who have developed tachycardia-related myopathies. Otherwise, the physical examination may be unremarkable. Findings during tachycardia will include a rapid rate if there is 1:1 AV conduction. If there is AV block, multiple A waves may be noted in the jugular venous pulsations. Other findings during tachycardia depend on the patients' clinical presentations.

THERAPY

Short bursts of AT require therapy only if the patient has intolerable symptoms. Reassurance of the benign nature of this rhythm as well as correction of potential precipitating factors may alleviate the symptoms. If medications are required, first-line therapy should be a β-blocker, if there are no contraindications. Digoxin is not likely to be effective; however, it may be useful in slowing the ventricular response during AT. The efficacy of calcium channel blockers is not known.

The use of type Ia, type Ic, or type III antiarrhythmic agents must be balanced with the potential risks of proarrhythmia associated with these agents. Both paroxysmal and incessant ATs are reported to be difficult to treat medically. A variety of agents including digoxin, β-blockers, calcium channel blockers, type Ia antiarrhythmic agents, type Ic antiarrhythmic agents, and type III antiarrhythmic agents, including amiodarone, have all been used, with varying success rates.

Digitalis compounds are frequently used, but predominantly to control the ventricular response during tachycardia. β-Blockers have been reported to control both paroxysmal and incessant tachycardias, but the overall success rates are low. Type Ia agents have limited efficacy in patients with AT.

The type Ic agents may be somewhat effective in treating these tachycardias, with efficacy rates of approximately 50%. Amiodarone has been reported to be efficacious in both reentrant and automatic ATs.

Direct current cardioversion may be considered in the patient with AT associated with hemodynamic compromise. Some cases of automatic AT may resolve spontaneously without requiring drug therapy. Other treatment options include catheter and surgical ablation. Although there have been many reports on the use of surgical therapy for automatic AT, long-term outcome is uncertain. Catheter ablation has also been used with a limited experience in these tachycardias.

Presently, if there is an urgent need to stop the tachycardia, i.v. administration of digoxin-specific antibodies should be strongly considered.

SUGGESTED READING

Agarwal B, Agrawal B. Digitalis induced paroxysmal atrial tachycardia with AV block. Br Heart J 1972;34:330–335.

Brodsky M, Wu D, Denes P, Kanakis C, Rosen K. Arrhythmias documented by 24 hour continuous electrocardiographic monitoring in 50 male medical students without apparent heart disease. Am J Cardiol 1977;39:390–395.

Corazza L, Pastor B. Cardiac arrhythmias in chronic cor pulmonale. N Engl J Med 1958;259:862–868.

Dhingra R, Wyndham C, Amat-Y-Leon F, Denes P, Wu D, Rosen K. Sinus nodal responses to atrial extrastimuli in patients without apparent sinus node disease. Am J Cardiol 1975;36:445–452.

Gillette P, Garson A. Electrophysiologic and pharmacologic characteristics of automatic ectopic atrial tachycardia. Circulation 1977;56:571–575.

Haines D, DiMarco J. Sustained intraatrial reentrant tachycardia: clinical, electrocardiographic and electrophysiologic characteristics and long-term follow-up. J Am Coll Cardiol 1990;15:1345–1354.

Kastor J. Multifocal atrial tachycardia. N Engl J Med 1990;322:1713–1717.

Rosen K, Rahimtoola S, Gunnar R. Pseudo AV block secondary to premature nonpropagated His bundle depolarizations. Documentation by His bundle electrocardiography. Circulation 1970;42:367–373.

Wu D, Amat-Y-Leon F, Denes P, Dhingra R, Pietras R, Rosen K. Demonstration of sustained sinus and atrial re-entry as a mechanism of paroxysmal supraventricular tachycardia. Circulation 1975;51:234–243.

16   Atrial Flutter and Fibrillation

ATRIAL FLUTTER

It is now appreciated that there are two types of atrial flutter: type I (classical) and type II (very rapid) (Fig. 16.1). They are distinguished by the fact that type I atrial flutter can always be influenced by rapid atrial pacing, whereas type II atrial flutter cannot. Differentiation between two types of atrial flutter is also made in terms of the range of atrial rates. In the absence of drug therapy, type I atrial flutter is characterized by a range of atrial rates from 240–340 beats/minute, and type II atrial flutter by a range of from 340–433 beats/minute, although there probably is overlap in the upper range of rates of type I with the lower range rates of type II.

Incidence and Clinical Setting

Atrial flutter infrequently is a persistent rhythm. Rather, it is primarily paroxysmal, lasting for variable periods of time, usually seconds to hours, but on occasion even 1 day or more. Persistent atrial flutter, i.e., atrial flutter as a stable, chronic rhythm, is unusual, because atrial flutter usually reverts to sinus rhythm or atrial fibrillation (AF), either spontaneously or as a result of therapy.

The incidence of atrial flutter is uncertain. From a series of hospital-reviewed ECGs, it has been variously reported from 0.4–1.2% of patients. Atrial flutter is said to be more common in men than in women, with a reported ratio of 4.7:1. It can occur in patients with ostensibly normal atria or with abnormal atria. A unique population in which atrial flutter occurs commonly is in patients in the first week after open heart surgery. Atrial flutter is also seen in association with chronic obstructive pulmonary disease, mitral or tricuspid valve disease, thyrotoxicosis, and following repair of certain congenital cardiac lesions in which the right atrium is considerably incised. It is also associated with enlargement of the atria for any reason, especially the right atrium. Atrial flutter is commonly associated with AF. In fact, the two rhythms are often noted to occur in the same patient, and they may go back and forth between each other. Also, in its paroxysmal form, atrial flutter is associated with antecedent premature atrial beats.

Significance

Atrial flutter is largely a nuisance arrhythmia. Its clinical significance lies largely in its association with a rapid ventricular response rate, which is difficult to control, and which is associated with symptoms and its frequent connection to AF. Furthermore, if the duration of the rapid ventricular response rate is prolonged, it may be associated with ventricular dilatation and congestive heart failure (CHF).

Also, when associated with an underlying bundle branch block or aberrant ventricular conduction, it must be differentiated from ventricular tachycardia (VT). And in the presence of the Wolff-Parkinson-White (WPW) syndrome, or a very

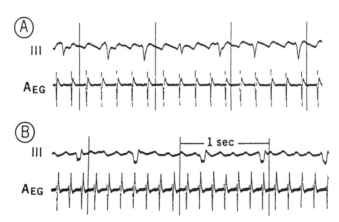

Figure 16.1. A and B. Both demonstrate the simultaneous recording of ECG lead III and a bipolar atrial electrogram (*AEG*) during type I atrial flutter with an atrial rate of 296 beats/min (*A*) and type II atrial flutter and a rate of 420 beats/minute (*B*). In each example, note the constant beat-to-beat cycle length, polarity, morphology, and amplitude of recorded atrial electrogram signal characteristic of atrial flutter. (Modified from Wells JL Jr, MacLean WAH, James TN, Waldo AL. Characterization of atrial flutter. Studies in man after open heart surgery using fixed atrial electrodes. Circulation 1979;60:665–673.)

short P-R interval (≤0.115 seconds) in the absence of a Δ wave (Lown-Ganong-Levine syndrome), it may be associated with 1:1 atrioventricular (AV) conduction.

Associated Symptoms and Hemodynamic Effects

The individual patient's symptoms associated with atrial flutter will depend considerably on the presence or absence of underlying heart disease as well as on the ventricular response rate during atrial flutter. A rapid ventricular rate will commonly be associated with palpitation, lightheadedness, dizziness, shortness of breath, weakness, faintness, and sometimes overt syncope. If the ventricular rate is very fast, angina may develop, particularly in the presence of underlying ischemic heart disease, but even in the absence of underlying ischemic heart disease if the rate is fast enough and the duration long enough. In patients with underlying heart disease, the presence of a rapid ventricular rate may induce signs and symptoms of CHF. Even in patients without underlying heart disease, if the rapid ventricular rate persists for prolonged periods, signs and symptoms of CHF may develop.

Hemodynamic effects depend on underlying disease, the ventricular rate, the duration of the rhythm, concurrent medications, and whether or not the patient is at rest or is exerting him- or herself. However, the hemodynamic effects of the arrhythmia are largely related to ventricular rate. At rapid ventricular rates, there is usually a decline in cardiac output. In addition, blood pressure can also be substantially reduced. The abrupt onset of increased rates is well known to reduce blood pressure, typically with an initial decline and subsequent rise. Actually, the response of the blood pressure depends in large measure on peripheral adaptation. The initial decline in blood pressure with the rapid rate associated with the onset of the tachycardia may be associated with presyncope and even with syncope in some cases. There may also be a significant reduction in coronary blood flow and a rate-related increment in myocardial oxygen consumption despite mainte- nance of baseline cardiac output.

Physical Examination

Commonly, during atrial flutter there is a regular ventricular response to the rapid atrial rate, either 2:1 or 4:1. Thus, during a paroxysm of atrial flutter, it is common for both the peripheral pulse and the rate auscultated from the pre- cordium to be regular and often rapid. However, atrial flutter also can be associ- ated with an irregular ventricular response rate. As a result, the findings at physical examination may mimic AF in that there may be an irregular ventricular rate ausculted at the precordium associated with an irregular peripheral pulse rate with dropped beats (i.e., the apical ventricular rate is greater than the peripheral ventricular rate). If neck veins are obvious, examination of the neck may reveal regular jugular venous pulsations occurring at a rapid rate (i.e., the atrial rate). The jugular venous pulsations will be more rapid than the peripheral or apical pulses, reflecting the degree of AV nodal blockade (e.g., 2:1, 4:1). Other signs dur- ing the physical examination relate primarily to the presence or absence of CHF.

ECG Manifestations and Diagnostic Features

Atrial flutter usually can be diagnosed from the ECG. Classically, there are "flut- ter waves," principally in ECG leads II, III, and aVF and in V1. Flutter waves appear as atrial complexes of constant morphology, polarity, and cycle length, in a rate range from 240–340 beats/minute. The atrial rate may be slower should the rhythm be present in the face of therapy with a Class I or III antiarrhythmic drug. The atrial rate may also be slower when there is significant disease of the atrial myocardium. In the inferior leads (II, III, and aVF), the flutter waves have the appearance of a picket fence (saw-tooth) because the leads are primarily negative (Fig. 16.2).

In contrast to classical flutter, atypical flutter has positive P waves in the inferior leads, and the atrial rate is sometimes slower than typical or classical flutter. Atypical atrial flutter is probably due to the same reentrant mechanism as typical atrial flutter, but the reentrant wave front travels in a clockwise direction instead of a counterclockwise direction around the reentrant circuit in the right atrium. If the ventricular response to atrial flutter is half that of the atrial flutter rate, it may, on occasion, be difficult to identify flutter waves in the ECG leads because they may be temporally superimposed on other ECG deflections, such as the QRS complex or the T wave.

Atrial flutter must be differentiated from sinus tachycardia, AV nodal reentrant tachycardia, AV reentrant tachycardia involving an accessory AV connection, an atrial tachycardia with 1:1 AV conduction, an accelerated AV junctional tachycar- dia, and sinus node reentrant tachycardia. Vagal maneuvers or other transient

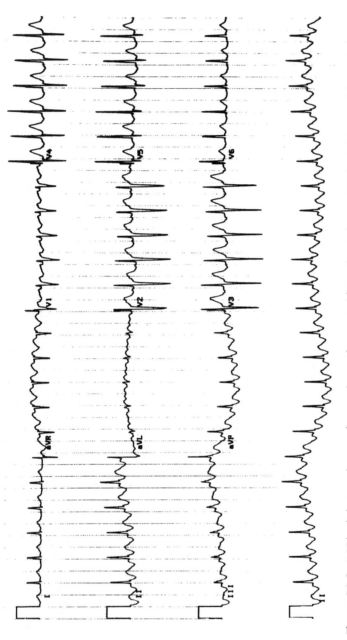

Figure 16.2. A 12-lead electrocardiogram of a typical case of type I atrial flutter. The atrial rate is 300 beats/minute and the ventricular rate is 150 beats/minute; 2:1 AV block is present. Notice how the atrial activity is best seen in leads II, III, and aVF and is barely perceptible in lead I. (From Waldo AL, Kastor JA. Atrial flutter. In: Kastor JA, ed. Arrhythmias. Philadelphia: WB Saunders, 1994:105–115.)

interventions are recommended to provide transient increased AV block while recording the ECG, thereby slowing the ventricular response rates, revealing the underlying flutter waves. In the presence of a wide QRS complex, atrial flutter must be differentiated from all the aforementioned rhythms when associated with an underlying bundle branch block or aberrant ventricular conduction as well as from VT or antegrade conduction over an accessory AV connection.

The ventricular response rate to the atrial flutter rate commonly is 2:1 or 4:1 and is therefore regular, but it may be irregular when there is variable AV conduction (a result of concealed and decremental conduction), and rarely it may even be 1:1 as in WPW syndrome, enhanced AV nodal conduction, or with sympathetic stimulation. Both the atrial flutter rate and ventricular response rate may be affected by drug therapy.

The QRS complex during atrial flutter most commonly is that of the QRS complex during sinus rhythm because atrial flutter is a supraventricular rhythm. However, atrial flutter beats may be conducted aberrantly to the ventricles, thereby manifesting a functional bundle branch block morphology, most commonly a right bundle branch. But, even when conducted normally, the QRS complex may be distorted by temporal superimposition of flutter waves on the QRS complex (Fig. 16.3). Thus, the QRS complex may "grow" a new R wave, S wave, Q wave, or a taller R or S wave.

If the diagnosis remains unclear following a vagal maneuver, and if permitted by

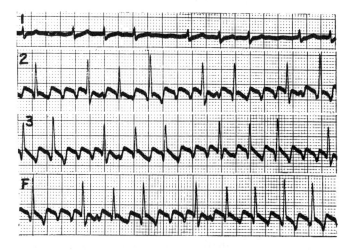

Figure 16.3. Atrial flutter with AV block varying between 2:1 and 4:1. Note the lack of evidence of atrial activity in lead I. Note also the superimposition of atrial flutter complexes on the QRS complexes, so that Q waves and S waves appear and disappear. (Adapted from Marriott HJL, ed. Practical electrocardiography. 3rd ed. Baltimore: Williams & Wilkins, 1962:119.)

the clinical situation, any of the following diagnostic maneuvers may be used: (a) an electrogram may be recorded directly from the atria by placement of an esophageal electrode, by transvenous placement of a catheter electrode, or by use of a temporary atrial epicardial wire electrode placed at the time of open heart surgery (mode of choice in patients following open heart surgery); or (b) a pharmacologic agent such as adenosine, esmolol, verapamil, diltiazem, or edrophonium may be administered intravenously to prolong or block AV conduction transiently, thereby revealing the atrial complexes in the ECG. However, it must be stressed that in the presence of a wide QRS complex tachycardia (which may represent a VT; or a supraventricular tachycardia with aberrant ventricular conduction, an underlying bundle branch block, an intraventricular conduction defect, or the presence of AV conduction over an accessory AV connection), drug intervention to establish the diagnosis of atrial flutter is fraught with difficulties and dangers and usually is contraindicated.

Clinical Electrophysiology

For patients with paroxysms of tachycardia in whom atrial flutter is suspected but has not been documented with an ECG, 24-hour ambulatory (Holter) monitoring is recommended. However, for some patients, the episodes of tachycardia are sufficiently infrequent that the documentation requires use of an event recorder such as a transtelephonic monitor.

Programmed electrical stimulation may induce atrial flutter, and the most reliable method is to pace the atria very rapidly to initiate AF, which then usually evolves to atrial flutter. Initiation of atrial flutter by introducing premature atrial beats after a train of 8 paced beats is much less reliable.

Mapping studies of atrial flutter are generally performed in an effort to identify the location of the reentrant circuit. Such a location is thought to be an isthmus between the tricuspid valve orifice and the orifice of the inferior vena cava or the coronary sinus in most cases of atrial flutter.

Management of Atrial Flutter

ACUTE TREATMENT OF ATRIAL FLUTTER

Three options are available to restore sinus rhythm: (a) administer antiarrhythmic drug therapy, (b) initiate DC cardioversion, or (c) initiate rapid atrial pacing to interrupt atrial flutter. Most often, the treatment depends on the clinical status of the patient. However, antiarrhythmic drug therapy may be initiated prior to performing either DC cardioversion or rapid atrial pacing (a) to slow the ventricular response rate (with a β-blocker or a calcium channel blocker, or digoxin); (b) to enhance the efficacy of rapid atrial pacing in restoring sinus rhythm (use of quinidine, procainamide, or disopyramide); or (c) to enhance the likelihood that sinus rhythm will be sustained following effective DC cardioversion (use of class Ia or a class Ic or class III antiarrhythmic agent).

The use of digoxin is still acceptable, but generally is not the treatment of choice. Whenever rapid control of the ventricular response rate to atrial flutter is desirable, this can usually and readily be accomplished by using either an intravenous (i.v.) calcium channel blocking agent (verapamil or diltiazem) or an i.v. β-blocking agent (esmolol, propranolol or metoprolol). Using an antiarrhythmic drug intravenously to convert atrial flutter to sinus rhythm may be attempted with procainamide or with newer arrhythmic drugs such as ibutilide. Success rates of conversion with ibutilide has been reported to approach 70%.

TECHNIQUES OF RAPID ATRIAL PACING TO INTERRUPT CLASSICAL (TYPE I) ATRIAL FLUTTER

Rapid atrial pacing is generally best initiated at a rate 120–130% of the spontaneous atrial flutter rate and continued for 15–30 seconds or until the atrial complexes in ECG lead II become positive. Then, pacing is either abruptly terminated or rapidly slowed to a desirable atrial pacing rate. If pacing at the initially selected rate does not interrupt atrial flutter, the atrial pacing rate should be increased by 5–10 beats/minute increments until atrial flutter is successfully interrupted. It is recommended that pacing be initiated with a stimulus strength of at least 10 mA. However, it is not unusual to require up to 20 mA and, on occasion, even stronger stimulus strength may be required.

Esophageal pacing may be used to interrupt atrial flutter. To capture the atria, the stimulus must be at least 9–10 msec in duration and up to 30 mA in stimulus strength.

DC CARDIOVERSION TO CONVERT ATRIAL FLUTTER TO SINUS RHYTHM

DC cardioversion of atrial flutter to sinus rhythm has a very high likelihood of success. It may also require as little as 25 J, although at least 50–100 J is generally recommended because it is more often successful.

DRUG THERAPY

For a long time, standard treatment consisted of administration of a class Ia antiarrhythmic agent (quinidine, procainamide, or disopyramide) in an effort to prevent recurrence. However, recent studies indicate that the class Ic antiarrhythmic agents (flecainide, propafenone) are as effective, if not more effective, than class Ia agents. In addition, they are better tolerated and have less organ toxicity.

Based on available long-term data, there appears to be a limited ability to maintain sinus rhythm without occasional to frequent recurrence of atrial flutter, even when multiple agents are used. Thus, when considering drug efficacy, an important measure should be the frequency of recurrence of atrial flutter rather than a single recurrent episode.

The risk of stroke associated with atrial flutter is uncertain. Although a recently published study found neither evidence of atrial clot formation nor stroke associated with atrial flutter in a relatively small cohort of patients following open heart surgery, no large systematic studies have been performed to confirm this.

Furthermore, atrial flutter may evolve from AF, and the rhythm may alternate between AF and atrial flutter. These factors further complicate this issue. Although there is no clear consensus on the use of anticoagulation in patients with atrial flutter (acute, recurrent, or chronic), daily aspirin therapy in patients under 75 years of age should be considered, and daily warfarin therapy to achieve an international normalized ratio (INR) of 2–3 should be considered on a case-by-case basis for all ages.

PERMANENT ANTITACHYCARDIA PACEMAKERS

In selected patients, consideration should be given to implantation of a permanent antitachycardia pacemaker to treat recurrent atrial flutter by interpreting the reentrant circuit.

CATHETER ABLATION THERAPY

Two types of catheter ablation have been used for the treatment of chronic or recurrent atrial flutter. One accepted clinical technique is His bundle ablation to create high-degree AV block (generally third-degree AV block), thereby eliminating rapid ventricular response rates to atrial flutter. For patients in whom antiarrhythmic drug therapy is not tolerated or in whom atrial flutter with a rapid and clinically unacceptable ventricular response rate recurs despite antiarrhythmic drug therapy, using catheter ablation to produce third-degree AV block or a high degree of AV block will provide a successful form of therapy without the need for further antiarrhythmic drugs. Such patients are then treated with a standard permanent pacemaker system.

A second type of catheter ablation therapy is still investigational. It involves first mapping the atria during atrial flutter to identify a critical area of slow conduction in the atrial flutter reentrant circuit. When this area is identified, ablative energy can be delivered through the catheter electrode to this area to destroy it. Recent reports have detailed a success rate of 50–80%.

SURGICAL THERAPY

Just as catheter ablation of a critical portion of the atrial flutter reentrant circuit remains controversial, acceptable surgical therapy awaits more definitive understanding of the mechanism of atrial flutter and the location of the critical portions of its reentry circuit. The Maze, which has been used primarily for the prevention of AF, should also be effective in the prevention of recurrent atrial flutter. In this operation, numerous incisions are made in both atria to prevent circulating reentrant wave fronts from developing. However, the total experience with the Maze operation to prevent atrial flutter is small, and the efficacy over time, the associated morbidity, and the associated mortality are not yet fully appreciated.

ATRIAL FIBRILLATION

Etiology and Pathogenesis

Atrial fibrillation (AF) is the most commonly sustained arrhythmia. The electrocardiographic manifestation of AF is "an irregular, disorganized, electrical activity of the atria. P waves are absent and the baseline consists of irregular wave forms which continuously change in shape, duration, amplitude and direction." Unfortunately, there is no uniform definition of the terms sustained, paroxysmal, or chronic when used to describe AF.

Review of the literature suggests that spontaneous reversion to sinus rhythm is uncommon after more than 1 week of continuous duration, and a cut-off of 1 week seems also to distinguish groups of patients with a higher and lower likelihood of pharmacological conversion to sinus rhythm with the use of antiarrhythmic agents.

RISK FACTORS

The Framingham Heart Study has clearly documented the relationship between age and AF, with a sharp increase in 2-year incidence in the 7th decade and older (Fig. 16.4). The most powerful predictor of risk of AF is the presence of rheumatic heart disease, followed by the presence of heart failure, hypertensive

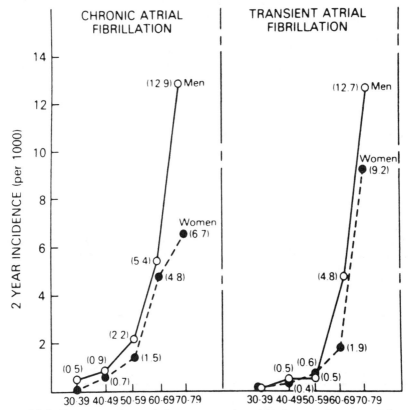

Figure 16.4. Two-year incidence of chronic sustained atrial fibrillation and transient AF from the Framingham Study. Transient atrial fibrillation includes single episodes such as those associated with acute MI. (From Kannel WB et al. Coronary heart disease and atrial fibrillation: the Framingham Study. Am Heart J 1983;106:389–396.)

heart disease (hypertension with left ventricular hypertrophy on the ECG or cardiomegaly), and coronary heart disease (Table 16.1).

Although rheumatic mitral valve disease is the strongest precursor of AF, its present-day rarity in developed countries makes it account for only a very small proportion of the total cases. Indeed, overt cardiovascular disease in the Framingham Heart Study accounted for only 25% of cases of AF. The remaining patients presumably developed the arrhythmia due to hypertension without either cardiomegaly or ECG evidence of hypertrophy or from other occult or noncardiac causes.

Histology and Gross Pathology

The cardiac and systemic disorders enumerated in Table 16.2 result in various pathological abnormalities without an obvious unifying physiopathologic finding to account for the presence of AF. Investigators have suggested that age is one of the most powerful predictors of AF, even in diseases such as rheumatic heart disease, in which this arrhythmia has the highest prevalence. The commonest abnormality found in patients with AF both during life and at postmortem examination is atrial enlargement.

Typical etiologies include ischemic heart disease (always associated with premortem signs of heart failure) in 25 (33.8%), rheumatic heart disease (24%), cor pulmonale (13.5%), hypertension (9.4%), and lone AF (8.1%). The history of CHF in all patients with ischemic heart disease is worth emphasizing, as it supports data from the Framingham Heart Study and from the Coronary Artery Surgery Study (CASS) that, in the absence of heart failure, chronic AF is relatively uncommon as a complication of coronary artery disease.

Table 16.1
Risk of Development of Atrial Fibrillation (AF) by Cardiovascular (CV) Disease Status in 2326 Men and 2866 Women after 24 Years of Follow-up in the Framingham Study[a]

Predisposing Cardiovascular Disease	Chronic AF		Transient AF	
	Men	Women	Men	Women
Coronary heart disease	2.2[b]	0.5[c]	2.1[b]	4.5[b]
Hypertensive CV disease	4.7[b]	4.0[b]	4.4[b]	4.6[b]
Cardiac failure	8.5[b]	13.7[b]	8.2[b]	20.4[b]
Rheumatic heart disease	9.9[b]	27.5[b]	7.6[b]	24.3[b]
Any cardiovascular disease	3.2[b]	4.8[b]	4.4[b]	5.4[b]

[a]Two-year age-adjusted risk ratio. All patients with coronary heart disease, defined as prior infarction and/or angina, are included regardless of coexistence of other risk factors such as hypertension. Hypertensive cardiovascular disease is defined as hypertension with either evidence of left ventricular hypertrophy by ECG, cardiomegaly on x-ray, or cardiac failure.
[b]P<.05.
[c]Not significant.

Table 16.2
Cardiovascular and Noncardiovascular Precipitants of Atrial Fibrillation

Atrial pressure elevation
  Mitral or tricuspid valve disease
  Myocardial disease (primary or secondary, leading to systolic or diastolic dysfunction)
  Semilunar valvular abnormalities (causing ventricular hypertrophy)
  Systemic or pulmonary hypertension (pulmonary embolism)
  Intracardiac tumors or thrombi
Atrial ischemia
  Coronary artery disease
Inflammatory or infiltrative atrial disease
  Pericarditis
  Amyloidosis
  Myocarditis
  Age-induced atrial fibrotic changes
Intoxicants
  Alcohol
  Carbon monoxide
  Poison gas
Increased sympathetic activity
  Hyperthyroidism
  Pheochromocytoma
  Anxiety
  Alcohol
  Exertion-induced
  Drugs
Increased parasympathetic activity
Primary or metastatic disease in or adjacent to the atrial wall
Postoperative
  Cardiac and pulmonary surgery
  Pericarditis
  Cardiac trauma
  Hypoxia
  Pneumonia
Congenital heart disease
  Particularly atrial septal defect
Neurogenic
  Subarachnoid hemorrhage
  ? Nonhemorrhagic, major stroke
Idiopathic

Electrophysiology

AF is a reentrant arrhythmia that is caused and maintained by a random series of multiple wavelets, independent of one another. The presence of areas of refractory tissue permits the persistence of these wavelets, which vary in size, direction, and duration.

Analysis of experimental mapping data suggests that the wavelets of AF tend to reenter an area recently depolarized by another wavelet. Neural effects on the atrium also affect inducibility of AF and possibly modify the activity of antiarrhythmic agents. There is a group of patients with paroxysmal AF in whom vagal activity precedes the onset of the arrhythmia. These patients generally have a structurally normal heart and have the arrhythmia precipitated by rest or following a large meal. Vagotonic maneuvers may provoke this type of AF, and digoxin may increase the frequency and duration of palpitations. Adrenergically triggered AF has also been described, with arrhythmias primarily occurring during activity.

Electrophysiology studies in patients with paroxysmal AF demonstrate prolonged and fragmented electrograms in recordings from multiple atrial sites.

EFFECT OF ATRIAL FIBRILLATION ON VENTRICULAR FUNCTION

An unusual effect of poorly controlled heart rate in AF is the development of ventricular dysfunction. Provocation of CHF by AF in the absence of clinical evidence of heart disease has been recognized. More rigid heart rate control after restoration of sinus rhythm is probably the leading mechanism of improvement of ventricular function. Normalization of ventricular function has been documented to be a function of restoration of sinus rhythm.

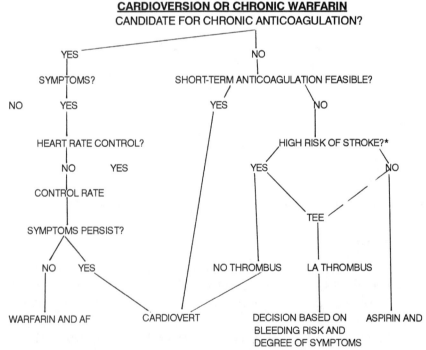

Figure 16.5. Outline of a potential decision process in the treatment of a patient with recent-onset AF. The broken line on the right side of the figure offers an alternative option in the low-risk stroke patient. Short-term anticoagulation is therapy for 3–4 weeks prior to electrical cardioversion, and 2–3 weeks thereafter. Asterisk, LV dysfunction, CHF, prior embolus, or hypertension. TEE, transesophageal echocardiogram.

Therapy of Atrial Fibrillation

Three major considerations play a role in the management of the patient with AF—heart rate control, antithrombotic therapy, and restoration of sinus rhythm (Fig 16.6 and 16.7). Heart rate control and antithrombotic therapy are always factors to be considered prior to cardioversion in patients for whom restoration of sinus rhythm is attempted.

CONTROL OF THE VENTRICULAR RESPONSE

An excessive heart rate with exertion, despite adequate resting heart rate with control with digoxin, is common in patients with chronic AF. Digoxin has some direct effect on AV nodal conduction, but the degree of rate slowing due to this mechanism is modest and may require oral doses in excess of those generally used to control resting heart rate, thus increasing the risk of toxicity (Table 16.3).

The predominant negative chronotropic effect of digoxin is to increase vagal tone at rest. Early in exercise, vagal tone is withdrawn, followed by an increase in sympathetic activity—a phenomenon that also occurs in the presence of digoxin. Thus, the benefits of the drug during exercise are virtually lost.

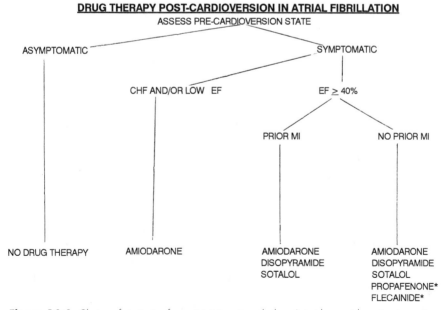

Figure 16.6. Choice of strategies for maintaining sinus rhythm. Asterisk, consider using in conjunction with a calcium channel blocker or β-blocker, particularly in patients with a history of atrial flutter. CHF, congestive heart failure; EF, ejection fraction; MI, myocardial infarction.

Table 16.3
Effective Agnets for Slowing Ventricular Rate in Atrial Fibrillation (in Absence of Preexcitation)

Drug	Acute Dose	Maintenance Dose
Digoxin	1.0–1.5 mg i.v. or oral over 24-hr in increments of 0.25–0.5 mg	0.125–0.5 mg daily
Propranolol	1–5 mg i.v. (1 mg every 2 min)	10–120 mg three times daily
Esmolol	0.5 mg i.v./kg/min	0.05–0.2 mg/kg/min i.v.
Xamoterol	No information	200 mg twice daily
Verapamil	5–20 mg in 5-mg increments i.v. boluses of 5–10 mg every 30 min	40–120 mg three times daily or 120–360 mg of the slow-release form once daily
Diltiazem	20–25 mg or 0.25–0.35 mg/kg i.v. followed by 10–15 mg infusion i.v./hr	60–90 mg three or four times daily or single dose 240–360 mg slow release form once daily

Tachycardia on mild exertion is associated with symptoms of palpitations, angina, dyspnea, or fatigue. Occasional patients with prolonged episodes of excessive heart rate may develop progressive left ventricular dysfunction.

The optimal heart rate in AF (either resting or during exertion) has not been determined. Loss of the atrial contribution to ventricular filling, particularly when left ventricular hypertrophy is present, may result in a reduction in stroke volume of 25% or more. Consequently, some degree of tachycardia is likely to be beneficial to maintain cardiac output, although the exact degree will vary from patient to patient. In addition, any advantage may be offset by excessive myocardial oxygen demand or elevation in atrial filling pressure.

Two main categories of drugs, the β-blockers and calcium channel blocking agents, are often utilized to control heart rate commonly in combination with digoxin. β-Blocker use is not associated with improved exercise tolerance, and some series actually show a decreased exercise tolerance. Impairment of exercise tolerance is most probably related to an excessive blunting of exertional tachycardia by β-blockade, although other mechanisms such as a negative inotropic effect or bronchoconstriction may play a role. In contrast to β-blockers, some studies of calcium channel blocking agents have demonstrated an improvement in exercise tolerance.

ACUTE HEART RATE CONTROL

The untreated patient presenting with AF most commonly has a ventricular rate of 110–150 beats/minute, although even in the absence of preexcitation or thyrotoxicosis, the ventricular response may show brief surges as high as 200 beats/minute. The urgency of ventricular rate control depends upon symptoms associated with the tachycardia. In the minority of cases (those with hemodynamic compromise or clear electrocardiographic changes of ischemia), restoration of sinus rhythm by urgent cardioversion may be indicated. At the other extreme, patients whose arrhythmia is either an incidental finding or is causing minimal discomfort and no other clinical abnormality, may need only digoxin for rate control, even though the maximum effect occurs after several hours.

The middle group comprises those in whom digoxin is likely to be ineffective because of a high sympathetic tone (e.g., fever, thyrotoxicosis, acute hypoxia) or in whom a more rapid control of ventricular rate is desired. For these patients, i.v. verapamil, diltiazem, or i.v. β-blockers (esmolol, propranolol, or metoprolol) are effective. As a general rule, calcium channel blockers are a better choice in this situation, as their use avoids the possibility of precipitating bronchospasm in susceptible patients. Intravenous β-blockade is preferable when AF complicates acute myocardial infarction (MI) or thyrotoxicosis.

CHRONIC HEART RATE CONTROL

Digoxin is frequently ineffective in preventing wide heart rate swings in AF. Thus, the combination of digoxin with a β-blocker, verapamil, or diltiazem is the mainstay of therapy. Although the negative chronotropic effect of these agents is desirable during waking hours, they may aggravate the nocturnal pauses commonly seen in AF. This phenomenon, if it occurs, may be minimized by substituting the chosen agent for digoxin rather than combining therapy or by using short-acting verapamil, diltiazem, or β-blocker given twice daily (morning and noon) to reduce nocturnal effects.

For patients who are intolerant of both calcium channel blockers and β-blockers, low-dose amiodarone may be effective in controlling heart rate. Symptomatic patients refractory to standard pharmacologic therapy should be considered for radiofrequency modification or ablation of the AV node.

RATE CONTROL IN PAROXYSMAL ATRIAL FIBRILLATION

Many patients with paroxysmal AF are very troubled by the palpitations, particularly at the onset of the arrhythmia.

Review of the available literature suggests that digoxin fails to adequately control heart rate at the onset of a paroxysm of AF. The apparent failure of digoxin to prevent excessive tachycardia at the onset of a paroxysm may be related either to the role of the sympathetic nervous system in triggering some episodes of AF or to sympathetic activation triggered by the sudden change in stroke volume produced by the arrhythmia.

There is a widespread practice among cardiologists to prescribe digoxin in conjunction with quinidine whenever the latter drug is used to prevent recurrent AF, in the belief that recurrence will occur at a slower ventricular rate. There are, however, no convincing data to suggest that AF occurring in a quinidine-treated patient will be conducted with an excessive ventricular response or that digoxin will slow this response. It is preferable to prescribe either a β-blocking drug or a calcium channel blocking agent in conjunction with quinidine for any patient in whom atrial flutter has been documented.

THROMBOEMBOLISM AND ANTICOAGULATION

It had long been recognized that AF occurring in patients with rheumatic heart disease, particularly mitral stenosis, was associated with autopsy and clinical evidence of systemic and cerebral thromboembolism (Table 16.4). Autopsy and epidemiology studies pointed to a significant risk of thromboembolism due to AF, regardless of etiology.

In the past few years, several major studies of warfarin anticoagulation for nonvalvular AF have clearly demonstrated a significant risk of stroke in untreated patients and a marked reduction in stroke risk with relatively low-dose warfarin use. These studies demonstrated that the incidence of events of presumed embolic etiology in nonvalvular AF was significant (4–7% per annum) and was reduced by 65–80% by low-dose warfarin anticoagulation with an acceptably low incidence of serious noncerebral bleeding and intracranial hemorrhage. A reasonable estimate of the risk of stroke in untreated chronic AF is 5% per annum. In contrast to previous belief, these studies clearly indicate that stroke risk is ongoing at a steady rate in AF without obvious clustering close to study entry.

Patients with paroxysmal AF have less of a stroke risk. Indeed, it is the progression to chronic arrhythmia that increases stroke risk. Warfarin anticoagulation is a reasonable treatment in patients whose paroxysmal AF is associated with clinical or echocardiographic evidence of underlying heart disease (Fig. 16.5).

Table 16.4
An Approach to Antithrombotic Therapy in Patients with Atrial Fibrillation

1. Chronic sustained and paroxysmal atrial fibrillation (PAF) should be considered equivalent in assessing risk of stroke in AF (unless PAF is very infrequent and short lasting).
2. All patients with rheumatic mitral valve disease or prosthetic heart valves should receive warfarin.
3. Warfarin therapy sufficient to maintain an INR of 2.0–3.0 should be prescribed for the following patients.[a]
   a. Prior stroke or transient ischemic attack
   b. Clinical heart failure or subclinical left ventricular systolic dysfunction
   c. Thyrotoxocosis-related atrial fibrillation
4. Warfarin therapy should be strongly considered in patients with a history of hypertension (and no CHF or stroke history) in conjunction with vigorous attempts to control blood pressure. Caution with poorly controlled hypertension, particularly in the elderly.
5. Aspirin therapy 325 mg daily (minimum dose) may be sufficient therapy for patients younger than 75 years, without diabetes, hypertension, heart failure, pr prior stroke/TIA.[b]
6. For patients younger than 60 years, without any of the above risk factors and a normal echocardiogram (lone atrial fibrillation), no increased risk of stroke has been shown to exist. Aspirin therapy may be considered.
7. Patients ≥75 years of age may benefit more from warfarin for embolic stroke reduction but have an increased intracranial bleeding risk. Either aspirin or warfarin may be prescribed, individualizing therapy based on other risk factors for stroke or bleed.

[a]Assuming no obvious contraindications such as active bleeding source, poor compliance, recurrent falls, etc.
[b]TIA, transient ischemic attack.

ASPIRIN THERAPY

Therapy with 75 mg of aspirin fails to reduce embolic events. The Stroke Prevention in Atrial Fibrillation 1 (SPAF 1) trial used aspirin (325 mg). The study had insufficient power to directly compare the benefit of aspirin and warfarin, but each was found to significantly reduce events when compared with placebo (warfarin reduction of 67% and aspirin reduction of 42%). Interestingly, aspirin appeared to show no benefit over placebo in patients 75 years and older, although the reason for this is unclear. In a follow-up study (SPAF 2), a direct comparison was made between warfarin and aspirin, with stratification of patients by age (<75 years or >75 years). In the younger subjects, both aspirin and warfarin therapy resulted in an annual incidence of systemic embolism and presumed ischemic stroke of less than 2% (1% from aspirin and 1% with warfarin). In patients 76 years or older, the primary event rate was higher than that in the younger group, being 4.8% with aspirin and 3.6% with warfarin. However, the benefits of warfarin in the older group were offset by an increased annual incidence of intracerebral bleeding, which was 1.8% in the warfarin group and 0.5% in the aspirin group. The incidence of disabling stroke in the older population was not reduced by warfarin (4.6% per annum), compared with aspirin (4.3% per annum).

RISK FACTORS FOR STROKE IN ATRIAL FIBRILLATION

Echocardiographic analysis of risk factors identified only mitral annular calcification, left ventricular dysfunction, and left atrial enlargement as risk factors. Clinical risk factors offer a simpler approach to risk stratification. In SPAF 1, the presence of systolic hypertension (>160 mm Hg), history of CHF, or previous stroke each identified a group of patients with a stroke risk 2.5 times that of subjects without any of these factors. A combination of two or three of these risk factors was a strong predictor of stroke risk, and the absence of any factors in nondiabetic patients identified a very low-risk population (Table 16.5). By multivariate analysis, the most powerful predictor of stroke was a prior stroke or transient ischemic attack followed by diabetes, history of hypertension (relative risk 2.5), heart failure history, and increasing age. Paroxysmal AF neither increased nor decreased the likelihood of stroke compared with that from chronic AF.

ROLE OF TRANSESOPHAGEAL ECHOCARDIOGRAPHY IN THE MANAGEMENT OF ATRIAL FIBRILLATION

The location of most thrombi in the left atrial appendage renders the vast majority invisible by standard transthoracic echocardiography. In contrast, transesophageal echocardiography allows excellent visualization of the whole of the left atrium, including the appendage, and is an ideal imaging tool for the visualization of intraatrial thrombi. The 1992 American College of Chest Physicians guidelines recommend that patients being cardioverted from AF of a duration of more than 2 days be anticoagulated for 3 weeks prior to cardioversion and 4 additional weeks following return of sinus rhythm to assure restoration of atrial mechanical func-

Table 16.5
Clinical Risk Factors for Stroke in Patients with Nonrheumatic Atrial Fibrillation[a]

Variable	Relative Risk	95% Confidence Intervals
History of hypertension	2.2	1.1–4.3
Prior thromboembolism	2.1	1.0–4.2
CHF within the past 100 days	2.6	1.2–5.4

[a]Modified from The Stroke Prevention in Atrial Fibrillation Investigators. Predictors of thromboembolism in atrial fibrillation. I. Clinical feature of patients at risk. Ann Intern Med 1992;116:6–12.

tion. Unfortunately, this approach is time consuming and frequently inconvenient. In an attempt to identify patients without atrial thrombi, transesophageal echocardiography has been performed in patients scheduled for cardioversion who were not receiving warfarin. Its precise role, however, remains uncertain.

ANTIARRHYTHMIC THERAPY

Electrical cardioversion of chronic AF is a simple and highly effective procedure. However, antiarrhythmic therapy is frequently prescribed following the procedure because of a high incidence of recurrence of AF in untreated patients. Although a number of drugs are effective in the maintenance of sinus rhythm, no agent is perfect. The decision to use a particular drug should, aside from personal preference, depend upon the side-effect profile and the characteristics of the patient being treated. Indeed, some patients may not require antiarrhythmic therapy at all (Fig. 16.6).

MAINTENANCE OF SINUS RHYTHM WITHOUT ANTIARRHYTHMIC DRUGS

It is well recognized that AF may be precipitated by transient noncardiac factors in susceptible subjects. These include infection, thyrotoxicosis, hypoxia, and alcohol. In addition, several acute cardiac conditions, such as acute MI, pericarditis, and exacerbation of heart failure, may provoke the arrhythmia. Frequently, correction of noncardiac precipitating factors will result in spontaneous reversion and, even in those patients with sustained arrhythmia who still require cardioversion, the correction of the initiating factor suggests a greater likelihood of continued sinus rhythm.

With use of antiarrhythmic drugs, sinus rhythm may be maintained in 50–60% of cases. The increased success must be measured against the cost and side effects of therapy. Drugs of benefit are the class Ia agents (quinidine, procainamide, and disopyramide), the class Ic agents (propafenone, flecainide), and the class III agents (sotalol and amiodarone) (Fig. 16.6).

Atrial Fibrillation and the Wolff-Parkinson-White Syndrome

Patients with the WPW syndrome have an increased risk of AF. The exact prevalence of this arrhythmia is unknown, but in specialized centers, from 10–35% of patients requiring therapy for preexcitation have experienced AF.

The ventricular response to AF in WPW syndrome is dependent upon properties of both the AV node and the accessory pathway. Electrocardiographic recordings during spontaneous AF frequently demonstrate narrow complexes representing conduction through the AV node with wide complexes of slightly varying morphology. These variations occur because of the varying degrees of fusion between beats arising from ventricular depolarization with the accessory pathway and the AV node. Although the shortest preexcited R-R interval during AF correlates with the anterograde refractory period of the accessory pathway, this interval is shortened by heightened sympathetic tone and possibly lengthened by retrograde concealed conduction into the accessory pathway from impulses conducted via the AV node. Sudden cardiac death is a recognized manifestation of WPW syndrome and is considered to be precipitated by AF in the majority of patients.

Atrial Fibrillation Following Cardiac Surgery

AF after cardiac surgery is a common disorder. Studies in patients undergoing coronary artery bypass grafting (CABG) have failed to consistently identify predisposing factors other than age, with an incidence of arrhythmia increasing from about 15% in patients under 65 years to 30% in those 65 years and older. Although usually transient and frequently self-limiting, hemodynamic deterioration may occur; an association with postoperative stroke has been recognized. Hospital stay is lengthened in patients with postoperative AF by 1–2 days. A metaanalysis of 24 studies of drug therapy to prevent post-CABG AF demonstrated a significant reduction in postoperative AF in patients treated with a variety of β-blockers. Digoxin has no clear effect in preventing postoperative AF. Although a few small trials have suggested a benefit, many fail to do so, and a metaanalysis showed no benefit over placebo.

SUGGESTED READING

Andrews TC, Reimold SC, Berlin JA, Antman EM. Prevention of supraventricular arrhythmias after coronary artery bypass surgery. Circulation 1991;84:(suppl III):236–244.

Arnold AZ, Mick MJ, Mazurek RP, Loop FD, Trohman RG. Role of prophylactic anticoagulation for direct current cardioversion in patients with atrial fibrillation or atrial flutter. J Am Coll Cardiol 1992;19:851–855.

Falk RH, Leavitt JI. Digoxin for atrial fibrillation: a drug whose time has gone? Ann Intern Med 1991;114:573–575.

Feld GK, Fleck P, Cheng P-S, et al. Radiofrequency catheter ablation for the treatment of human type I atrial flutter. Identification of a critical zone in the reentrant circuit by endocardial mapping techniques. Circulation 1992; 86:1233–1240.

Kannel WB, Abbott RD, Savage DD, McNamara PM. Epidemiologic features of atrial fibrillation. The Framingham Study. N Engl J Med 1982;306:1018–1022.

Manning WJ, Silverman DI, Gordon SPF, Krumholz HM, Douglas PS. Cardioversion from atrial fibrillation without prolonged anticoagulation with use of transesophageal echocardiography to exclude the presence of atrial thrombi. N Engl J Med 1993;328:750–756.

Stroke Prevention in Atrial Fibrillation Investigators. Stroke prevention in atrial fibrillation study final results. Circulation 1991;84: 527–539.

The Boston Area Anticoagulation Trial for Atrial Fibrillation Investigators. The effect of low-dose

warfarin on the risk of stroke in patients with non-rheumatic atrial fibrillation. N Engl J Med 1990;323:1505–1511.

Waldo AL, MacLean WAH, Karp RB, Kouchoukos NT, James TN. Entrainment and interruption of atrial flutter with atrial pacing: studies in man following open heart surgery. Circulation 1977;56:737–745.

17   AV Node and AV-Reciprocating Tachycardia and Wolff-Parkinson-White Syndrome

ATRIOVENTRICULAR NODE REENTRANT TACHYCARDIA

In patients with PSVT without ventricular preexcitation in sinus rhythm, AV node reentry is the most common mechanism of tachycardia, accounting for 60% or more of unknown tachycardias. A hypothetical model of how dual AV nodal pathways can give rise to a tachycardia is shown in Figure 17.1. AV reentrant tachycardia using a concealed accessory pathway is the mechanism for PSVT in most of the remaining patients. Rarely is the mechanism sinus node reentry or atrial tachycardia. Clinically, atrioventricular node reentrant tachycardia (AVNRT) can strike at virtually any age. Cases of children younger than 10 years old and of octogenarians have been described, but the onset of arrhythmia is most often beyond the fourth decade. In one study the average age at presentation was 55 years, with a range of 24–81. This finding demonstrated a statistically older group than other patients with PSVT due to reentry over a concealed bypass tract. In general, there is a minor female predilection. Multiple authors have also reported that there is no significant association with other structural heart disease.

Palpitations are the primary symptom during AV node reentry. The rate of the tachycardia is usually from 150–200 beats/minute, although rates of up to 250 beats/minute can occur. Rapid ventricular rates may be associated with complaints of dyspnea, weakness, angina, lightheadedness, or even frank syncope. Some symptoms, for example, neck pain, are related to the simultaneous contraction of the atria and ventricles against closed mitral and tricuspid valves. Episodes may last from seconds to hours, and many patients with sustained reentry require treatment to terminate the arrhythmia. Patients often relate various methods they have discovered that will terminate their arrhythmia. These include the Valsalva maneuver, carotid sinus massage, quiet deep breathing while lying down, and coughing. In essence, most successful maneuvers rely on enhanced vagal tone, discussed in detail later.

The physical examination is remarkable for the rapid, regular heart rate. Because of the simultaneous contraction of the atrium and ventricle, cannon A waves may be seen in the jugular venous waveform, i.e., prominent jugular venous pulsations. Because most often there is a 1:1 regular relationship between atrial and ventricular activation, these cannon waves are regular. Infrequently there is retrograde V-A block and in such situations the cannon A waves will be irregular.

Electrocardiographic and Electrophysiologic Considerations

The resting electrocardiogram (ECG) is usually normal in patients with AVNRT. On rare occasions, a patient may spontaneously show two distinct P-R intervals, suggestive of dual AV pathways. ECG documentation of the initiation of

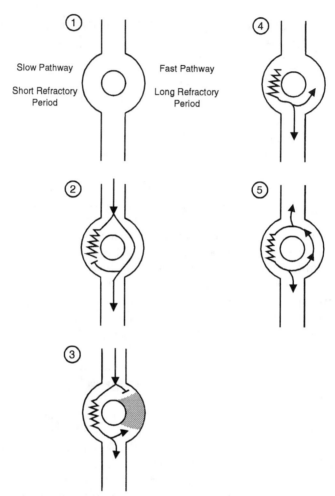

Figure 17.1. Hypothetical model of a dual AV nodal transmission system proposed by Mendez and Moe. In this model, two AV nodal pathways are represented, one with fast conduction and a relatively long refractory period, and a second with slower conduction but shorter refractory period (1). A sinus impulse conducts over both pathways, but reaches the bundle of His first via conduction over the fast pathway (2). A premature atrial depolarization finds the fast pathway still refractory and conducts over the slower AV nodal pathway (3). If the fast pathway has enough time to recover excitability, the impulse may reenter the fast pathway retrogradely and establish sustained reentry (4 and 5).

AVNRT usually shows a premature atrial beat that conducts with marked delay to the ventricle, followed by the generation of a regular narrow QRS complex tachycardia (Fig. 17.2). Atrial and ventricular activation are nearly simultaneous; thus, distinct P waves are not usually visible. However, close inspection of lead V1 often reveals a pseudo r-prime pattern due to deformation of the terminal portion of the QRS complex by the retrograde P wave (Figs. 17.2 and 17.3). It is rare for the

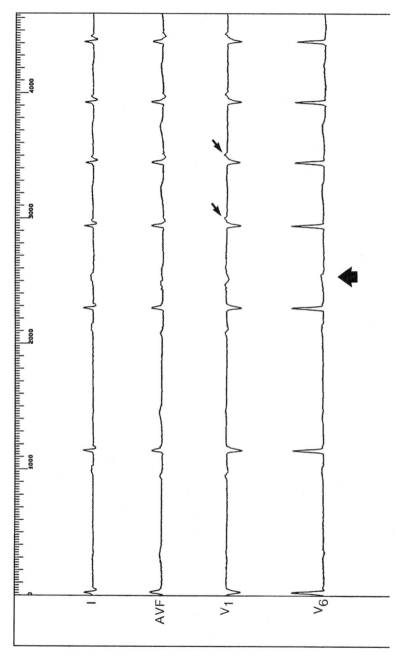

Figure 17.2. Initiation of AVNRT by a premature atrial beat. A premature atrial beat (large arrow) occurs, which presumably blocks in the fast pathway and conducts with marked delay over the slow pathway to the ventricle. This initiates AVNRT. Also noted is the pseudo r-prime in lead V1 (small arrows) representing retrograde depolarization of the atrium.

AVN Reentry

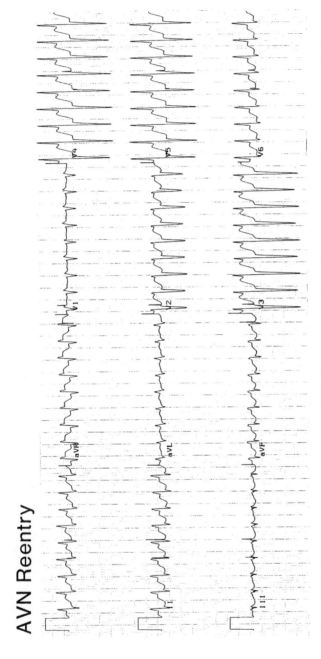

Figure 17.3. Twelve-lead electrocardiogram of AVNRT. This is a typical 12-lead electrocardiogram taken from a patient with AVNRT. Again note the pseudo rprime in lead V1 representing retrograde atrial activation. Distinct P waves in the ST segment are not present.

usual (slow anterograde/fast retrograde conduction) form of AVNRT to be initiated by a spontaneous premature ventricular complex. If PSVT is induced by a single PVC, one should suspect AV reentry, or the unusual (fast anterograde/slow retrograde conduction) variety of AV nodal reentry when the P-R:R-P ratio is less than one.

AV node reentry most often occurs with a narrow QRS morphology similar to the QRS morphology recorded during normal sinus rhythm. On occasion, functional right or left bundle branch block aberrancy may be present. In rare instances AV node reentry may coexist with ventricular activation of an accessory pathway. In this case the accessory pathway is an innocent bystander, and the tachycardia will have a preexcited appearance, similar to the QRS morphology noted in sinus rhythm. Differentiation of antidromic AV reentrant tachycardia from AVNRT with a bystander accessory pathway requires electrophysiologic testing.

The purported electrophysiologic circuit of AV nodal reentry includes two conducting pathways in the AV node, one with fast conducting characteristics but a long refractory period, and the second with slower conduction and a shorter refractory period (Fig. 17.1). However, there has been considerable debate over whether the reentrant circuit is confined to the AV node or whether it also includes atrial tissue. Additionally, it is unclear whether dual AV nodal pathways are ubiquitous, but unrecognized in most patients, or are a distinct pathologic entity. As stated previously, we think that most individuals have the capability of conduction over a slow pathway, but it is concealed.

Demonstration of dual AV nodal physiology using premature atrial stimuli in patients with PSVT is suggestive but not diagnostic of AV nodal reentry as the mechanism of tachycardia. In fact, dual AV nodal physiology may occur in patients with AV reentry, and the slow pathway may be used for anterograde conduction during AVRT. Premature atrial stimulation involves the introduction of a series of atrial extrastimuli at progressively earlier intervals during sinus rhythm or atrial pacing. The hallmark of dual AV nodal physiology is a "jump" or discontinuity in either the AV nodal function curve (A1–A2/H1–H2) or the AV nodal conduction curve (A1–A2/A2–H2) by at least 50 msec in response to a 10-msec decrement in the A1–A2 coupling interval. The 50-msec increase is rather arbitrary and may differ, depending on the paced rate used. A continuous AV nodal function curve does not exclude AVNRT. For example, if a premature atrial complex blocks in the fast pathway and conducts over the slow pathway, but conduction over the slow pathway is only slightly longer than that of the fast pathway, AVNRT could be initiated without a discontinuous curve. Importantly, changes in the atrial paced cycle length may cause unpredictable changes in the ERP of the fast and slow pathways. Although the AV node ERP will generally increase in response to a faster paced cycle length, the degree of increase in the ERP of the fast and slow pathway may differ at various heart rates. Thus, dual AV nodal physiology and discontinuous AV nodal function curves may be present at one cycle length and absent at a another.

In some patients with PSVT, dual AV nodal physiology is demonstrated, but neither echo beats nor tachycardia is initiated. Assuming AVNRT is the mechanism of the tachycardia, then either a critical AV nodal delay has not been achieved to allow recovery of the fast pathway or retrograde conduction over the fast pathway is poor. Generation of greater AV nodal delay can often be accomplished with more closely coupled atrial extrastimuli or the use of two closely coupled atrial extrastimuli. Facilitation of retrograde AV nodal conduction can usually be accomplished with pharmacologic measures. Isoproterenol and atropine can enhance both anterograde and retrograde AV nodal conduction and allow the induction of sustained tachycardia.

Differential Diagnosis

Certain features are useful to diagnose the usual form of AV node reentry:

1. Atrial activation occurs simultaneously with or immediately after ventricular activation. The earliest V-A interval is therefore usually less than 60 msec and the V to high right atrial (V-HRA) interval is typically less than 90 msec. P waves are not clearly visible but may occur at the end of the QRS complex, leading to the pseudo r-prime in V1 (Figs. 17.2 and 17.3);
2. Retrograde atrial activation is concentric with the earliest atrial activation recorded in the interatrial septum;
3. A critical A-H interval is necessary to initiate the tachycardia,
4. Because the reentrant loop is small and at least partly intranodal, only very early premature atrial or ventricular extrastimuli can penetrate the tachycardia circuit to reset it or terminate tachycardia. Often AVNRT is a diagnosis of exclusion.

AVNRT of the unusual variety (fast anterograde/slow retrograde) also has a concentric retrograde atrial activation sequence; however, the R-P interval is longer than the P-R interval. The differential diagnosis of this long R-P tachycardia also includes atrial tachycardia and various forms of AV reentry using a slowly conducting accessory pathway for retrograde conduction. Differentiation among these mechanisms of tachycardia may be difficult and is beyond the scope of this chapter. Several other features are characteristic of the unusual form of AVNRT. These include (a) retrograde dual AV nodal function curves; (b) reproducible initiation with premature ventricular beats, more common than with atrial premature beats; and (c) initiation dependent on a critical H-A interval during retrograde slow pathway conduction.

AVNRT must be differentiated from other forms of narrow complex supraventricular tachycardia with 1:1 AV conduction, including sinus node reentry, atrial tachycardia, and AV reentry. Certain clinical features can be helpful; however, the analysis of the surface ECG and invasive electrophysiologic studies can almost always distinguish among these mechanisms.

Sinus node reentrant tachycardia has a high-low atrial activation sequence and the P wave morphology is identical or very similar to the sinus P wave. Atrial tachycardias may be caused by abnormal automaticity, triggered automaticity, or reentry. Because they may occur from many locations within either atria, the P wave morphology is variable, and the sequence of atrial activation will depend on the site of tachycardia origin. Consequently, a high-low or eccentric, that is, not in the septum, atrial activation sequence distinguishes this tachycardia from AV nodal reentry. Continuation of the tachycardia in the presence of AV nodal block is typical for atrial tachycardia, but rare for AVNRT. Drugs such as adenosine or verapamil often cause AV node block without termination of atrial tachycardia or just prior to termination. Introduction of closely coupled premature ventricular stimuli during tachycardia, which terminate the tachycardia without conduction to the atrium, effectively rules out atrial tachycardia.

In orthodromic AV reentry, the AV node is part of the anterograde limb of the tachycardia circuit, and the accessory pathway forms the retrograde limb. The P waves are usually seen following the QRS deflection in the early ST segment. The earliest V-A interval during tachycardia is typically greater than 70 msec, and the V-HRA is >95 msec. Thus, very short V-A intervals are incompatible with AVRT. Atrial activation may be eccentric when the pathway is located either on the right or left free wall, and this finding excludes AVNRT as the mechanism of an unknown tachycardia. In patients with septal accessory pathways and longer V-A conduction times, the differentiation of AV node from AV reentry is considerably more difficult. Preexcitation of the atria during tachycardia with ventricular extrastimuli introduced when the His bundle is refractory, confirms the presence of an accessory pathway, but does not prove AVRT. AVRT is diagnosed when infra-AV nodal structures are demonstrated to be part of the tachycardia circuit. Examples are (a) increases in the V-A interval during tachycardia with bundle branch block; (b) an increase in the H-V interval associated with an increase in the H-A interval; and (c) termination of the tachycardia with a premature ventricular complex that occurs with the His electrogram visible and unperturbed and does not conduct to the atria.

Pharmacologic Therapy

Digoxin and β-adrenergic blocking agents can be used clinically in the termination and prevention of AVNRT. As noted earlier, these agents predominantly act via the autonomic nervous system on the slow anterograde pathway. Other agents may act directly on this pathway. Verapamil is a calcium channel blocking agent that can terminate and prevent the induction of AVNRT. Verapamil slows conduction and prolongs refractoriness in the fast and slow pathways. Interestingly, the termination of AVNRT is usually due to anterograde block, but not infrequently also occurs because of block in the retrograde fast pathway.

Adenosine is a relatively new agent that can acutely and transiently cause AV nodal blockade. The effect is usually short-lived, as endogenous enzymes rapidly metabolize adenosine. Adenosine also exhibits a dose-related effect on AV nodal conduction. At lower doses, a gradual prolongation in the A-H interval is noted. At higher doses, complete AV nodal block may be achieved. Multiple studies have shown that adenosine is nearly 100% effective to terminate AV nodal dependent arrhythmias. Usually, prolongation of the A-H interval occurs immediately prior to tachycardia termination. Because of its dramatic effect on AV nodal conduction, adenosine has been proposed as a diagnostic tool to differentiate AV nodal dependent from AV nodal independent tachycardias. Clearly, the development of AV block with perpetuation of the tachycardia indicates that the AV node is not a requisite part of the tachycardia circuit. However, adenosine can also terminate some types of atrial tachycardia.

Many other agents have been employed in the therapy of AVNRT. In general, most sodium channel blocking agents can prevent AV nodal reentry. These include the class Ia agents quinidine, procainamide, and disopyramide, the class Ic agents, including flecainide, encainide, propafenone, ethmozine, and ajmaline, and the class III agents. Most commonly these agents depress retrograde fast pathway conduction. Based on these observations, it has been speculated that the anterograde slow pathway is composed of slow channel tissue, while the retrograde pathway contains a mixture of fast and slow channel tissue.

Nonpharmacologic Therapy

Electrophysiologic studies demonstrate that AVNRT may be terminated by atrial and ventricular pacing techniques that interfere with the reentrant circuit. Implantable antitachycardia pacemakers were previously used—albeit infrequently—for the chronic therapy of some patients with AVNRT. However, this form of therapy is rarely prescribed anymore with the advent of radiofrequency ablation to cure AVNRT.

For many years, a significant controversy has existed concerning the anatomic boundaries of the reentrant circuit. The observation of AVNRT with two to one block below the bundle of His is well described and has been used as evidence to confirm that the ventricle is not part of the AVNRT circuit. Whether a very proximal part of the His bundle is used in the circuit cannot be excluded, but we do not think it is. However, the role of the atrium remains more contentious. In rare cases, the tachycardia may be initiated in the absence of an atrial echo and may persist in the presence of AV dissociation. These observations do not rule out the possibility that a small rim of atrial tissue near the AV node participates in the reentrant tachycardia, with intraatrial block preventing atrial activation.

Several observations favor the atrium being part of the reentrant circuit. In a microelectrode study in the rabbit, the reentrant circuit was mapped to the perinodal region and used the coronary sinus as a mechanical obstacle around which the AVNRT occurred. Further data on this issue relate to a patient with AV node reentry in when AV nodal in when AV nodal surgical ablation was attempted. However, anterograde conduction persisted postoperatively, with AV conduction being slower and markedly impaired in both the anterograde and retrograde directions. This resulted in cure of the arrhythmia. The authors concluded that conduction in the fast and slow pathways was anatomically distinct, and that it was possible to abolish AVNRT with operations on specific components of the AV conduction system.

In one study, using a canine model, cryolesions were strategically placed in the peri-AV nodal region of the right atrium to modify AV nodal conduction. AV nodal conduction was slowed anterogradely and retrogradely without the development of AV block. Additional studies showed that this cryosurgical procedure was capable of selectively ablating only one of the pathways of AV conduction, thus leaving some degree of conduction intact, and disrupting the anatomic substrate necessary for AV node reentry. Cure of AV nodal reentrant tachycardia with this technique in humans has been reported. In 10 patients with AVNRT, cure was obtained with cryosurgical ablation of perinodal tissue. Five of seven patients additionally had dual AV nodal physiology abolished. In another report, eight patients with classic AV node reentry and dual AV node curves preoperatively were described. Postoperatively, the patients had no AVNRT, and none had dual AV node function curves. Thus, it became clear that modification of the perinodal atrial tissue could result in cure of AVNRT.

Despite the intuitive appeal of "curing" AV node reentrant tachycardia by surgical modification of the AV node and its atrial input, this procedure did not receive widespread acceptance. However, catheter ablation to cure AVNRT has permanently changed the therapeutic approach to this arrhythmia. It has also offered compelling data implicating the atrium as part of the tachycardia circuit.

Fast and slow AV nodal pathways have different retrograde exit points into the right atrium. Thus, it has been hypothesized that delivery of direct current energy at the site of earliest retrograde atrial activation can abolish preferentially the atrial insertion of the retrograde fast pathway. During tachycardia, this region can be consistently localized to an area in the atrial septum, just anterior to the AV node. An early report of results of direct current catheter ablation in this region involved 21 patients with AV node reentrant tachycardia. Treatment resulted in the preferential ablation or impairment of retrograde AV nodal conduction in all patients. Anterograde conduction was modified in 19 patients, and complete heart block occurred in two. Sixteen patients remained free of arrhythmia over a mean follow-up of 14 months. Similar results using this technique were reported in nine patients with drug refractory AVNRT. Six of the nine patients had complete cure over a mean follow-up of 12.3 months. No patient required permanent pacing, although one patient developed complete AV block, which persisted for several months. Interestingly, three patients had complete retrograde block in the fast pathway, but three other patients had attenuation of only slow pathway conduction, suggesting that it might be possible to modify selectively the slow pathway.

A prominent limitation to the use of direct current modification of the AV node was the uncontrolled delivery of an abrupt shock to the perinodal atrial region. Consequently, other energy sources for catheter ablation were investigated. An early report described the use of catheter-delivered radiofrequency energy for the controlled modification of the anterior fast pathway in 39 patients who underwent this therapy. The ablation catheter was positioned anteriorly with a large atrial electrogram and very small His electrogram (<100 μV) recorded. The endpoints of energy delivery were either first-degree AV block or the impairment of ventriculoatrial conduction. A cure of the tachycardia was achieved in 32 of 39 patients and the development of complete AV block in three patients. In successfully treated patients, the mean A-H interval increased from 74 to 146 msec, and retrograde V-A conduction was eliminated in all but one patient. In 17 patients with dual AV nodal physiology before the procedure, 14 had continuous AV nodal function curves postprocedure. It may be concluded that the delivery of radiofrequency energy can modify the AV node and successfully ablate the fast AV nodal pathway. However, the rather high incidence of complete heart block in this region led other investigators to develop radiofrequency techniques for the ablation of the slow pathway.

These observations suggested that atrial tissue, located posteriorly near the os of the coronary sinus, may be part of the AVNRT circuit. Detailed mapping of this posterior space and in variable posterior locations were able to identify a unique potential, termed Asp. This potential was shown to be distinctly different from local atrial activation, and is felt to represent the activation of the atrial insertion of the slow pathway. We do not think that this potential is activation of the slow pathway per se, but it may represent depolarization of atrial tissue overlying or adjacent to the slow pathway. Perhaps it is caused by anisotropic conduction in this region. Delivery of radiofrequency energy to this region in 80 patients with AVNRT and dual AV nodal pathways resulted in abolishment or modification of the slow pathway in 78 patients. In one patient the fast pathway was ablated, and in one patient complete heart block resulted. Similar results with high success rates and a low incidence of complications have been reported by several other groups. In one histologic study of a patient who underwent cardiac transplant shortly after slow pathway modification, the lesion extended from the septal portion of the tricuspid annulus to the posterior border of the AV node, but did not include the compact AV node. Thus, it appears that the slow pathway is composed of posterior approaches to the AV node, but is distinct from the compact AV node. A caveat must be inserted here: the anatomical arrangement of the fast and slow pathways are not identical in different patients. Intraoperative ice mapping of the AV nodal region and detailed mapping of the recorded area of the Asp potential have identified variable posterior locations where destructive lesions can abolish or modify anterograde conduction over the slow pathway. These studies have demonstrated that the slow pathway is at least, in part, anatomically separated from the fast pathway and that modification of perinodal atrial tissue can selectively affect changes in one or the other pathway. Figure 17.4 depicts our concept of the anatomic circuit of AVNRT.

Approach to Therapy

AV nodal reentrant tachycardia is the most common mechanism of PSVT. The AV node, rather than acting as a simple passive electrical conduit between the atrium and ventricle, has unique anatomic and electrophysiologic properties that allow it to be a critical part of the reentrant circuit. Pharmacologic and nonpharmacologic therapy are directed to selected components of the tachycardia circuit.

Patients without ventricular preexcitation who have very infrequent, self-terminating episodes of ECG-documented PSVT causing minimal symptoms may not

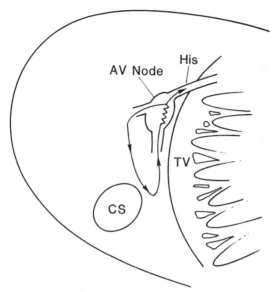

Figure 17.4. A schematic of the AVNRT reentrant circuit. In this simplified model, the AV node has anterior and posterior atrial inputs. Based on the available data, we think that in most cases the anatomic substrate of AVNRT includes a small rim of posterior atrial tissue. As we learn more about AVNRT, this model will undoubtedly become more complex. CS=coronary sinus; TV=tricuspid valve. (From Prystowsky EN, Klein GK. Cardiac arrhythmias: an integrated approach for the clinician. New York: McGraw-Hill, 1994:326. Reproduced with permission of McGraw-Hill.)

require further workup or treatment. We recommend electrophysiologic testing to diagnose the mechanism of PSVT in other patients with more frequent or symptomatic episodes of tachycardia. Acute therapy should begin with methods to increase vagal tone such as carotid sinus massage or the Valsalva maneuver. The patient should be in a resting, supine position to enhance parasympathetic tone. If PSVT persists, intravenous (i.v.) adenosine or verapamil is given, which almost always restores sinus rhythm. Chronic treatment can be palliative with drugs or curative with endocardial catheter ablation. We prefer to cure patients, and therefore recommend ablation as first-line therapy for almost all adult patients who have significant symptoms with AVNRT. Alternatively, one can prescribe drugs to try to prevent AVNRT. β-Adrenergic blockers, as well as verapamil and diltiazem are often quite effective, usually more so than digitalis. Quinidine, disopyramide, flecainide, propafenone, and sotalol may also be given.

**ATRIOVENTRICULAR-RECIPROCATING TACHYCARDIA AND WOLFF-
PARKINSON-WHITE SYNDROME**

Orthodromic AV-Reciprocating Tachycardia

Orthodromic AV reciprocating tachycardia (OAVRT) comprises 95% of the reciprocating tachycardias associated with the Wolff-Parkinson-White (WPW) syndrome (Fig. 17.5). Because OAVRT incorporates the entire heart within its macroreentrant circuit, tachycardia initiation, termination, and perturbation are easily invoked by spontaneous or induced APDs, VPDs, or rapid atrial and ventricular pacing. Intracardiac recordings during EPS show that the APD-inducing OAVRT is conducted with an increased AH interval compared with the AH intervals during the preceding atrial drive train. The tachycardia QRS complexes following the APD will be nonpreexcited with either normal HV intervals and QRS durations or, not uncommonly, initially prolonged HV intervals and/or QRS durations. Following the first nonpreexcited QRS complex, retrograde atrial activation occurs in a pattern consistent with the bypass tract's site of atrial insertion. Initiation of OAVRT in the presence of a concealed accessory pathway follows the same rules except that preexcitation is not present during the preceding atrial drive train or sinus rhythm (Fig. 17.6).

When a VPD induces OAVRT, the AV node/His-Purkinje system must have a longer retrograde refractory period than the AV bypass tract. The tachycardia-inducing VPD conducts retrogradely and activates the atria in a pattern consistent with the atrial insertion point of the accessory pathway. A nonpreexcited QRS complex then follows as a result of antegrade AV node/His-Purkinje system conduction.

OAVRT tends to be a rapid tachycardia with rates ranging from 150 to over 250 beats/min. A beat-to-beat oscillation in QRS amplitude (QRS alternans) may be present in up to 38% of cases. The mechanism for QRS alternans is not clear but may in part result from oscillations in the relative refractory period of the His-Purkinje system. "Ischemic"-appearing ST segment depression may also occur during OAVRT, even in young individuals who are unlikely to have coronary artery disease. In these cases, the ST segment depression results from autonomic nervous system influences and intraventricular conduction disturbances. However, ST segment depression occurring during OAVRT in an older patient mandates considering the possibility of coexisting coronary disease.

The relationship and timing of atrial and ventricular activation are important diagnostic features of OAVRT. Since the atria and ventricles are part of a macroreentrant circuit and have a 1:1 relationship with each other, observing AV dissociation or intermittent AV block during a tachycardia excludes an AV-reciprocating mechanism. The ECG during tachycardia will show P waves inscribed within the ST-T wave segment with an R-P interval that is usually less than half the tachycardia R-R interval (Fig. 17.6). The R-P interval remains constant, regardless of the tachycardia cycle length.

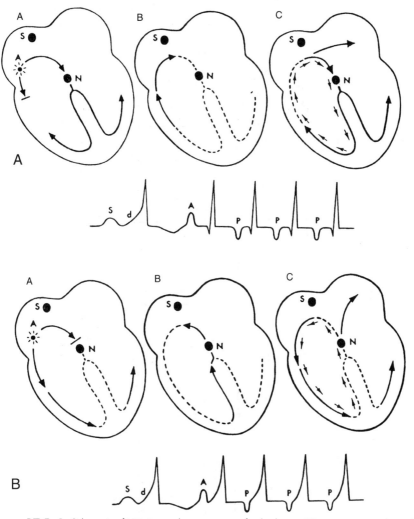

Figure 17.5. A. Schematic of initiation and maintenance of orthodromic AV-reciprocating tachycardia. A diagrammatic ECG recording is also displayed with the first P wave of sinus node (S) origin yielding a preexcited QRS complex with a Δ wave (d) and short P-R interval. In A, an ectopic atrial premature depolarization (A) blocks antegradely in the bypass tract but still conducts through the AV node (N) and His-Purkinje system to the ventricles. This causes the second QRS complex to appear nonpreexcited as it follows the premature A with a longer P-R interval. In B, the premature impulse continues to conduct retrogradely through the bypass tract because the latter has had time to recover excitability during the preceding period of antegrade impulse conduction through the AV node and His-Purkinje system. In C, the retrogradely conducted impulse has activated the atria from the bypass tract's atrial insertion point and generated the first retrograde P wave (P) of OAVRT. Reentrant penetration of the impulse into the AV node and His-Purkinje system then occurs with maintenance of OAVRT determined by the conduction velocities and refractory periods of all tissues comprising the reentrant circuit as well as the circuit length. **B.** Schematic of initiation and maintenance of antidromic AV reciprocating tachycardia (AVRT). In A, the premature atrial depolarization blocks antegradely in the AV node but still conducts through the bypass tract to the ventricles. The second QRS complex following the premature A is therefore fully preexcited with a short PR interval. In B, the premature impulse continues to conduct retrogradely through the His-Purkinje system and the AV node because these tissues have recovered excitability. In C, the retrograde-conducted impulse has activated the atria starting from the centrally located AV node's atrial insertion point. Reentrant penetration of the impulse into the bypass tract then occurs with maintenance of AAVRT. (From Chung EK. Wolff-Parkinson-White syndrome–Current views. Am J Med 1977;62:261.)

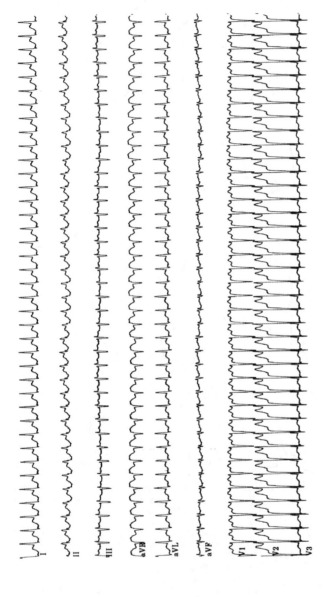

Figure 17.6. ECG recording during OAVRT obtained from a patient with a concealed right free wall accessory pathway (leads V4 and V6 are not recorded). The tachycardia cycle length is 250 msec. Retrograde-conducted P waves during tachycardia having an R-P interval less than half of the tachycardia's RR interval are most readily seen in lead V1; the early portion of the ST-T segment in this lead is negative, giving the T wave a biphasic appearance. This results from the superimposition of the tachycardia's retrograde P wave on the ST-T segment.

Spontaneous or induced functional bundle branch block occurring during OAVRT can yield a diagnostically useful phenomenon. If bundle branch block exists ipsilateral to a free wall bypass tract, the reentrant impulse is compelled to traverse a greater distance from the ventricular insertion of the conducting His-Purkinje fibers to the ventricular insertion of the bypass tract. As a result, the global V-A time interval during the tachycardia must increase, usually by at least 35 msec. The tachycardia cycle length may also increase, although little or no change may occur because of an offsetting decrease in the AH interval. In contrast, bundle branch block occurring contralateral to a free wall AV bypass tract exerts no effect on the V-A interval and the tachycardia cycle length.

During OAVRT, the ability to reset by advancing the next atrial activation with a properly timed VPD, the next ventricular activation with an APD, and the next tachycardia cycle with either an APD or VPD indicates that the entire heart is involved in the tachycardia circuit. Furthermore, a VPD delivered late in the diastolic interval of OAVRT (when the His bundle is refractory) that advances the next set of atrial electrograms without altering the retrograde atrial activation pattern and also advances the next tachycardia cycle proves that a bypass tract is present and is necessary for maintenance of the tachycardia; retrograde conduction of such a VPD could occur only over an accessory pathway because the His bundle is still refractory.

Termination of OAVRT results when block occurs within either the AV node/His-Purkinje system or the accessory pathway. An APD usually terminates the tachycardia by blocking antegradely (in the orthodromic direction) within the AV node and colliding retrogradely (in the antidromic direction) with the previous tachycardia impulse, usually within the atria or bypass tract. Tachycardia termination by a VPD usually occurs when the extrastimulus blocks orthodromically within the bypass tract and collides antidromically with the tachycardia's previous impulse in the AV node/His-Purkinje system.

Spontaneous tachycardia termination after a retrograde P wave on the surface ECG and an atrial electrogram not followed by a His bundle potential on the intracardiac recording indicates that block occurred within the AV node. Tachycardia termination after a QRS complex and ventricular electrogram not followed by a retrograde P wave and atrial electrogram implies that block occurred within the bypass tract. In most instances, spontaneous block occurs within the AV node. Cycle length alternans may be seen immediately preceding AV node block and tachycardia termination, during which, long-to-short oscillations occur in the tachycardia's cycle length and AH interval while the HV and V-A intervals remain constant. Spontaneous block occurring within the AV bypass tract is uncommonly observed during very rapid OAVRT. However, accessory pathways exhibiting slow, decremental retrograde conduction may be the site of block and tachycardia termination following the same autonomic and pharmacologic perturbations that affect the AV node.

The Permanent Form of Junctional Reciprocating Tachycardia (PJRT)

This tachycardia occurs at rates between 120 and 200 beats/min with a usually normal QRS duration; distinguishing features are its tendency for incessant behavior and the QRS/P wave relationship. The arrhythmia is actually an OAVRT mediated by a concealed AV bypass tract with slow and decremental conduction properties. The bypass tract is usually located within the posteroseptal region, although other portions of the AV groove may also harbor this unique pathway. Slow retrograde conduction over the pathway causes the RP interval during PJRT to be long and usually greater than half the tachycardia's RR interval. P waves resulting from retrograde conduction are easily seen on the ECG (Fig. 17.7). Since the accessory pathway is anatomically separate from the AV node/His-Purkinje system, a ventricular extrastimulus delivered late in diastole when the His bundle is refractory can easily reset the next atrial activation and tachycardia cycle. This response cannot occur during uncommon "fast-slow" AVNRT or atrial tachycardia and is useful for differentiating between these three forms of "long R-P" supraventricular tachycardia. Because the accessory pathway conducts decrementally during PJRT, the atrial and tachycardia cycle reset response to the VPD may actually be one of delayed activation, rather than advancement.

The reason for the incessant nature of PJRT is not clear. Its onset and rate are quite sensitive to changes in autonomic tone and prior sinus rhythm rate. Spontaneous PJRT initiation and induction during EPS often occur after only trivial increases in the rate of sinus rhythm or atrial overdrive pacing. Tachycardia termination occurring spontaneously or following vagomimetic maneuvers frequently results from block in the accessory pathway; the ECG and intracardiac recordings show the last tachycardia event as a QRS complex and ventricular electrogram without a subsequent P wave and atrial electrogram. Chronic suppression of PJRT is usually not possible with drugs, and ablation of the accessory pathway is often necessary to achieve arrhythmia control. The tachycardia frequently occurs in infants and children, and its incessant behavior may result in dilated cardiomyopathy and congestive heart failure; the latter are potentially reversible if the accessory pathway can be successfully ablated.

Antidromic AV-Reciprocating Tachycardia (Fig. 17.5B)

AAVRT is the least common arrhythmia associated with WPW syndrome, occurring in only 5–10% of patients. The tachycardia is characterized by a wide QRS complex that is fully preexcited and with usually regular RR intervals, occurring at rates of up to 250 beats/min. AAVRT can result in considerable diagnostic and therapeutic uncertainty because the differential diagnosis includes all other wide QRS tachycardias; i.e., VT, any supraventricular tachycardia conducted aberrantly, and tachycardias of atrial and junctional origin with "bystander" accessory pathway activation of the ventricles (Fig. 17.8). During intervening sinus rhythm, preexcitation may be relatively inapparent because AAVRTs frequently utilize left-sided bypass tracts as the antegrade route for conduction. Demonstrating an identical preexcited QRS morphology during AAVRT and atrial pacing near the atrial insertion of the accessory pathway is diagnostically helpful if additional antegrade-conducting accessory pathways are not present. However, the prevalence of multiple accessory pathways in patients who experience AAVRT may range from 33 to 60%.

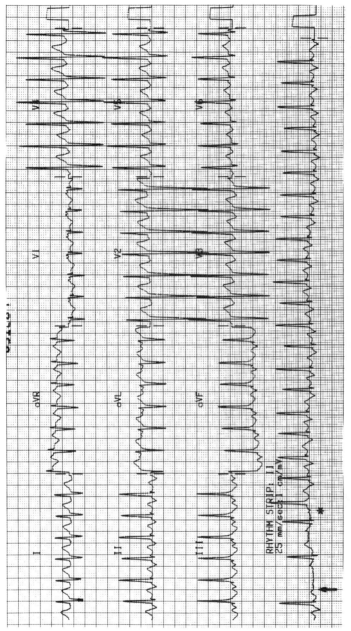

Figure 17.7. A 12-lead ECG and lead II rhythm strip recording obtained from a patient with the permanent form of junctional reciprocating tachycardia. Arrhythmia termination occurs after the first QRS complex because spontaneous block develops in the accessory pathway; the arrow marks where the next retrograde-conducted P wave would have been inscribed if block and tachycardia termination had not occurred. After two sinus depolarizations, a spontaneous APD (asterisk) reinitiates PJRT.

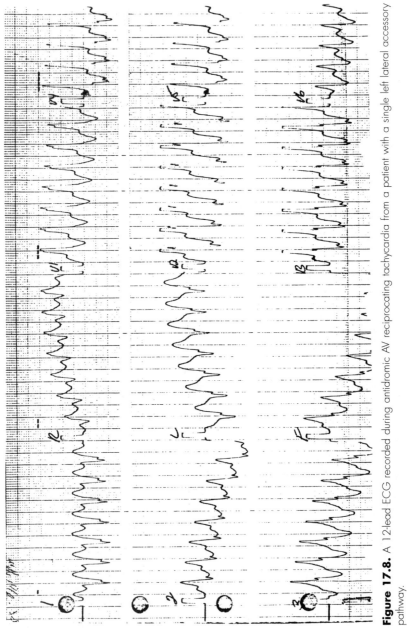

Figure 17.8. A 12-lead ECG recorded during antidromic AV reciprocating tachycardia from a patient with a single left lateral accessory pathway.

If only one antegrade-conducting AV bypass tract exists, the AV node/His-Purkinje system must be the route for retrograde atrial activation during AAVRT. During tachycardia, earliest retrograde atrial activation is inscribed at the His bundle recording site; the sequence of retrograde atrial activation is normal and identical to that during ventricular pacing. A one-to-one V-A conduction relationship exists since there is obligatory participation of the atria and ventricles in the reentrant circuit. Atrial and ventricular extrastimuli will advance, respectively, the next set of ventricular and atrial electrograms as well as the entire tachycardia cycle while preserving the tachycardia's electrogram activation sequence since the atria and ventricles are necessary for tachycardia maintenance. The width of the preexcited QRS complex and the amplitude of the ST-T wave segment usually obscure the retrograde P wave on the surface ECG. The H-V interval is negative with a retrograde His potential either immediately preceding the local ventricular electrogram of the His bundle recording or, alternatively, occurring simultaneously with and obscured by the larger amplitude ventricular electrogram. As with OAVRT, tachycardia termination can occur following properly timed atrial and ventricular extrastimuli or spontaneously when block occurs within either the accessory pathway or the AV node/His-Purkinje system.

Atrial Tachycardias Including Atrial Fibrillation and Atrial Flutter

AF may be the index arrhythmia in up to 20% of patients with WPW syndrome. It is usually paroxysmal rather than chronic and persistent. Patients with bypass tracts causing overt preexcitation seem to be more prone to AF than patients whose bypass tracts are concealed. The accessory pathway's ability to mediate a rapid and hemodynamically unstable preexcited ventricular response is what determines the clinical mode of presentation with AF in the WPW syndrome. It should be emphasized that ventricular fibrillation resulting from AF is rare as the first presenting arrhythmia in an individual not previously known to have WPW syndrome. Furthermore, the majority of patients with WPW syndrome who have AF have had preexisting episodes of AVRT. Paroxysmal and chronic AFL are less common than paroxysmal AF in WPW syndrome. This may result from the low incidence of associated structural heart disease in WPW syndrome.

The ECG during preexcited AF will exhibit an irregularly irregular ventricular response; however, a sustained rapid ventricular rate more than 180–200 beats/min will often create "pseudoregularized" RR intervals when the ECG is recorded at 25 mm/sec. The atrial electrograms recorded during preexcited AF are not different in appearance from those recorded in the absence of preexcitation. Not uncommonly, AF may secondarily develop from degeneration of rapid OAVRT. The ventricular rate during preexcited AF can vary considerably; the important rate-modulating effects of autonomic tone and the interplay between refractoriness and conduction in the AV node/His-Purkinje system versus the bypass tract have already been discussed. Repetitive retrograde concealed conduction into the bypass tract during preexcited AF may result in a slower ventricular response than predicted on the basis of the bypass tract's antegrade refractory period and shortest atrial pacing cycle length maintaining 1:1 preexcited conduction. These factors also influence the degree to which QRS complexes will be totally preexcited or variably exist as fusions of normal and preexcited complexes. Detecting the presence of more than one preexcited QRS morphology during AF also aids in identifying multiple AV bypass tracts. The total absence of preexcited QRS complexes during AF despite the presence of (often intermittent) preexcitation during sinus rhythm is also a reassuring sign that the antegrade refractory period of the bypass tract is long and the pathway unlikely to mediate a rapid ventricular response during spontaneous AF.

THERAPY OF ARRHYTHMIAS ASSOCIATED WITH THE WPW SYNDROME

A number of treatment options exist for patients with the WPW syndrome. These include pharmacologic agents, antitachycardia devices, catheter and surgical ablation, and combinations of these therapies.

Pharmacologic Therapy

The rational choice of an antiarrhythmic drug depends on making a correct arrhythmia diagnosis and defining the electrophysiologic properties of the tachycardia. When treating AVRT, a drug should be chosen that has its most potent depressant action on the "weak link" of the tachycardia circuit. Performing atrial and ventricular pacing at incremental rates above the tachycardia's rate and noting the paced cycle lengths leading to block in, respectively, the antegrade and retrograde limbs of conduction, can define a "safety factor" for conduction over these routes. During AVRT, the antegrade or retrograde conduction pathway having the greater difference between the tachycardia cycle length and the paced cycle length causing block in that pathway can be considered the "strong" limb of conduction. The "weak" limb of the AVRT circuit will contain tissue with the longest refractory period and/or most tenuous conduction properties. The drug may also lengthen the strong limb's refractory period in the direction opposite to that over which the tachycardia impulse propagates. If this tissue is the site of unidirectional block that helps to initiate reentry, the result may be widening of the tachycardia induction zone, an increased probability that spontaneous APDs and VPDs will trigger AVRT, and a reentrant circuit that maintains a more frequently occurring, if not incessant, tachycardia with a slower rate.

Orthodromic AV-Reciprocating Tachycardia

The AV node is usually the weak link in this arrhythmia. Relatively specific therapies that lengthen nodal refractoriness and depress conduction are therefore desirable to cause the reentrant impulse to block in the node and terminate the tachycardia. The resultant depression of AV node function from carotid sinus massage and Valsalva's maneuver may also be sufficient to cause AV node block and tachycardia termination.

Intravenous verapamil is probably the optimum drug for acute termination of OAVRT, provided that the patient is not profoundly hypotensive and/or suffering from congestive heart failure associated with severely depressed ventricular systolic function. Intravenous adenosine is equally effective for acutely terminating OAVRT. Its ultra-short duration of action is preferable for the patient whose hemodynamic state is more tenuous before resorting to emergent DC cardioversion. However, adenosine's proclivities to transiently increase atrial vulnerability to AF and cause atrial ectopy that can reinitiate OAVRT after acute tachycardia termination are potential disadvantages compared with verapamil.

Agents of second choice include the β-blockers approved for i.v. administration: propranolol, metoprolol, and esmolol. Intravenous digoxin's prolonged times to onset of action and peak effect coupled with low potency make it a less attractive treatment alternative.

Intravenous procainamide is also an important alternative drug choice. Unlike the other agents listed, procainamide depresses conduction in all cardiac tissues and prolongs refractoriness in the atria, ventricles, bypass tract, and the His-Purkinje system while having no effect or causing slight shortening of the AV node refractory period. Procainamide is the drug of choice if the OAVRT presents as a wide QRS complex tachycardia due to functional or preexisting chronic bundle branch block and the diagnosis of OAVRT is in doubt. Intravenous procainamide is the safest, if not most efficacious, drug to administer for acute treatment of an unknown wide QRS tachycardia.

An antiarrhythmic drug's efficacy in preventing OAVRT is predicated on its ability to alter the electrophysiologic properties of the reentrant circuit so as to render reentry incapable of sustaining itself. Antiectopic activity is also desirable to decrease the number of arrhythmia-triggering APDs and VPDs. Chronic drug therapy usually requires continuous dosing at regular intervals. However, occasional patients with infrequent episodes of OAVRT that are not overly symptomatic or hemodynamically destabilized may be served equally well by an intermittent, acute oral drug regimen. Patients requiring chronic drug treatment are potentially committed to indefinite antiarrhythmic drug prophylaxis. The optimum drug must not only have a high efficacy rate but also a low risk for causing adverse effects and noncardiac organ toxicity. Cardiac toxicity is less of an acute concern in the absence of structural heart disease, but the risk may ultimately need to be confronted as the patient ages.

Presently, the class IC antiarrhythmic drugs possess the most favorable efficacy record. Only flecainide has received approval for chronic suppression of paroxysmal supraventricular tachycardia including OAVRT. Propafenone is probably equally efficacious and its β-blocking activity may provide ancillary benefit.

Second line drugs for chronic suppression of OAVRT include agents with AV node-specific activity, i.e., β-blockers, calcium channel blockers, and digoxin. These agents may be inadequate as monotherapy because of their inability to directly slow conduction and increase retrograde refractoriness in the accessory pathway; they also do not reduce the frequency of arrhythmia-triggering APDs and VPDs and do not increase antegrade refractoriness in the bypass tract. However, a β-blocker or verapamil may be a useful adjunct to a class I drug, preventing catecholamine reversal of drug effect.

The class IA drugs were previously the agents of choice for suppressing OAVRT before the advent of the class IC drugs because they lengthened antegrade and retrograde refractoriness and slowed conduction in the accessory pathway. However, these compounds are less potent than the class Ic drugs, minimally lengthen AV node refractoriness, and have a substantial risk of causing serious organ toxicity and intolerable noncardiac adverse effects.

Amiodarone has multiple electrophysiologic effects that make it effective in suppressing OAVRT. These include antiadrenergic activity, prolongation of repolarization and voltage-dependent refractoriness, and blockade of the fast and slow inward currents. These effects result in slowing of conduction and lengthening of refractoriness in both the bypass tract and the AV node/His-Purkinje system. Combined with its excellent antiectopic activity, amiodarone would seem to be an "ideal" drug for suppressing OAVRT. Despite the drug's well-known array of adverse effects, life-threatening pulmonary and hepatic toxicity necessitating drug discontinuation during long-term therapy is uncommon, particularly when low maintenance doses of 200–300 mg/day are used. However, less "serious" adverse effects that at least limit quality of life eventually occur in 30–93% of patients and lead to amiodarone withdrawal in 9–28%.

Sotalol has also been shown to have clinical efficacy in preventing OAVRT. An incidence of torsade de pointes as high as 4% raises concern about the drug's long-term safety. This risk seems greatest during the acute dose-titration phase of therapy in patients with advanced structural heart disease and life-threatening ventricular arrhythmias.

Antidromic AV Reciprocating Tachycardia

Although retrograde AV node conduction is usually the "weak link" during AAVRT, intravenously administered AV node-specific blocking drugs such as β blockers, calcium channel blockers, adenosine, and digoxin should be avoided. Unless the tachycardia is known to be AAVRT with certainty before treatment is initiated, the patient should be considered to have an undiagnosed wide QRS tachycardia. AAVRT could also degenerate into AF following drug administration, especially if adenosine is administered. Since bypass tracts capable of supporting AAVRT usually have short antegrade refractory periods, the resultant ventricular response during preexcited AF might be hemodynamically even more destabilizing. The i.v. drug of choice for acute treatment to terminate AAVRT is therefore procainamide. Even if it does not cause outright tachycardia termination, i.v. procainamide may at least slow the tachycardia rate and can improve the hemodynamic state.

The accessory pathway mediating antegrade conduction during AAVRT is also capable of serving as the limb for antegrade preexcited conduction during AF. Drugs that are useful must affect the accessory pathway. The class Ic drugs are the agents of choice in the absence of contraindications; class Ia drugs and amio-darone would be less desirable second choices for reasons previously mentioned.

Atrial Fibrillation

The goals of acute drug therapy for preexcited AF are prompt control of the ventricular response and stabilization of the patient's hemodynamic state. Treatment of preexcited AF requires a parenteral drug with rapid onset of action that lengthens antegrade refractoriness and slows conduction in both the AV node/His-Purkinje system and the accessory pathway. Flecainide and propafenone are highly efficacious when used for these purposes, but the parenteral formulations of these drugs are not approved for use in the United States. Intravenously administered procainamide is therefore the drug of choice.

AV node-specific antiarrhythmic drugs that are normally used to control the ventricular rate during nonpreexcited AF are contraindicated. Intravenous β blockers when used alone do not increase bypass tract refractoriness. β-Blocker-mediated inhibition of AV node conduction may also enhance the preexcited ventricular rate response by decreasing the degree of concealed retrograde conduction into the bypass tract. A bypass tract with a short intrinsic antegrade refractory period that was initially competing with the AV node could become the dominant route for antegrade conduction.

Intravenous digoxin is also contraindicated because of its unpredictable effect on bypass tract refractoriness. Digoxin's vagomimetic action also lengthens AV node refractoriness and reduces concealed retrograde conduction into the bypass tract. A comparatively slow time to onset of action and peak effect also make digoxin an unacceptable drug to use when rapid ventricular rate control is required.

Verapamil is the most dangerous AV node blocker to administer during preexcited AF. Intravenous verapamil lengthens AV node refractoriness, decreases concealed conduction into the accessory pathway, and has no direct effect on the accessory pathway. Myocardial contractility and systemic vascular resistance are also reduced; these latter effects may cause a reflex increase in already elevated sympathetic tone that in turn further shortens accessory pathway refractoriness. Precipitation of cardiac arrest by degeneration of preexcited AF to ventricular fibrillation has been reported after i.v. verapamil administration. Intravenous adenosine causes a similar effect.

The drug selected for suppressing paroxysmal AF in WPW syndrome should possess antiectopic activity to suppress both APDs and VPDs that can induce AF as well as AVRT since the latter can subsequently degenerate into AF. The drug must also provide adequate background protection against a rapid ventricular response should AF intermittently "break through" by lengthening refractoriness in both the accessory pathway and the AV node/His-Purkinje system. Class Ic drugs again possess the best electrophysiologic profile for achieving these goals if no cardiac contraindications exist. Class Ia drugs are less potent and have greater noncardiac adverse effect and organ toxicity risks as previously noted. Amiodarone is again useful in instances where class IC/Ia drugs are ineffective and/or not tolerated and where ablation therapy is inappropriate or has failed.

Antitachycardia Devices

Antitachycardia device therapy includes the use of external DC cardioverters, temporary pacemakers, and permanently implanted antitachycardia pacemakers that can be manually or automatically activated. External DC cardioversion may be emergently necessary when the patient presents with serious hemodynamic symptoms or when initially prescribed therapy is either ineffective or leads to abrupt worsening of the patient's condition.

AVRTs lend themselves well to pacemaker termination because the entire heart is involved in a reentrant circuit. Temporary pacemaker stimulation of the right atrium or ventricle or transesophageal pacing are alternatives to DC cardioversion if an AVRT episode persists following initial attempts to terminate it with an i.v. antiarrhythmic drug; this approach assumes that the patient''s hemodynamic state permits time to insert a transvenous pacing catheter. The risk of inadvertently inducing preexcited AF with a rapid ventricular response is particularly likely when delivering multiple atrial extrastimuli at close coupling intervals or when rapidly pacing the atrium at rates in excess of 250 beats/min. This risk may be reduced by first administering i.v. procainamide to slow the tachycardia rate and lengthen bypass tract refractoriness. Type I atrial flutter that is conducted with preexcitation can also be pace-terminated after the ventricles have been drug-protected from one-to-one AV conduction and the atrial flutter rate decreased. Pacemaker stimulation is not effective for termination of atrial fibrillation.

Permanent antitachycardia pacemakers are contraindicated for patients with WPW syndrome who have manifest preexcitation due to accessory pathways with short antegrade refractory periods because a rapid ventricular rate can occur if AF were inadvertently precipitated during automatic antitachycardia pacing. Antitachycardia pacemakers do not prevent AVRT and frequently have relatively poor long-term efficacy. Permanent antitachycardia pacing is also undesirable for patients who experience severe symptoms during their tachycardia episodes, especially if the episodes occur frequently and/or require multiple pacing attempts before termination finally occurs.

Ablation Therapy

Ablation therapy is playing an increasingly prominent role in the management of patients with WPW syndrome. Prior to the advent of radiofrequency energy catheter-mediated ablation, surgical ablation of AV bypass tracts was the standard technique that provided a true cure for patients suffering from drug-refractory WPW syndrome. The success rate for WPW surgery is now near 100% with an operative mortality rate of less than 1%.

Radiofrequency energy catheter-mediated ablation is now achieving success rates that rival those of surgery with a comparable or lower mortality risk and a lower acute morbidity risk. Recent compilations of the results from a number of large centers have disclosed success rates of 90–95%, acute morbidity and mortality rates of less than 1%, and recurrence rates of 5–6%. A compelling argument has been made for the cost-effectiveness of the procedure compared with prolonged periods of therapy with multiple antiarrhythmic drugs.

As a cautionary counterpoint, appropriate concerns have been raised about the mutagenic and carcinogenic risks to patients and personnel resulting from the often lengthy fluoroscopic exposure times required for successful completion of the procedure. The long-term risk of future arrhythmias occurring as a result of the lesions created during radiofrequency ablation of AV bypass tracts is unknown. However, animal studies and the accumulated clinical experience over the past 5 years suggest that this risk may be low.

Patients who experience only infrequent and minimally symptomatic OAVRT are encouraged to consider "cocktail" treatment, i.e., large single-dose pharmacologic therapy, taken on basis along with properly taught self-performed vagomimetic maneuvers to assist in terminating arrhythmia episodes. However, these patients should first undergo an EPS to assure that their accessory pathway's antegrade conduction properties are not potentially malignant (although performing atrial pacing using a transesophageal electrode might offer a less invasive method for performing this assessment). WPW syndrome patients whose life expectancy is severely limited by other diseases and/or who are elderly are probably best treated with chronic antiarrhythmic medical therapy, including amiodarone. However, relatively healthy elderly patients should not be denied radiofrequency energy catheter ablation therapy because of their age alone if they experience highly symptomatic arrhythmia that responds poorly to medical treatment. Although surgical ablation has been relegated to a "third-line" position, it still can offer benefit to good surgical risk patients suffering from highly symptomatic and hemodynamically unstable, drug-refractory arrhythmias when radiofrequency energy catheter ablation has failed at centers with a proven track record of success in performing the procedure. Finally, patients with symptomatic arrhythmia who undergo cardiac surgery for other indications may be candidates for having concomitant bypass tract resection performed if the added surgical trauma and cardiopulmonary bypass time are not likely to substantially increase the operative mortality risk.

SUGGESTED READING

Rosen KM, Mehta A, Miller RA. Demonstration of dual atrioventricular nodal pathways in man. Am J Cardiol 1974;33:291–294.

Sung RJ, Styperck JL, Myerburg RJ, Castellanos A. Initiation of two distinct forms of atrioventricular nodal reentrant tachycardia during programmed ventricular stimulation in man. Am J Cardiol 1978;42:404–415.

Josephson ME. Preexcitation syndromes. Clinical cardiac electrophysiology. Philadelphia: Lea & Febiger, 1993:311–416.

Milstein S, Sharma AD, Guiraudon GM, Klein GJ. An algorithm for the electrocardiographic localization of accessory pathways in the Wolff-Parkinson-White syndrome. PACE 1987;10: 555–563.

Krahn AD, Manfreda J, Tate RB, Mathewson FAL, Cuddy TE. The natural history of electrocardiographic preexcitation in men. The Manitoba follow-up study. Ann Intern Med 1992;116:456–460.

Akhtar M, Lehmann MH, Denker ST, Mahmud R, Tchou P, Jazayeri M. Electrophysiologic mechanisms of orthodromic tachycardia initiation during ventricular pacing in the Wolff-Parkinson-White syndrome. J Am Coll Cardiol 1987;9:89–100.

Wellens HJJ. The wide QRS tachycardia. Ann Intern Med 1986;104:879.

18 Ventricular Premature Beats Depolarizations and Nonsustained Ventricular Tachycardia

VENTRICULAR PREMATURE DEPOLARIZATIONS

Prevalence

The prevalence of ventricular premature depolarizations (VPDs) is directly related to the methods that are used to detect them and to the patient population that is studied. On a resting 12-lead ECG, patients with no known heart disease have been noted to have VPDs less than 5% of the time. However, studies using 24-hour ambulatory monitoring have found VPDs to be present in 50% of a healthy population.

Aging increases the prevalence of VPDs independent of the presence of heart disease. In patients with coronary artery disease (CAD), the prevalence of VPDs is 14% on a 12-lead ECG and up to 90% on 24-hour monitoring. Within a CAD population, the degree of left ventricular dysfunction correlates closely with the number of VPDs, independent of the severity of anatomic stenoses. Similarly, patients with larger areas of infarction will have a greater number of VPDs in the periinfarct period. Following hospital discharge, there appears to be an increase in the amount of ventricular ectopy during the recovery phase, with a greater incidence of VPDs and nonsustained ventricular tachycardia (NSVT) 1 month after the acute event compared with a predischarge evaluation.

There is an increased incidence of VPDs in patients with nearly every other form of structural heart disease as well. There is diurnal variability of VPD frequency, i.e., they are more common in the morning than during the night. The hourly and absolute number of VPDs on an ambulatory ECG recording can show wide hourly and daily fluctuations when serial 24-hour monitoring recordings are compared. The longer the time interval between monitoring, the greater is the variability. As a result, deciphering whether a change in VPD frequency is secondary to a drug effect or to the arrhythmia's inherent variability can be difficult. Most investigators recognize that a reduction in VPD frequency by 75% probably represents a true clinical effect.

Clinical Evaluation

The most frequent symptoms resulting from VPDs are palpitations secondary to the hypercontractility of the post-VPD beat or a feeling that the heart has stopped secondary to the post-VPD pause. Less commonly, frequent VPDs can result in a pounding sensation in the neck, lightheadedness, or near syncope. There is great variability as to when the symptoms are most prominent, although a quiet environment may make a patient more aware of the ectopy. The palpitations that the patient feels invariably provoke significant anxiety, often causing a vicious cycle of palpitations, anxiety, catecholamine surges, and more ectopy. Patients thus affected may report dizziness that is not related to any fall in cerebral perfusion pressure or blood flow.

On physical examination, atrioventricular (AV) dissociation or a change in P-R interval, if present, will result in a changing intensity of the first heart sound (secondary to the changing P-R interval) as well as the production of cannon "A" waves of variable intensity. The splitting of the second heart sound (S2) will vary, depending on whether the VPD has a right or left bundle branch morphology; a delayed S2 should be appreciated if a right bundle block VPD occurs. Finally, an auscultated fully compensatory pause is present with most VPDs, identified by the prolonged pause following the premature beat itself.

The electrocardiographic (ECG) characteristics of a VPD include duration of >120 msec, bizarre morphology, T wave in the opposite direction from the main QRS vector, and usually a fully compensatory pause (Fig. 18.1). This pause results from an inability of the VPD to reset the sinus node, either from slow or absent ventriculoatrial conduction or secondary to the VPD occurring late in the cardiac cycle. The sinus node fires on time, but the impulse is unable to conduct antegradely through the AV node, hence causing a compensatory pause (i.e., the R-R interval surrounding the VPD is twice the sinus R-R interval).

However, the ECG manifestations of VPDs can be quite variable. An interpolated VPD does not affect the underlying ventricular rate because it occurs so early that the function of the sinus node and AV conduction system is not disturbed (Fig. 18.2). In essence, the VPD is unable to conduct retrogradely and

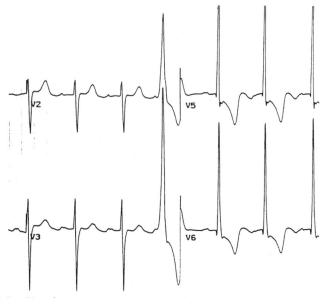

Figure 18.1. VPD with a compensatory pause.

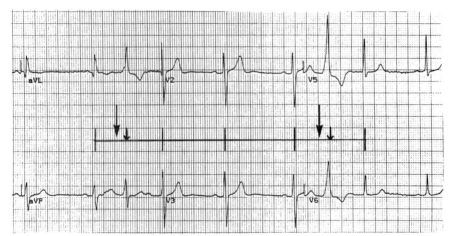

Figure 18.2. Sinus arrhythmia with interpolated VPDs. The underlying sinus rate is unaffected by the presence of the VPD (arrows).

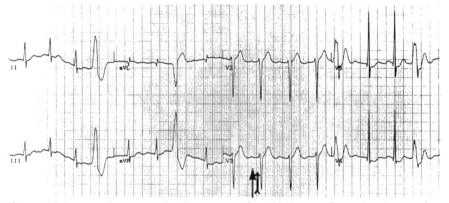

Figure 18.3. Ventricular parasystole. The presence of exit block is manifest as the absence of an ectopic complex determined by the prior interectopic intervals (arrow).

affect conduction of the next sinus impulse. Multifocal PVCs may originate from various sites or may originate from one site if there are differing exit points into the ventricular myocardium or changes in the pattern or direction of myocardial activation. VPDs classically have fixed coupling intervals to the preceding beat, while variable coupling suggests a parasystolic focus. This focus is usually associated with entrance block, whereby the prevailing cardiac rhythm cannot penetrate nor interfere with the parasystolic autonomy. Parasystole may be caused by an automatic or triggered mechanism, may be modulated by other coincident cardiac rhythms, or may be irregularly manifest due to exit block (Fig. 18.3). Beats that

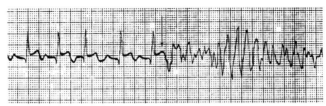

Figure 18.4. R-on-T phenomenon with initiation of an episode of ventricular fibrillation.

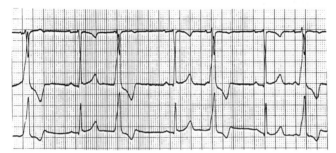

Figure 18.5. Ventricular bigeminy.

begin at or near the apex of the T wave are said to illustrate the "R-on-T" phenomenon (Fig. 18.4).

Several specific VPD patterns have been described. Ventricular bigeminy refers to a persistent alternation of normal and premature beats (Fig. 18.5). The coupling intervals between normal and ectopic beats are constant. When bigeminy occurs in patients with compromised ventricular function, especially in patients with an intrinsically slow sinus rate, the alternating loss of an effective contraction can cause hemodynamic embarrassment. This is one of the few situations in which VPDs can provoke hypotension. Trigeminal and quadrigemal patterns have also been described but rarely cause severe symptoms and have no known independent prognostic importance.

VPDs may facilitate the diagnosis of certain cardiac conditions. For example, patients who have hypertrophic obstructive cardiomyopathy will have an increase in their outflow tract gradient during the more forceful contraction that follows the compensatory pause. Dubbed the "Brockenbrough" sign, it can be responsible for an increase in the intensity of the heart murmur characteristic of this entity, as well as for an increase in the gradient as measured either in the echocardiography or catheterization laboratory. VPDs may precipitate pulsus alternans, a marker of severe left ventricular dysfunction. Also, a post-VPD pause may allow for normal conduction of the subsequent supraventricular beat in patients with rate-dependent bundle branch and may permit the diagnosis of otherwise covert infarctions. Finally, VPDs with a QR pattern may uncover an infarction otherwise not obvious in beats that have been conducted from above the AV node .

Classification of VPDs

There have been several attempts to characterize VPDs to better characterize their prognostic significance. The oldest is the Lown grading system (Table 18.1). Perhaps a more clinically relevant schema considers VPDs within the context of the type and severity of the underlying heart disease, as well as by their own complexity. The more complex the arrhythmia and the worse the heart disease, the greater the likelihood of an untoward event.

Clinical Significance

VPDs have clinical impact either because they cause symptoms or because they signal an increased risk of sudden cardiac death. The latter has been defined in large clinical trials, most of which have focused on the myocardial infarction (MI) survivor. The presence of VPDs has also been shown to be associated with an increased total mortality in some patient subgroups, suggesting that VPDs are a marker of a more severe disease process rather than the provocateur of a terminal electrical event.

Patients with a history of CAD and MI have a diminished long-term survival if VPDs have been documented (Fig. 18.6). This increased death rate is obvious if frequent and complex ectopy is considered, especially in subgroups with a recent MI.

In patients without clinically evident heart disease, there is no relationship between simple VPDs and sudden cardiac death. The significance of frequent and complex ventricular ectopy in patients with apparently normal hearts is also debatable.

Patients with poor left ventricular function have a higher prevalence of ventricular ectopy. The proportion of deaths in such patients that are sudden has varied in the literature, but 50% may be an accurate estimate. This does not imply that all sudden cardiac death in this population is a result of a ventricular tachyarrhythmia, as bradyarrhythmias account for an appreciable number, perhaps as many as 25% according to some authors. As a result, there is controversy concerning the prognostic significance of ventricular ectopy in this population.

Table 18.1
The Lown Classification of Ventricular Ectopy

Grade	Observed
0	No ventricular ectopic beats
1	Occasional, isolated VPDs
2	Frequent VPDs (>1/min or 30/hr)
3	Multiform VPDs
4	Repetitive VPDs
a	Couplets
b	Salvos
5	Early VPDs

From Lown B, Wolf M. Approaches to sudden death from coronary heart disease. Circulation 1971;44:130–142.

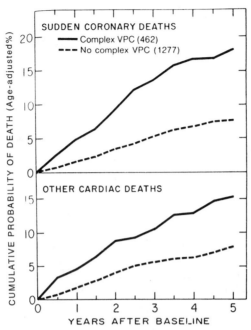

Figure 18.6. Increased risk of sudden death and cardiac mortality in postinfarction patients with complex VPDs throughout a 5-year observation period. (From Ruberman W, Weinblatt E, Goldberg JD, Frank CW, Chaudhary BS, Shapiro S. Ventricular premature complexes and sudden death after myocardial infarction. Circulation 1981;64:297–305.)

Patients with left ventricular hypertrophy (LVH), especially if ECG evidence of repolarization abnormalities is also present, have more ventricular ectopy and are at increased risk of sudden cardiac death compared to individuals with hypertension and no hypertrophy.

Treatment of Ventricular Ectopy

The two goals in the treatment of VPDs are to reduce symptoms and to prolong life; however, the eradication of VPDs in obtaining the former goal cannot be at the expense of the latter. As mentioned earlier, the presence of ventricular ectopy has independent prognostic importance for the patient with heart disease. Intuitively, the successful suppression of this asymptomatic ectopy should improve a patient's prognosis. However, this is yet to be demonstrated. Indeed, the Cardiac Arrhythmia Suppression Trial (CAST), which involved post-MI patients, reported results to the contrary. The study was interrupted at 22 months after documenting a 2.4 times higher risk of death and a 3.6-fold greater risk of nonfatal cardiac arrest and arrhythmic death, despite successful reduction in VPD frequency (Fig. 18.7).

A number of studies have almost uniformly documented the lack of benefit of prophylactic class I antiarrhythmic therapy postinfarction (Table 18.2).

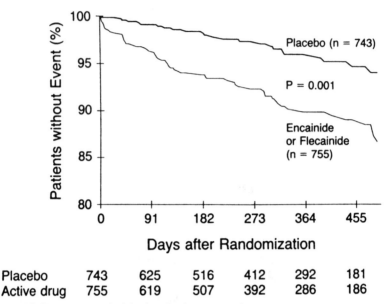

Figure 18.7. Increasing risk of death or cardiac arrest in the active treatment versus placebo groups during a >1-year follow-up. (From Echt DS, Liebson PR, Mitchell B, et al. Mortality and morbidity in patients receiving encainide, flecainide, or placebo. N Engl J Med 1991;324:781-788.)

Clearly, however, in the patient with organic heart disease and diminished left ventricular function, it appears wise to avoid antiarrhythmic therapy for the suppression of asymptomatic VPDs. Exceptions may be amiodarone and β-blockers. β-Blocker therapy has been shown to reduce postmyocardial infarction mortality by approximately 20% and is well accepted as part of a standard postinfarction therapeutic regimen (Table 18.3). Amiodanone is now being evaluated in large trials, after some encouraging results in preliminary analyses.

Some alternative techniques employed for VPD suppression include antianxiety agents, biofeedback, exercise, and stress reduction. The use of antiarrhythmic therapy for relief of severe symptoms may be reasonable. β-Blockers and anxiolytics are usually first-line agents for these patients. The lowest dose of β-blockers that relieves symptoms should be used to minimize side effects. Although patients who fail the aforementioned measures may require class I or III drugs, this strategy should be reserved for the most symptomatic patients.

NONSUSTAINED VENTRICULAR TACHYCARDIA

Electrocardiographic Characteristics

NSVT is most commonly defined as a run of three or more consecutive ventricular complexes at a rate greater than 100 beats/minute that terminates spontaneously within 30 seconds.

Table 18.2
The Failure of Class I Antiarrhythmic Therapy to Reduce Postinfarction Mortality

Agent (No. of Trials)	Allocation No. Deaths/No. Randomized		Odds Ratio (95% CI[a])	P
	Active Treatment	Control		
Class Ia				
Quinidine (2)	10/94	6/113	2.05 [0.73–5.78]	.17
Procainamide hydrochloride (5)	15/182	19/182	0.77 [0.38–1.56]	.46
Disopyramide (7)	104/460	98/1452	1.06 [0.80–1.41]	.68
Imipramine hydrochloride (1)	7/102	6/100	1.15 [0.38–3.54]	.80
Moricizine (3)	117/1454	88/1443	1.39 [1.04–1.87]	.02
Subtotal (18)	253/3292	217/3290	1.19 [0.99–1.44]	.07
Class Ib				
Lidocaine (i.v.) (10)	103/1379	76/1261	1.23 [0.91–1.68]	.18
Lidocaine (i.m.) (7)	53/3737	47/3738	1.02 [0.68–1.53]	.94
Tocainide (6)	20/721	23/725	0.87 [0.47–1.60]	.66
Phenytoin (2)	41/359	40/359	1.04 [0.65–1.65]	.88
Mexiletine hydrochloride (7)	89/872	89/862	0.99 [0.72–1.36]	.94
Subtotal (32)	306/7068	275/6945	1.06 [0.89–1.26]	.50
Class Ic				
Aprindine (3)	28/258	37/255	0.72 [0.53–1.22]	.22
Encainide hydrochloride (3)	45/619	24/56	1.82 [1.12–2.97]	.02
Flecainide (2)	24/426	13/418	1.82 [0.94–3.53]	.07
Subtotal (8)	97/1303	74/1235	1.31 [0.95–1.79]	.10
Quin/Dis/Mex (1)	4/49	5/47	0.75 [0.19–1.79]	.68
Total (59)	660/11712 (5.6%)	571/11517 (5.0%)	1.14 [1.01–1.28]	.03

From Teo KK, Yusuf S, Furberg CD. Effects of prophylactic antiarrhythmic drug therapy in acute myocardial infarction. An overview of results from randomized controlled trials. JAMA 1993;270:1589–1595.

[a]CI, confidence interval; Quin/Dis/Mex, quindine, disopyramide, and mexiletine.

Table 18.3
Sudden Death Reduction Postinfarction with β Blocker Therapy

Study	Study Drug	No. of Patients	Follow-up (mo)	Sudden Death Reduction (%)
BHAT, 1982	Propranolol	3837	25	25% (P < .05)
Wilhelmsson et al., 1974	Alprenolol	230	24	2-fold (P < .05)
Ahlmark et al., 1974	Alprenolol	162	24	7-fold (P < .05)
Multicentre Int. Study, 1977	Practolol	3053	12	55% (P < .01)
Norwegian Multicenter Study Group, 1981	Timolol	1884	12	2-fold (P < .001)
Hansteen et al., 1982	Propranolol	560	12	2-fold (P < .038)
Julian et al., 1982	Sotalol	1456	12	15% (P = NS)
European Infarction Study, 1984	Oxyprenolol	1741	12	0%

Adapted from Yusuf S, Peto R, Lewis J, Collins P, and Sleight P. Beta blockade during and after myocardial infarction: an overview of the randomized trials. Prog Cardiovasc Dis 1985;27:335-371

Most episodes of NSVT are discovered during "routine" screening with Holter monitoring or in-hospital telemetry. Episodes of NSVT typically are brief, lasting 3–10 beats. Ventricular rates usually range from 100–200 beats/minute.

The frequency with which episodes of NSVT occur seems to be influenced by the type of underlying heart disease. The majority of patients with CAD and prior MI have infrequent episodes of NSVT: one or two daily. This also appears to be true of patients with hypertrophic cardiomyopathy. In contrast, in patients with nonischemic dilated cardiomyopathy, NSVT tends to occur with a higher frequency. It is interesting to note that patients with NSVT tend to have a higher frequency of isolated ventricular premature depolarizations when compared with patients without NSVT.

The electrocardiographic morphology of NSVT may be uniform and constant (Fig. 18.8), or polymorphic, varying constantly during individual episodes (Fig. 18.9). There does not appear to be any relationship between the morphologic characteristics and the type of underlying heart disease, with two exceptions. First, when episodes of NSVT arise during acute myocardial ischemia, they often appear polymorphic. Episodes of VT associated with the long Q-T syndrome are also typically polymorphic.

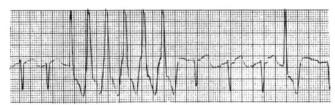

Figure 18.8. Typical episode of nonsustained VT in a patient with chronic CAD. The tachycardia appears to have a uniform morphology in this single monitor lead. The initial complex of the arrhythmia is a late-coupled ventricular premature beat.

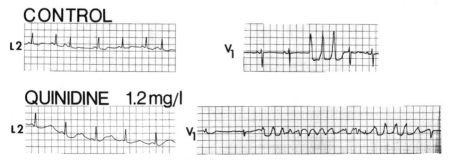

Figure 18.9. Polymorphic VT resulting from quinidine-induced long Q-T syndrome. The top tracings were recorded in the baseline state, in the absence of antiarrhythmic drugs. The patient had asymptomatic, brief runs of NSVT that appeared monomorphic in lead V_1. After initiation of quinidine therapy, the patient developed longer runs of polymorphic VT. ECG recordings from leads 2 (L2) and V_1 are shown in the baseline state and after initiation of quinidine. Note the marked prolongation of the Q-T interval in the presence of quinidine.

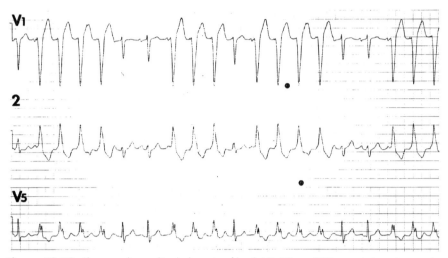

Figure 18.10. Electrocardiographic rhythm strip of leads V1, V2, and V5 recorded simultaneously. The morphology is typical of tachycardia originating in the right ventricular outflow tract in a patient without structural heart disease: left bundle branch pattern with an inferiorly directed frontal plane QRS axis. The pattern is typical of repetitive monomorphic VT. Note that the sinus QRS complexes have a normal pattern.

Second, a unique subtype of NSVT, which usually appears in persons without obvious structural heart disease, has a left bundle branch block pattern with an inferior frontal plane axis (Fig. 18.10). These patients exhibit a range of arrhythmias, including isolated ventricular premature ventricular complexes, NSVT episodes, and rarely, sustained VT, all having this same morphology. Consistent with this electrocardiographic appearance is the endocardial catheter map, which demonstrates that this tachycardia originates in the right ventricular outflow tract.

Prevalence

The prevalence of NSVT depends on the presence, the type, and the severity of underlying heart disease (Table 18.4). In apparently healthy asymptomatic subjects, the prevalence of NSVT is reported to be 0–3%, without a significant difference between men and women. One recent study suggests that the prevalence is increased (11%) in asymptomatic elderly subjects.

NSVT also occurs infrequently in patients with hypertensive LVH (2–12%) and rheumatic heart disease (7%), when these processes are not complicated by congestive heart failure. Interestingly, NSVT occurs much more often (17–28%) in patients with idiopathic hypertrophic cardiomyopathy (Table 18.5), but the highest prevalence of NSVT is seen in patients with nonischemic dilated cardiomyopathy. In this case, about half the patients have asymptomatic NSVT, (Table 18.5). Some of these studies have correlated an increased prevalence with more advanced disease.

Table 18.4
Prevalence of Nonsustained Ventricular Tachycardia in Asymptomatic Subjects

Study	Type of Subjects	Frequency (%)
Hinkle et al., 1969	Middle-aged men	3.2
Califf et al., 1982	All had coronary angiography	0
Romhilt et al., 1984	Healthy women	1
Pilcher et al., 1983	Healthy runners	1
Kantelip et al., 1986	All elderly (age >80 years)	2

Table 18.5
Prevalence of Nonsustained Ventricular Tachycardia in Patients with Cardiomyopathy

Study	Type of Subjects	Frequency (%)
Savage et al., 1979	HCM[a]	19
Mulrow et al., 1986	HCM	22
Huang et al., 1983	DCM	60
Suyoma et al., 1986	DCM	46
Neri et al., 1986	DCM	43
Olshausen et al., 1988	DCM	42

[a]HCM, hypertrophic cardiomyopathy; DCM, idiopathic dilated cardiomyopathy.

In patients with CAD referred for cardiac catheterization (i.e., primarily an ambulatory population), NSVT is observed in 5% of patients. The highest prevalence of NSVT is seen in the first 24 hours after the onset of acute MI, where up to 45% of patients have been reported to have this arrhythmia. During the late hospital phase after MI (1–4 weeks after onset), the prevalence drops to 7–16% (Table 18.6). The incidence then remains fairly constant over the first year after infarction.

There is an increased prevalence of NSVT associated with a lower ejection fraction in the setting of CAD. Likewise, the prevalence of NSVT is increased in patients with multivessel disease, with increasing severity of regional wall-motion abnormalities, the presence of ventricular aneurysm, and in the presence of abnormal hemodynamics.

Symptoms/Presentation

As noted previously, most episodes of NSVT are incidentally found during inpatient monitoring or outpatient Holter studies. Although NSVT may be discovered during the evaluation of palpitations, presyncope, chest pain, and syncope, most episodes of NSVT do not correlate with those symptoms. Occasionally, one can document an association between NSVT and dizziness, palpitations, angina, or syncope during Holter recordings. The lack of associated symptoms is undoubtedly related in part to the brief duration of the arrhythmia.

Table 18.6
Prevalence of Nonsustained Ventricular Tachycardia in Myocardial Infarction:
Late Hospital Phase

Study	VT Frequency[a] (%)	Time of Recording from Onset of MI (days)
Vismara et al., 1975	8	11
Schulze et al., 1975	19	14–28
Anderson et al., 1978	7	~14
Kleiger et al., 1981	12	28
Bigger et al., 1981	12	10–20

[a]VT, ventricular tachycardia; MI, myocardial infarction.

Electrophysiology of Nonsustained Ventricular Tachycardia

PROGRAMMED ELECTRICAL STIMULATION

The response to programmed stimulation may also provide information on the mechanisms causing NSVT. VT due to automaticity cannot be induced by programmed stimulation, while the presence of inducible VT supports either a reentrant mechanism or triggered activity. The likelihood of inducing sustained VT depends on the presence and type of underlying heart disease in patients who have presented with spontaneous NSVT.

Patients without structural heart disease who have NSVT rarely have VT inducible by programmed electrical stimulation, except in the case of patients with right ventricular outflow tract tachycardia. In patients with nonischemic dilated cardiomyopathy who have NSVT, rates for the induction of sustained VT have ranged between 0–20%. In patients with hypertrophic cardiomyopathy and NSVT, inducible sustained VT has been reported in 40–75% of patients. Unlike patients with CAD, sustained VT induced during programmed electrical stimulation is polymorphic up to 80% of the time in these patients.

Induction rates for patients with NSVT and CAD have been reported between 20–50%. Increased induction rates are seen in subjects with depressed ejection fractions and in subjects with left ventricular aneurysm. Little is known about the relationship between spontaneous NSVT and the induced tachycardias.

Prognostic Significance of Nonsustained Ventricular Tachycardia Documented on Monitoring

The prognostic significance of NSVT depends on the presence and type of underlying heart disease. However, it is important to remember that it is not clear in most cases whether episodes of NSVT bear a cause-and-effect relationship with the sustained VTs that are documented to precipitate sudden death, or whether they merely reflect an epiphenomenon indicating overall poor cardiac function.

The presence of NSVT in apparently healthy individuals does not correlate with an increased risk for sudden death. This lack of association extends to the elderly as well.

In general, patients with dilated cardiomyopathy are at considerable risk of sudden death and overall cardiac mortality, with 1-year mortality rates reported as high as 40–50%. The prognostic significance of NSVT is variable, with little evidence that the occurrence of NSVT is related specifically to an increased risk for sudden death, although it does correlate with increased overall cardiac mortality (Table 18.7).

Sudden death is a significant cause of mortality in patients with hypertrophic cardiomyopathy, with a yearly incidence reported of 2–3% in selected referral populations. There is a 70% chance of discovering NSVT in patients who have experienced syncope or survived cardiac arrest, compared with a 20% prevalence in those without such a history. Furthermore, in patients with hypertrophic cardiomyopathy and NSVT, the yearly sudden death mortality rate is reported to be 8–10%, compared with 1% in patients without NSVT.

The prognostic significance of NSVT with underlying CAD depends on the time the arrhythmia is discovered in the course of the disease. The occurrence of NSVT during the first 24 hours of acute MI does not carry an increased risk for subsequent overall cardiac mortality or sudden death, either while in the hospital or long term. In contrast, the occurrence of this arrhythmia in the late hospital phase of MI more than doubles the risk of subsequent sudden death when compared with patients without NSVT. NSVT has been shown repeatedly to be an independent risk factor for both overall cardiac death and sudden death. NSVT detected 3 months to 1 year post-MI is also associated with a significantly higher mortality rate.

It is important to note that although the overall incidence of cardiac mortality and sudden death is both higher in patients with NSVT, the proportion of sudden death compared with overall cardiac mortality is not increased in the setting of NSVT (Table 18.8). This observation raises the question of the specificity of NSVT as a marker for subsequent arrhythmic events rather than as a marker for overall poor cardiac function.

Table 18.7
Prognostic Significance of Nonsustained Ventricular Tachycardia in Idiopathic Dilated Cardiomyopathy

Study	Patients with NSVT:[a] % of Cardiac Deaths That Were Sudden	Patients without NSVT: % of Cardiac Deaths That Were Sudden
Huang et al., 1983	50	100
Unverferth et al., 1984	100	100
Neri et al., 1986	9	143
Olshausen et al., 1988	33	80

[a]NSVT, nonsustained ventricular tachycardia.

Studies in the postthrombolytic era have also reported that NSVT was indeed associated with a significantly increased risk of sudden death and overall cardiac mortality with a follow-up of 180 days after MI. Contrary to what one might expect, multiple analyses demonstrate that the association of NSVT and subsequent mortality is not influenced by the frequency, duration, or rate of NSVT.

Prognostic Significance of the Response to Programmed Electrical Stimulation in Patients with Nonsustained Ventricular Tachycardia

A recent metaanalysis of programmed electrical stimulation in patients with NSVT found an overall induction of sustained VT of 27%. Because of the heterogeneous nature of the populations, the positive predictive accuracy was only 18%, while noninducible patients had a 93% chance of remaining event free.

In patients with nonischemic dilated cardiomyopathy who have NSVT, studies have failed to demonstrate any correlation between inducibility of sustained VT and subsequent arrhythmic events or total cardiac mortality.

The presence of inducible VT in patients with hypertrophic cardiopathy carries a poorer prognosis over a 28-month follow-up period. In the subset of patients with NSVT on Holter monitoring, those who did not have induction of sustained VT had a 3% mortality, compared with a 20% mortality in inducible patients. However, this was a highly selected population of patients, with the majority having survived episodes of cardiac arrest or syncope or having a strong family history for sudden death. Thus it is not clear whether the results of programmed stimulation have any prognostic utility in asymptomatic patients with a negative family history for sudden death.

Patients with coronary artery disease with NSVT whose ejection fraction is greater than 40% have a low incidence of sudden death. Thus, there appears to be little need for programmed electrical stimulation in patients with well-preserved systolic ventricular function. However, results from many studies suggest that programmed electrical stimulation may have a valuable role in risk stratification in

Table 18.8
Prognostic Significance of Nonsustained Ventricular Tachycardia in Patients with Coronary Artery Disease: Recent Infarction

Study	Patients with NSVT:[a] % of Cardiac Deaths That Were Sudden	Patients without NSVT: % of Cardiac Deaths That Were Sudden
Anderson et al., 1978	73	64
Kleiger et al., 1981	33	64
Bigger et al., 1981	58	75
Bigger et al., 1986	70	58

[a]NSVT, nonsustained ventricular tachycardia.

patients with CAD and NSVT whose left ventricular ejection fraction is 40% or less.

Prognostic Significance of the Signal-Averaged Electrocardiogram in Patients with Nonsustained Ventricular Tachycardia

In studies of mixed populations of patients with NSVT and/or complex ventricular ectopy, the presence of an abnormal signal-averaged ECG has predicted inducibility of sustained VT with 92–100% sensitivity and 75–88% specificity. The negative predictive accuracy in predicting inducibility has been reported to be up to 91%.

In patients with NSVT and idiopathic dilated cardiomyopathy, the presence of late potentials has correlated with induction of sustained VT by programmed electrical stimulation, with a sensitivity and specificity of 66 and 86%, respectively. No study has examined the potential correlation between the signal-averaged ECG and sudden death in patients with NSVT and nonischemic dilated cardiomyopathy.

Several studies suggest that the signal-averaged ECG may identify patients with prior MI likely to have VT inducible by programmed stimulation. Nevertheless, the utility of the signal-averaged ECG to predict future arrhythmic events has not been tested prospectively in this population. Thus, it is not clear what utility the signal-averaged ECG may contribute beyond the results of programmed stimulation.

Treatment

The first step in deciding whether to initiate therapy is to determine whether significant symptoms attributable to NSVT are present. If symptoms are clearly caused by NSVT, regardless of the presence or type of underlying heart disease, treatment may be appropriate—not to improve survival, but to make the patient feel better. In general, no antiarrhythmic agent can be considered to be specific for the treatment of symptomatic NSVT. Repetitive monomorphic VT originating in the right ventricular outflow tract may respond to β-blockade in up to 50% of patients tested. Verapamil, propafenone, and amiodarone have also been used with variable success. More recently, severely symptomatic patients that have not responded to pharmacologic therapy have been treated successfully with radiofrequency catheter ablation.

The second potential indication for treatment is to reduce the risk of sudden death that has been associated with the presence of NSVT in certain patients with structural heart disease. The prophylactic use of antiarrhythmic agents in patients with nonischemic dilated cardiomyopathy has been discouraging, having no clear benefits. Whether or not antiarrhythmics are beneficial in the setting of hypertrophic cardiomyopathy is also unclear. Pharmacologic therapy guided by Holter monitoring has been used in an attempt to reduce the risk of sudden death in the setting of NSVT and CAD, but data are not conclusive.

SUGGESTED READING

Bigger JT, Fleiss JL, Kleiger R, Miller JP, Rolnitzky LM, and The Multicenter Post-Infarction Research Group. The relationships among ventricular arrhythmias, left ventricular dysfunction, and mortality in the 2 years after myocardial infarction. Circulation 1984;69: 250–258.

Brodsky M, Wu D, Denes P, Kanakis C, Rosen KM. Arrhythmias documented by 24 hour continuous electrocardiographic monitoring in 50 male medical students without apparent heart disease. Am J Cardiol 1977;39:390–395.

Buxton AE, Marchlinski FE, Waxman HL, Flores BT, Cassidy DM, Josephson ME. Prognostic factors in nonsustained VT. Am J Cardiol 1984;53:1275–1279.

Chakko CS, Gheorghiade M. Ventricular arrhythmias in severe heart failure: incidence, significance, and effectiveness of antiarrhythmic therapy. Am Heart J 1985;109:497–504.

Kennedy HL, Whitlock JA, Sprague MK, Kennedy LJ, Buckingham TA, Goldberg RJ. Long-term follow-up of asymptomatic healthy subjects with frequent and complex ventricular ectopy. N Engl J Med 1985;312:193–197.

Kligfield P, Levy D, Devereux RB, Savage DD. Arrhythmias and sudden death in mitral valve prolapse. Am Heart J 1987;113:1298–1307.

Kowey PR, Taylor JE, Marinchak RA, Rials SJ. Does programmed stimulation really help in the evaluation of patients with nonsustained VT? Results of a meta-analysis. Am Heart J 1992; 123:481–485.

Levy D, Anderson KM, Savage DD, Balkus SA, Kannel WB, Castelli WP. Risk of ventricular arrhythmias in left ventricular hypertrophy: the Framingham Heart Study. Am J Cardiol 1987; 60:560–565.

Maggioni AP, Zuanetti G, Franzosi MG, et al., on behalf of GISSI-2 Investigators. Prevalence and prognostic significance of ventricular arrhythmias after acute myocardial infarction in the fibrinolytic era: GISSI-2 results. Circulation 1993;87:312–322.

Maron BJ, Savage DD, Wolfson JK, Epstein SE. Prognostic significance of 24 hour ambulatory electrocardiographic monitoring in patients with hypertrophic cardiomyopathy: a prospective study. Am J Cardiol 1981;48:252–257.

Meinertz T, Hofmann T, Kasper W, et al. Significance of ventricular arrhythmias in idiopathic dilated cardiomyopathy. Am J Cardiol 1984;53:902–907.

Wilber DJ, Olshansky B, Moran JF, Scanlon PJ. Electrophysiologic testing and nonsustained ventricular tachycardia: use and limitations in patients with coronary artery disease and impaired ventricular function. Circulation 1990;82:350–358.

19 Sustained Monomorphic Ventricular Tachycardia

DEFINITION AND ELECTROCARDIOGRAPHIC DIAGNOSIS

Ventricular tachycardia (VT) is defined as a wide complex tachycardia of greater than three successive ventricular complexes. When the tachycardia lasts for less than 30 seconds, it is termed nonsustained; if it lasts for more than 30 seconds or requires termination because of hemodynamic instability, it is considered sustained. If the QRS morphology is relatively constant, it is termed monomorphic or uniform VT; if the QRS complexes manifest multiple morphologies during each episode, it is termed polymorphic or multiformed. There are various forms of monomorphic VT largely classified by the rate at which they occur. Most often, sustained VT has a rate of 100–220 beats/minute. If the rate is <100 beats/minute, it is termed accelerated idioventricular rhythm (AIVR); when the rate is >220 beats/minute, it is known as ventricular flutter.

On the ECG, the QRS morphology is bizarre, and the QRS width is greater than 0.12 seconds. Based on the morphology in lead V1, the VT is said to have either a left or right bundle morphology. However, this does not always correlate with or predict the site of origin of the VT. During monomorphic VT, the QRS morphology is fairly constant, but there may be slight changes in morphology as the result of changes in the direction of impulse conduction through the ventricle and differences in ventricular activation sequence. An important finding on the ECG is the presence of atrioventricular (AV) dissociation. Although it is not obvious in all cases, when seen it is generally diagnostic of VT. In some cases, obvious P waves can be seen, dissociated from the QRS complex. This is most often observed when the VT rate is slower. When P waves are not obvious, AV dissociation can be established by the presence of fusion or capture (Dressler) beats, which represent partial or complete activation of the ventricle from the atrium via the AV node and His-Purkinje system. Capture does not terminate the tachycardia but does alter the QRS morphology and may alter the R-R interval. In some cases, the presence of dissociation may be presumed when there is variability in the ST and T waves, a result of superimposed P waves.

In some cases of VT, retrograde V-A conduction is present. There may be 1:1 retrograde conduction or there may be second-degree retrograde block (Mobitz I or II), and retrograde P waves may be seen after some but not all of the QRS complexes. The R-P interval may be fixed (if there is Mobitz II block) or variable (in Mobitz I block). However, the presence of intermittent retrograde block, similar to complete retrograde block or AV dissociation, is diagnostic of VT. When there is 1:1 retrograde V-A conduction, a P wave follows each QRS complex with a fixed R-P interval.

The 12-lead surface electrocardiogram (ECG) during VT has been touted by some as a way to localize the endocardial site of origin. The surface ECG data are less useful for localization in patients with prior myocardial infarction (MI) who also have wall motion abnormalities. However, Josephson has stated that one can use the ECG to determine an "area," if not the specific site, from which VT arises in a majority of cases.

Electrophysiologic testing is the gold standard in establishing the mechanism of VT. The study will often reveal AV dissociation even when not apparent on the surface ECG. Atrial activity is frequently independent of, and slower than, ventricular activity. Because the initial activation is within the ventricle, there is retrograde activation of the bundle of His simultaneously with, or after, ventricular activation. Hence the His (H) electrogram may be absent, may follow, or may be dissociated from the electrogram. In contrast, there is a constant and fixed H-V interval seen with supraventricular tachycardia because activation originating in the atrium or AV junction is always conducted via the His-Purkinje system to the ventricular myocardium.

SYMPTOMS AND PHYSICAL EXAMINATION

Severity of the symptoms resulting from VT range from none or mild to cardiovascular collapse and sudden death. The patient may be aware of only palpitations or rapid heart action or may have symptoms of reduced cardiac output and hypotension, including lightheadedness, dizziness, altered mentation, visual disturbances, diaphoresis, presyncope or syncope. In some patients, new or exacerbated congestive heart failure occurs. In patients with underlying coronary artery disease, angina may be provoked and it may be unstable and unresponsive to medication. If the blood pressure cannot be maintained during VT, cardiovascular collapse and cardiogenic shock may occur. Lastly, VT may degenerate into ventricular fibrillation (VF) and cause sudden death.

The physical examination during VT may be normal in some patients, reflecting the maintenance of a good cardiac output. However, most often the physical examination demonstrates hypotension and evidence of AV dissociation, i.e., independent atrial and ventricular activity. The patient may be conscious, unconscious, or have waxing and waning mentation, reflecting frequent changes in stroke volume and cardiac output. Even when patients initially experience syncope and loss of consciousness, there may be some restoration of cerebral blood flow once they are recumbent, despite the continuation of the arrhythmia. The blood pressure may be normal, low, or even unobtainable. If measurable, it is often labile, reflecting changes in stroke volume and cardiac output, the result of AV asynchrony. The jugular venous pulsations demonstrate cannon waves, i.e., intermittent augmented pulsations due to atrial contraction against a closed AV valve. The carotid pulse is often diminished in amplitude and may be variable in intensity, reflecting changes in cardiac output. The lung examination may reveal evidence of congestive heart failure.

The cardiac examination is usually abnormal. In addition to the rapid heart rate, there may be abnormal chest wall pulsations, resulting from contraction abnormalities of either right or left ventricle. These may be caused by an altered pattern of ventricular contraction or the development of ischemia and myocardial dysfunction. There may be variability in the intensity of the first heart sound, reflecting AV dissociation, although this is difficult to appreciate when the rate is rapid. Additionally, the first and second heart sounds may be variably split, and third and fourth heart sounds may be intermittently heard. New murmurs may develop and old murmurs may change. This great variability results in a "cacophony" of heart sounds, reflecting disordered contraction and AV asynchrony. It can be clearly distinguished from the very regular heart sounds heard during any supraventricular rhythm when ventricular activation is normal and the association between atrial and ventricular contraction is constant.

SPECIFIC ENTITIES ASSOCIATED WITH MONOMORPHIC VENTRICULAR TACHYCARDIA

Myocardial Infarction

Myocardial ischemia and infarction offer an electrophysiologic milieu that is especially favorable for the initiation and maintenance of VT. Ventricular arrhythmia seen in the earliest stages of acute MI has generally been attributed to reentry, whereas after 6–8 hours, the mechanism probably is abnormal automaticity. The vast majority of sustained monomorphic VTs occur late after infarction and arise at the periphery of the site of the acute infarction. They also appear to be mechanistically related to reentry, although triggered automaticity is a possibility in some cases. The characteristic features of reentry—a reentrant pathway, dispersion of refractoriness, and an area of slow conduction—can be demonstrated in patients with prior infarction and sustained VT. Furthermore, intraoperative mapping has demonstrated activation sequences that may represent definable reentrant circuits. Pressure or myocardial lesions applied to the site of mid-diastolic activity has resulted in termination of tachycardia. Endocardial catheter mapping in sinus rhythm has demonstrated the presence of markedly fractionated low amplitude potentials. Signal-averaged ECGs have also demonstrated the presence of "late potentials" consistent with areas of slow conduction in the infarcted ventricle. The ability to define an area of slow conduction within the infarct zone forms the basis for curative interventions (Right Ventricular Tachycardia), such as surgical or catheter ablation.

Exercise-Related Ventricular Tachycardia

Exercise-related or catecholamine-facilitated VT frequently arises from the right ventricular outflow tract and may be easily evaluated with catheter mapping techniques. The patients usually are women who have no definable structural heart disease. An ECG during the episodes manifests, in general, a left bundle branch block configuration with a right inferior axis. The pathologic basis for this arrhythmia is not completely known, although one must be certain to exclude right ventricular dysplasia. Detailed cardiologic studies generally do not reveal any significant abnormality, although signal-averaged ECGs may show a late potential, and subtle anatomical abnormalities may be seen on magnetic resonance imaging

(MRI) or two-dimensional echocardiography. The electrophysiologic mechanism of this tachycardia is not completely clear, but the preponderance of evidence favors triggered activity due to delayed afterdepolarizations. Several features are in favor of such a mechanism including initiation dependent upon catecholamines or burst pacing, occurrences mainly during wakefulness, prevention with β-blockers and calcium channel blocking agents, unreliable initiation with programmed stimulation, and termination with adenosine.

The first choice for chronic therapy for this arrhythmia has been β-adrenergic blocking drugs. This treatment has a high success rate and generally has been well tolerated. Calcium channel blocking drugs have not been as well studied but may work in select cases. In the last several years, multiple investigators have reported excellent short-term results using radiofrequency ablation techniques. Long-term results, especially recurrence rates, need to be determined.

Left Ventricular Tachycardia

This clinical arrhythmia occurs in young people, predominantly in men. The characteristic ECG features are a right bundle branch block morphology with superior axis deviation. In contrast to tachycardias arising from the right ventricular outflow tract, this arrhythmia generally is readily initiated with ventricular (and occasional atrial) pacing or extrastimulation. As with tachycardia from the right ventricular outflow tract, detailed diagnostic studies have demonstrated no significant cardiac abnormalities. The electrophysiologic mechanism of this tachycardia appears to be reentry possibly involving the posterior division of the left bundle branch. Activation mapping during the tachycardia suggests the earliest activation may be in the inferior mid-septal region in the left ventricle. There are, however, no fragmented electrograms recorded in contrast to studies of a similar nature in patients with coronary artery disease. Signal-averaged ECGs are, in general, negative.

Of most interest is the observation that this tachycardia is often sensitive to verapamil or other calcium channel blocking agents, making these the therapies of choice. Generally, β-adrenergic blockers are not useful. Resistant arrhythmias may require type I antiarrhythmic drug therapy. Radiofrequency ablation may have a role. Mapping frequently localizes the VT to the inferior mid-septal region where ablation lesions may prevent recurrence.

Ventricular Tachycardia Associated with Arrhythmogenic Right Ventricular Dysplasia

This arrhythmic entity was first described by Fontaine and colleagues in 1977. Pathologic abnormalities include severe muscular displacement with fat and fibrous tissue involving the right ventricle and, in unusual cases, the left as well. The findings are similar but pathologically different from Uhl's anomaly in which the right ventricular wall is described as having a parchment-like quality without fatty deposition. The right ventricle functions reasonably well, at least early in the course of arrhythmogenic right ventricular dysplasia, but heart failure is frequently seen in Uhl's anomaly. Clinically, the entity has a male preponderance, with an average age at presentation of 40 years. ECGs frequently show T-wave inversion in the right precordial leads, with many patients having incomplete right bundle branch block during sinus rhythm (Fig. 19.1). Cardiac MRI studies have been very helpful in establishing the diagnosis of arrhythmogenic right ventricular dysplasia, but these studies generally require gating to obtain the highest quality data. Other studies that may be useful in evaluating and/or diagnosing patients with suspected right ventricular dysplasia include transthoracic echocardiography, which may demonstrate an increase in right ventricular diastolic diameter and aneurysmal abnormalities; right ventricular angiography showing a large right ventricle with segmental wall motion abnormalities and/or aneurysmal abnormalities; and right ventricular wall motion studies with nuclear imaging techniques with a depressed right ventricular ejection fraction (frequently less than 25%). The left ventricule is generally normal by routine testing procedures, but in some cases can be involved as well.

The associated monomorphic VT usually has a left bundle branch block morphology with a superior or inferior axis. Depending on the degree of right ventricular abnormality, multiple morphologies may be observed. The signal-averaged ECG is usually abnormal and frequently correlates with a fragmented prolonged right ventricular electrogram during endocardial mapping. This tachycardia is usually easily initiated with ventricular pacing and extrastimulation, suggesting that it has a reentrant mechanism.

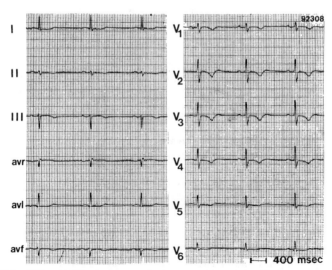

Figure 19.1. 12-lead ECG during sinus rhythm in a patient with arrhythmogenic right ventricular dysplasia and recurrent VT. Note the prominent T-wave abnormalities in the precordial leads. (From Metzger JT, de Chillou C, Cheriex E, Rodriguez L-M, Smeets JLRM, Wellens HJJ. Value of the 12-lead electrocardiogram in arrhythmogenic right ventricular dysplasia, and absence of correlation with echocardiographic findings. Am J Cardiol 1993;72:964–967.)

These patients frequently present a management dilemma. Their tachyarrhythmias may not respond to any antiarrhythmic drug therapy, including amiodarone. A surgical approach has been developed that essentially involves disconnection and "autotransplantation" of the right ventricular free wall. Radiofrequency ablation has been attempted, but the diffuse nature of the disease does not permit a high success rate. The use of an implantable defibrillator or even cardiac transplantation may be required in some patients.

Bundle Branch Reentry

This arrhythmia is seen almost exclusively in patients with a dilated cardiomyopathy. The surface QRS during sustained VT has a left bundle branch block morphology, generally with a superior axis deviation. The tachycardia utilizes the right bundle branch as the anterograde limb and the left bundle branch as the retrograde limb of this reentrant pathway. The characteristic features of this tachycardia include the presence of a His bundle deflection prior to each QRS; tachycardia cycle length changes preceded by changes in the H-H interval; H-V intervals equal to or greater than the H-V intervals in sinus rhythm; a critical V-H delay at the initiation of the tachycardia; a His deflection that precedes the right bundle deflection with an H-RB interval in sinus rhythm longer than during VT; and right ventricular activation that always precedes left ventricular activation.

The incidence of this tachycardia is uncertain but clearly depends upon the population studied. Interestingly, a fairly high incidence of bundle branch reentry of brief duration (1–2 complexes) has been observed by many investigators during routine electrophysiologic studies, but the incidence of sustained bundle branch reentry appears low in most series.

The recognition of this form of VT has greater significance since the advent of radiofrequency ablation because this tachycardia appears to be highly amenable to "cure" with ablation of the proximal right bundle branch. Some patients may require permanent pacing if they also have preexisting disease of other portions of the intraventricular conduction system.

Accelerated Idioventricular Arrhythmia

AIVR or "slow VT" is caused by an abnormal focus within the ventricular myocardium that becomes dominant and assumes pacemaker control (Fig. 19.2). It is defined as a wide complex ventricular rhythm at a rate of 60–100 beats/minute. Usually the ventricular rate is close to the sinus rate, and often the pacemaker focus alternates between sinus (narrow QRS complexes preceded by a P wave) and ventricular (wide QRS complexes with dissociated P waves). Because the rate is slow, capture beats, fusion beats, and 1:1 retrograde V-A conduction are often seen. AIVR may be the result of an accelerated focus in the ventricular myocardium or may be an escape rhythm due to slowing of impulse generation from more proximal pacemakers (sinus or AV nodal). AIVR may also arise because of failure of higher pacemaker tissue to generate an impulse or failure of the AV node to conduct an impulse.

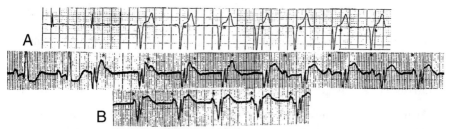

Figure 19.2. Examples of accelerated idioventricular rhythm. In A, there are two sinus beats at a rate of 68 beats/minute, followed by a pause due to sinus node arrest. Following this is the development of an escape idioventricular rhythm at a rate of 64 beats/minute. Noted are retrograde P waves (asterisk) at the end of the QRS complex and within the first part of the ST segment. In B, there are two sinus beats at a rate of 58 beats/minute. This is followed by a premature ventricular beat, which initiates an idioventricular rhythm at a rate of 62 beats/minute. Noted are sinus P waves (asterisk) that are dissociated from the ventricular complexes. The lower rhythm strip shows P waves that precede each QRS complex, and the atrial and ventricular rates are almost identical. However, the P-R interval is short and variable because AV dissociation is still present.

When the AIVR is due to an enhanced ventricular focus, it is treated like any other VT. Indications for therapy are symptoms of hemodynamic impairment or association with or provocation of other serious ventricular arrhythmias. However, if the AIVR is an escape rhythm due to failure of other pacemakers, it should not be treated, as it may represent a stable rhythm and the only available pacemaker for the patient. This is often the case in patients with an acute MI.

Ventricular Tachycardia Associated with Dilated Cardiomyopathy

Patients with sustained monomorphic VT and dilated cardiomyopathy represent a very high risk group. The sudden death incidence may be as high as 50%, but the majority of deaths are associated with VF, rather than sustained monomorphic VT. Generally, patients with dilated cardiomyopathy and sustained VT have abnormal signal-averaged ECGs. Although most patients are not inducible to sustained VT, the vast majority of patients who do have provocable tachycardia have had similar arrhythmias spontaneously. Bundle branch reentry is a more common finding in this patient group (see previous discussion). Endocardial mapping studies in these patients have documented abnormal electrograms but not as consistently as in patients with VT who have coronary artery disease and a prior infarction. Nevertheless, the most common mechanism for VT in this patient group appears to be reentry based on the presence of abnormal signal-averaged electrograms, abnormal endocardial electrograms, and inducibility by standard electrophysiologic protocols.

Many patients with recurrent VT and cardiomyopathy are ultimately candidates for cardiac transplantation, which may be considered either because of recurrent VT not responsive to drug therapy or recalcitrant and progressive heart failure. In this group of patients, implantation of a cardioverter-defibrillator may be considered as a "bridge to transplantation." The ICD is especially useful because its use may permit a significant reduction or elimination of antiarrhythmic agents with potential negative hemodynamic effects while preventing sudden death, which is a most frequent cause of death in those awaiting transplant.

Ventricular Tachycardia Associated with Hypertrophic Cardiomyopathy

Symmetric or asymmetric hypertrophy of the left ventricle without dilation is the pathologic hallmark of this disease state. Although the hemodynamic deterioration with this disease is slowly progressive, unexpected sudden death occurs with a reported frequency of up to 3% per year. This is especially important in considering therapy of a patient with the familial form of hypertrophic cardiomyopathy in which sudden death is particularly frequent. The incidence of monomorphic VT appears to be very low. In many of these patients, polymorphic VT can be reproducibly induced, even with unaggressive protocols of programmed simulation. The electrophysiologic mechanism of the arrhythmia is unknown, but marked muscular fiber disarray lends itself well to the development of reentry, perhaps because of a dispersion in refractoriness. Some experimental data suggest that triggered activity may also play a role.

Drug therapy when initiated may have two potential benefits, including arrhythmia reduction/prevention and reduction in the obstructive phenomenon. Antiarrhythmic drugs that have a negative inotropic effect such as β-blockers, disopyramide, sotalol, and amiodarone may be particularly helpful. For drug-resistant patients, the cardioverter-defibrillator may have the most usefulness, based on its good efficacy and safety in small trials.

Miscellaneous Entities

There are a number of other entities that have been associated with monomorphic VT, including infiltrative diseases of the myocardium such as sarcoidosis or amyloidosis. Cardiovascular involvement in sarcoidosis has been well recognized for at least 60 years with an autopsy incidence of at least 20% in patients who were diagnosed antemortem. However, sustained monomorphic VT has only rarely been described. Treatment with antiarrhythmic drug therapy has not been very successful, and the use of implantable cardioverter-defibrillators has been advocated. This may be particularly important in those cases in which conventional antiinflammatory therapy has had limited success in controlling disease progression.

ELECTROPHYSIOLOGY STUDIES FOR VENTRICULAR TACHYCARDIA INDUCTION

There has been considerable debate with regard to the best stimulation protocol to induce monomorphic VT in the electrophysiology laboratory. A number of variables have been considered over the years in an attempt to maximize the yield without increasing the changes of provoking a nonclinical arrhythmia. These have included the length and rate of the drive train, the number of extrastimuli and their current strength, site of stimulation (including usefulness of left ventricular stimulation), the advantage of burst pacing or infusion of isoproterenol, and the number of times stimulation should be repeated. What has emerged from this cauldron of controversy is a consensus regarding an "optimal" testing protocol. Most clinicians would now agree that drive trains of 450–600 msec with up to three extrastimuli at energies of twice threshold delivered at two right ventricular sites constitutes a fair protocol, likely to have a reasonable yield and a fairly low false-positive rate. What has also become clear is that employing these techniques in a stepwise hierarchy of "aggression" will maximize the yield while limiting non-clinical events. It is also recognized that special clinical situations exist, such as in patients who have had recent cardiac surgery in whom temporary epicardial pacing wires can be used for postoperative testing. Similarly, patients with implanted tiered cardioverter-defibrillators can undergo electrical testing using noninvasive stimulation via their device with the expectation of obtaining useful clinical data.

A major clinical concern has been raised with regard to the reproducibility of VT induction. This is especially important in the use of electrophysiologic studies for the evaluation of antiarrhythmic drug effectiveness. The majority of investigators agree that there is day-to-day variability in the mode of induction of monomorphic VT. There are some reports that there is also variability in the ability to induce the arrhythmia. This is seen during baseline as well as during drug therapy. The variability may occur because of the many modulating factors (ischemia, electrolyte abnormalities, catecholamines) that can alter the reentrant circuit and hence affect the ability to activate it and induce the VT. However, most also agree that this variability does not totally preclude a practical assessment of drug efficacy in patients whose arrhythmias can be reproduced during their initial drug-free study.

PACING MANEUVERS DURING VENTRICULAR TACHYCARDIA

Resetting

Resetting implies that an induced (or spontaneous) ventricular extrastimulus is able to enter the reentrant circuit, traverse the circuit in an anterograde fashion, and produce a less than compensatory return cycle. The return cycle length has been observed to be a function of the coupling interval of the induced premature complex. The three responses that have been observed are flat, increasing, and flat and then increasing.

The flat response of the return cycle suggests the presence of an area of fully excitable tissue within the reentrant circuit. An increasing response, inversely related to the premature coupling interval, probably represents a reentrant circuit with only a partially excitable gap. The resetting of a VT does not conclusively prove that reentry is the mechanism because tachycardias caused by triggered activity and automatic arrhythmias may be reset. In isolated tissue studies, however, the response curves do permit some discrimination between triggered and reentrant arrhythmias. Although a flat response curve may be seen in both reentry and triggered activity, a decreasing curve may be specific for triggered activity and an increasing curve more consistent with a reentrant mechanism.

Fusion

Fusion of programmed premature beats with sustained VT suggests a reentrant mechanism. By necessity, the reentrant circuit would have a separate entrance and exit as well as a zone of slow conduction. Furthermore, the probability of fusion during sustained VT is a function of activation time from the pacing site; the longer the activation time the more likely fusion will occur. In addition, the return cycle after the ventricular premature beat (with fusion) is significantly shorter than the return cycle observed in VT that is reset without fusion. This implies that the functional distance between the entrance and exit sites, reset with fusion, is relatively long.

Entrainment

Overdrive pacing during monomorphic VT may result in the phenomenon of entrainment. This phenomenon has the following characteristics: the rate of the tachycardia is accelerated to the paced rate with constant fusion complexes on the surface ECG except for the last captured beat, which is captured but not entrained. In other words, it has the same ECG morphology as the tachycardia before the overdrive and progressive degrees of fusion as the overdrive rate is increased. Overdrive at a critical rate terminates the tachycardia after pacing is terminated.

ENDOCARDIAL MAPPING TECHNIQUES

Ventricular endocardial mapping was developed initially for identification of the site of origin of VT for purposes of surgical ablation. Subsequently, the technique has been expanded as catheter ablative techniques have developed. It is generally necessary to induce the index arrhythmia reproducibly or have it occur spontaneously to allow adequate endocardial mapping. A major problem with mapping ventricular arrhythmias has been hemodynamic instability. Therefore, antiarrhythmic drug administration such as intravenous procainamide has been utilized to slow the VT so that the patient can tolerate longer episodes of VT. Alternatively, multilead mapping systems have been used to localize the site or origin using only a few beats of the tachycardia. Although finding the earliest site of ventricular activation is the point of major interest, other important findings include electrograms with systolic and diastolic components, continuous diastolic activity, and double potentials (Fig. 19.3).

If VT cannot be initiated or if the tachycardia is hemodynamically unstable, endocardial catheter mapping during sinus rhythm to search for fractionation of the electrograms or late electrograms has some utility. However, the correlation between these abnormal electrograms and successful tachycardia termination, either with catheter ablation or endocardial resection techniques, has been poor, essentially negating this recording modality as a useful tool. Another technique in those without readily inducible monomorphic VT is pacing at multiple locations in

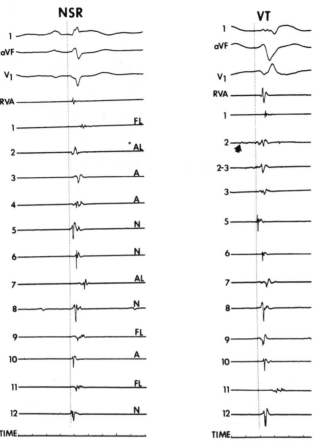

Figure 19.3. Electrograms recorded from a patient during sinus rhythm (*left panel*) and during VT (right panel). Surface leads 1, aVF, and V1 as well as recordings from 12 standard left ventricular sites and from the right ventricular apex. Fractionated abnormal or late electrical activity is noted at multiple left ventricular sites. The earliest site during the VT is LV site 2. It is important to note that during sinus rhythm, left ventricular site 2 is neither late nor abnormal. (From Josephson ME, ed. Clinical cardiac electrophysiology. 2nd ed. Philadelphia: Lea & Febiger, 1992.)

an effort to produce a QRS morphology that is "identical" to the spontaneous VT. This technique, known as pace mapping, has been used very effectively in tachycardias originating in the outflow tract of the right ventricle, especially in anticipation of catheter ablation.

SUGGESTED READING

Brugada P, Brugada J, Mont L, Smeets J, Andries EM. A new approach to the differential diagnosis of a regular tachycardia with a wide QRS complex. Circulation 1991;83:1649–1659.

Brugada P, Wellens HJJ. Entrainment as an electrophysiologic phenomenon. J Am Coll Cardiol 1984;3:451–454.

Kuchar DL, Ruskin JN, Garan H. Electrocardiographic localization of the site of origin of ventricular tachycardia in patients with prior myocardial infarction. J Am Coll Cardiol 1989;13:893–900.

Poll DS, Marchlinski FE, Buxton AE, Josephson ME. Usefulness of programmed stimulation in idopathic dilated cardiomyopathy. Am J Cardiol 1986;58:992–997.

Stevenson WG, Weiss JN, Wiener I, et al. Fractionated endocardial electrograms are associated with slow conduction in humans: evidence from pace-mapping. J Am Coll Cardiol 1989;13:369–376.

20 Torsade de Pointes and Other Forms of Polymorphic Ventricular Tachycardia

TORSADE DE POINTES

Definition

Torsade de Pointes (TdP) is a relatively rare form of ventricular tachycardia (VT), originally described by its peculiar electrocardiographic pattern of continuously changing morphology of the QRS complexes that seem to twist around an imaginary baseline. Over the years TdP has been reinterpreted and redefined by many investigators who contributed to the identification of additional electrocardiographic features. They include Q-T or Q-T-U prolongation, cycle length changes in the beats immediately preceding the onset of the tachycardia, and frequent spontaneous termination.

No agreement has yet been achieved on which is the most accurate definition of TdP that may help clinical diagnosis. For example, some have suggested that the diagnosis requires the initiation of tachycardia by a late extrasystole, while others have proposed that the arrhythmia must be suppressible by an increase in heart rate. Even in the absence of the twisting morphology of the QRS, some have opined that a tachycardia associated with T and U wave abnormalities could still be called TdP. Among so many conflicting opinions, it has even been advocated that "the term torsade de pointes has now become a chimera and should be abandoned." Besides upsetting every man and woman in France, this attitude has been refuted by pressing clinical needs. In fact, among the arrhythmias classified as polymorphic ventricular tachycardia, TdP still holds its separate profile because it presents very specific precipitating factors not shared by other ventricular tachyarrhythmias, and it responds to treatments different from those effective with the more common types of VT.

Another issue that has been raised is whether TdP is an arrhythmia and should therefore be defined as such or whether it would be better to consider it as a syndrome. Indeed, when Q-T prolongation and bradycardia dependence are included as part of the definition of TdP, we are in fact defining a syndrome and not merely describing an arrhythmic event. We believe that TdP should be defined as the typical arrhythmia of prolonged repolarization syndromes and that its definition should include those characteristics that may significantly contribute to the clinical diagnosis. The following definition is a possible clarification: "TdP is a polymorphic ventricular tachycardia often presenting with a typical 180° twisting of the QRS axis, associated with prolonged Q-T interval and amenable to suppression by fast pacing rate."

Diagnostic Criteria of Torsade de Pointes

As already mentioned, no agreement has yet been achieved on the diagnostic criteria for TdP. We will briefly discuss those aspects more frequently linked to TdP and that should be considered when dealing with an episode of polymorphic VT, which may possibly be a TdP.

ELECTROCARDIOGRAPHIC PATTERN

If TdP would always occur with its most typical electrocardiographic aspect, its diagnosis would be straightforward. The typical rotation of the QRS axis around an imaginary baseline leading to a complete 180°-twist in 10–15 beats is, however, observed only in a minority of cases. Moreover, even when it does occur, it is often evident in only a few electrocardiogram (ECG) leads. In a very interesting test, a set of ECG tracings were sent with the request to identify episodes of TdP to several investigators with specific experience in the field of ventricular arrhythmias and TdP. The very low level of agreement in the diagnosis among the investigators showed clearly that the electrocardiographic identification of TdP is often confusing and difficult, and even when cardiologists are not under the pressure of an urgent diagnosis in the coronary care unit, disagreement in the identification of "real" TdP does exist. It may therefore be of some help to base the diagnosis not only on the morphology of the tachycardia but also on the additional features of TdP, such as the rate dependence of the arrhythmia and the concomitant T-U wave abnormalities.

RATE DEPENDENCE OF TORSADE DE POINTES

TdP has a typical rate dependence. Profound sinus bradycardia, bradyarrhythmias such as complete atrioventricular (AV) block, and even abrupt prolongation of the R-R interval have been reported to trigger its onset. Accordingly, fast heart rates, such as those obtained by atrial or ventricular pacing or with pharmacologic interventions, have been shown to interrupt TdP and to prevent its recurrence. A peculiar aspect of the rate dependence of TdP should be considered the association of TdP onset with a typical initiating pattern, the "long-short sequence." The long-short sequence is now considered a major diagnostic criterion (Fig. 20.1). As discussed later in this chapter, the link between long cycle length and development of TdP is one of the major aspects in favor of the hypothesis that early afterdepolarizations (EADs) are the electrophysiologic mechanism underlying TdP.

T-U WAVE ABNORMALITIES

The concomitant presence of Q-T prolongation and Q-T-U abnormalities (often with a prominent U wave) in the sinus beats immediately preceding the development of TdP has been well described. Along the same lines, polymorphic VT, sometimes morphologically indistinguishable from TdP, may be differentiated from TdP by the lack of Q-T interval prolongation.

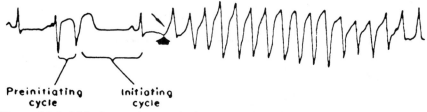

Figure 20.1. ECG of a typical paroxysm of quinidine-induced torsade de pointes demonstrating the typical cycle length changes just before an episode. The tachycardia starts (*thin arrow*) after the apex of the T wave (*heavy arrow*). In the vast majority of instances of quinidine-induced torsade de pointes, the initiating cycle is markedly prolonged and is longer than the preinitiating cycle. (From Roden DM, Woosley RL, Primm RK. Incidence and clinical feature of the quinidine associated long QT syndrome: implication for patients care. Am Heart J 1986;11:1088–1094.)

Clinical Conditions Associated with TdP

Prolongation of ventricular repolarization may be secondary to several conditions associated to the development of TdP (Table 20.1), which can be divided into two major groups: (*a*) idiopathic, or long Q-T syndrome, which includes the Jervell and Lange-Nielsen and the Romano-Ward variants; and (*b*) acquired forms, which are mainly iatrogenic, as those secondary to treatment with antiarrhythmic drugs, tricyclic antidepressants, phenothiazines, macrolide antibiotics, liquid diets, and a miscellaneous group of drugs.

IDIOPATHIC LONG Q-T SYNDROME

The idiopathic long Q-T syndrome is characterized by the presence of marked prolongation of the Q-T interval and T-wave morphological abnormalities, and by the occurrence of syncopal episodes and sudden cardiac death mostly triggered by the activation of the adrenergic nervous system. The arrhythmia responsible for the syncope is usually TdP. To obtain an accurate estimate of the prevalence of the long Q-T syndrome and to further characterize clinical aspects and prognosis of these patients, the International Study and Registry for long Q-T syndrome was initiated in 1979. Since then the registry has become an invaluable source of clinical and epidemiological information on the patients affected by their puzzling disease.

ACQUIRED PROLONGED Q-T SYNDROMES

The acquired forms of prolonged Q-T interval are discussed, according to the cause of Q-T interval prolongation.

Antiarrhythmic Agents

TdP may develop in association with antiarrhythmic drugs that prolong the Q-T interval. Quinidine is the most widely recognized antiarrhythmic agent favoring development of TdP. The prevalence of TdP in the group of quinidine-treated

Table 20.1
Clinical Conditions Associated with Repolarization Abnormalities and Torsade de Pointes

Congential forms
    Jervell and Lange-Nielsen syndrome
    Romano-Ward syndrome
Drugs and chemicals
    Antiarrhythmic agents (mainly K+ channel blockers)
    Neuroleptics (tricyclic antidepressant, thioridazine)
    Phenothiazines
    Antibiotics (erythromycin, pentamidine, trimethoprim-sulfamethoxazole, ampicillin, spyramycin)
    Organophosphate compounds
    Nonsedating antihistamines (astemizole, terfenadine)
Miscellaneous drugs
    Probucol
    Terodiline
    Ketanserine
    Cocaine
    Adenosine
    Papaverine
Metabolic disturbances
    Hypokalemia
    Hypocalcemia
    Hypomagnesemia
Nutritional disorders
    Anorexia
    Liquid diet
Bradyarrhythmias
    Sinus node dysfunction
    Atrioventricular block

patients has been evaluated by different authors to range from 1.5–8%. It is therefore a significant clinical problem, and TdP is regarded as a potential adverse reaction to quinidine therapy. Incessant TdP induced by quinidine has been terminated by isoproterenol infusion and by a bolus injection of 5 mg of verapamil administered at the rate of 1 mg/minute. Isolated reports have described TdP induced by disopyramide and procainamide. During therapy with these agents, the possibility of development of TdP should be considered and they should be used with extreme caution in patients with a prolonged Q-T interval in the absence of drug treatment.

Potassium channel blockers are considered by many as the most promising group of compounds for the treatment of ventricular arrhythmias, especially because sodium channels blockers have lost favor as a consequence of the results of the CAST study. The clinical use of these agents is expected to increase in the next few years. Thus, it is important that the risk of proarrhythmic events in general and the specific incidence of TdP are carefully evaluated. Although this information is available for compounds such as racemic d,l-sotalol, d-sotalol, and amiodarone, only limited data have been reported for the most recently developed agents such as dofetilide or ambasilide.

An analysis of the Bristol-Myers Squibb database on the incidence of TdP in more than 3200 patients receiving racemic sotalol for the treatment of ventricular and supraventricular arrhythmias was presented recently. The overall incidence of proarrhythmic events was 2.4%, and the vast majority of events (75 cases) consisted of TdP. When the subgroup of patients with concomitant structural heart disease was considered, the incidence of TdP increases to 4.5%. TdP development appeared to be dose related, as the arrhythmia occurred in about 1% of subjects treated with a daily dose of 320 mg, while the incidence rose to 4% in the group of patients receiving about 600 mg/day. Risk factors associated with TdP development were female gender, prolonged baseline Q-T interval, history of sustained ventricular arrhythmias, left ventricular impairment, and higher dosage. Most of the episodes of TdP occurred within the first week of treatment, but 12% of cases developed as late as 1 month after the start of therapy. The incidence of proarrhythmic events in a study population of about 1000 patients treated with d-sotalol or dofetiline was also about 1.5%, and TdP was the most frequent type of arrhythmia observed.

It should be noted, however, that not all antiarrhythmic agents that prolong repolarization favor development of TdP to the same extent. Amiodarone, despite significantly prolonging the Q-T interval, is very rarely associated with onset of TdP. It is even more intriguing to recall that amiodarone has even been shown to be safe in patients with TdP induced by sodium channel blockers. Despite its extensive use, only a few reports have described amiodarone-induced TdP, and most cases occurred in patients receiving therapy concomitant with other drugs. Because this evidence is in contrast with the common assumption that prolongation of repolarization is the major risk factor for the development of TdP, further investigation is needed to explain this apparent discrepancy.

Prolonged repolarization, as measured by the Q-T interval, is associated with increased risk for sudden death and cardiac mortality and is regarded as a gross index of electrical instability. It has recently been suggested that dispersion of repolarization might represent a better index of susceptibility to arrhythmias. Dispersion of repolarization can be assessed on the surface ECG by comparing the duration of Q-T interval in all 12 leads or in the six precordial leads. Two indexes have been proposed to quantify dispersion of repolarization. The first consists of the difference between the longest and the shortest Q-T interval. The second is based on the relative dispersion of Q-T ((standard deviation/mean) $\times$ 100). Evidence has been provided that increased dispersion of repolarization is a reliable index to predict the risk of TdP development during therapy with sodium channel blocking agents. Prolongation of the Q-T interval induced by amiodarone is rather uniform throughout the 12 leads and results in a modest dispersion of repolarization. This finding may explain the low incidence of TdP induced by this agent, despite the extensive lengthening of repolarization. Its multiple electrophysiologic properties make amiodarone a uniquely effective agent and may account for the low incidence of proarrhythmic effects. In fact, besides blocking potassium currents, amiodarone has a β-blocking activity and exerts a sodium channel blocking action and a calcium channel blocking effect. Therefore, all these rather complex antiarrhythmic actions may be involved in the clinical effectiveness and lack of proarrhythmic activity of amiodarone. It has been suggested that the inhibitory actions on sodium and calcium currents may have a suppressant effect on afterdepolarizations in the setting of prolonged repolarization.

Psychoactive Drugs

Unexpected sudden cardiac deaths have been described in patients treated with phenothiazines and tricyclic antidepressants. The analysis of ECG recordings preceding the episodes of sudden death showed electrocardiographic alterations, including Q-T prolongation and T wave abnormalities. TdP has been recognized as the most common type of ventricular tachyarrhythmia developing during therapy with psychoactive drugs. The proarrhythmic activity appears to be enhanced at the highest dosages, although patients receiving treatment at moderate dosages for several years may also experience Q-T-U prolongation, T-wave alternans, and syncopal episodes due to TdP.

The presence of structural heart disease, particularly dilated cardiomyopathy, and a history of alcohol abuse have been considered risk factors for TdP in individuals treated with psychoactive agents. Patients receiving psychoactive agents, and who are concomitantly treated with diuretics, should be carefully monitored for the risk of developing hypokalemia, which may greatly enhance the chances of TdP development.

Metabolic Disturbances and Altered Nutritional States

The most frequent metabolic disturbance that gives rise to TdP is hypokalemia. Low extracellular K^+ prolongs action potential duration (APD) in ventricular myocytes. A typical ECG pattern has been identified in hypokalemic patients that includes prolongation of Q-T interval and prominent U waves. The concomitant presence in the same patient of two predisposing conditions, such as hypokalemia and treatment with drugs that prolong repolarization, greatly increases the risk of TdP. Excessive use of diuretics as well as altered nutritional states due to anorexia, liquid diets, and starvation may lead to hypokalemia and hypomagnesemia and favor development of TdP in otherwise healthy subjects. Besides diuretic therapy, transfusion of a large volume of blood may cause severe hypomagnesemia. In fact, Q-T interval prolongation and recurrent episodes of TdP associated with severe magnesium depletion have been reported in an adult subject following a major blood transfusion.

Hypocalcemia is a relatively rare cause of TdP, whereas it is frequently associated with prolongation of Q-T interval mainly caused by ST segment prolongation with minor changes in T-wave or U-wave duration. Interestingly, acute hypocalcemia as a complication of subtotal thyroidectomy may be a cause for unexpected syncopal episodes caused by TdP.

Macrolide Antibiotics

Clinical reports have shown that several antiinfective agents may induce Q-T interval prolongation, leading to the development of TdP. Macrolides represent the group of antibiotics more frequently associated with proarrhythmic events.

Intravenous erythromycin has been shown by several investigators to produce Q-T interval prolongation and T-wave alternans in individuals with no structural heart disease and to exacerbate repolarization alterations in patients affected by the idiopathic long Q-T syndrome. A case of TdP and acquired long Q-T syndrome due to a cross-sensitivity between quinidine and erythromycin has been reported. Action potential duration is increased, combined with a reduction in Vmax in canine Purkinje fibers exposed to erythromycin, suggesting that it exerts electrophysiological effects similar to class I antiarrhythmic drugs.

Recently, the case of a newborn child who had Q-T interval prolongation and experienced a cardiac arrest during oral therapy with the macrolide agent spiramycin has been reported. After resuscitation, Q-T interval prolongation persisted for 3 weeks, while spiramycin therapy was maintained. The return of Q-T interval to normal after spiramycin withdrawal suggest a causal relationship between antibiotic treatment and cardiac arrest, probably due to TdP.

Limited data are available to explain the mechanism by which macrolide antibiotics prolong repolarization and favor TdP. Myocardial K^+ transport is inhibited by some antibiotics, and this effect causes a prolongation in the Q-T interval, leading to the development of VT. Along the same lines, erythromycin induces prolongation of action potential duration in Purkinje fibers, suggesting that this effect on repolarization may be the consequence of the inhibition of the repolarizing potassium currents. Erythromycin prolongs action potential duration to a greater extent in M cells as compared with endocardial or epicardial cells and induces early afterdepolarizations in M cells only. Such a disparate electrophysiologic effect in myocardial layers is likely to result in a large dispersion of repolarization, which may lead to the development of U waves and TdP.

Besides macrolides, several other antibiotics have been reported to produce Q-T interval prolongation. These include trimethoprim-sulfamethoxazole, ampicillin, and pentamidine. Inhaled pentamidine is largely used in AIDS patients to treat *Pneumocystis carinii* pneumonia, one of the most frequently observed opportunistic infections in HIV-positive patients. Multiple episodes of TdP refractory to conventional therapy have been reported in patients receiving pentamidine in the absence of cardiac disease, electrolyte abnormalities, or baseline Q-T interval prolongation. In one case report, arrhythmias induced by pentamidine, both TdP and VT, recurred repeatedly for 13 days after pentamidine therapy discontinuation. In this case, pentamidine-induced TdP responded to treatment with magnesium, lidocaine, and isoproterenol. The similarity in the molecular structure of pentamidine and procainamide has suggested that the two agents may share a similar mechanism for their proarrhythmic effects.

Antihistaminic Agents

An increasing number of reports have shown that the administration of the anti-histaminic agents terfenadine and astemizole, especially when used in patients with baseline prolonged Q-T interval or at high dosages, or concomitantly with the antifungal agents ketoconazole or itraconazole, may precipitate TdP. Ketoconazole alters the metabolism of terfenadine, resulting in the accumulation of the drug, which induces a marked prolongation of ventricular repolarization. Terfenadine exerts a block of the delayed rectifier potassium current similar to that of quinidine, thus resulting in a prolongation of action potential duration.

A case of a 25-year-old woman treated with terfenadine and itraconazole, who experienced a syncopal episode due to TdP was recently reported (Fig. 20.2). The Q-T interval was markedly prolonged (536 msec; Fig. 20.2A), and the Q-T interval dispersion, calculated as the difference between the longest and the shortest Q-T interval in the 12-leads ECG, was 94 msec. After discontinuation of drug therapy, both the Q-T interval and the Q-T interval dispersion returned to normal values (Q-T interval, 367 msec; Q-T interval dispersion, 28 msec; Fig. 20.2B). This observation suggests that combined treatment with terfenadine and itraconazole is associated with nonhomogeneous prolongation of ventricular repolarization, which results in a larger than normal dispersion of the Q-T interval likely to be responsible for the development of TdP.

Miscellaneous Drugs

Therapy with several drugs not belonging to one of the major groups discussed in the previous sections has been associated with the development of TdP. Use of terodiline in the management of urinary incontinence has been associated with the development of Q-T interval prolongation and TdP. This has led to the withdrawal of terodiline from the worldwide market and to investigations on the causal relationship between this drug and ventricular tachyarrhythmias. Again, the structural similarity of terodiline to the sodium channel blocker prenylamine, already known to cause TdP, suggests the importance of this mechanism in the development of TdP. It would be important to evaluate whether structural similarity with a drug known to prolong repolarization and induce ventricular arrhythmias should call for caution in the use of a compound and should require careful evaluation of its safety profile. Other drugs associated with occurrence of TdP are the cholesterol-lowering agent probucol, adenosine, papaverine, ketanserin, and cocaine.

Bradyarrhythmias

Severe bradycardia observed in patients with sinus node dysfunction or complete AV block has been associated with the development of TdP. An intriguing aspect of this cause of TdP is that in susceptible individuals arrhythmias are precipitated at heart rates that can be well tolerated by the majority of individuals. To address this question, 14 patients with AV block were entered into a study and were divided into two groups: six patients with TdP and eight patients without.

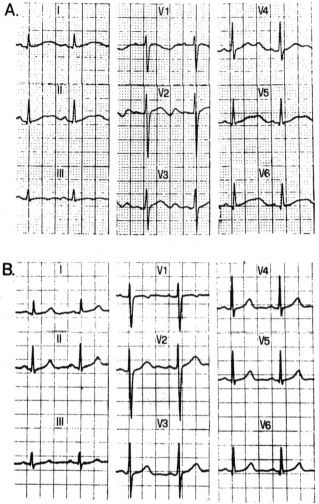

Figure 20.2. Surface ECG recording in a 25-year-old woman. A. During pharmacologic treatment with terfenadine and itraconazole, excessive Q-T interval dispersion (Q-Tmax − QT-min = 94 msec) and prolonged Q-T interval (Q-T = 536 msec) were observed; the patient presented in the emergency room with TdP. B. After a 3-month washout period, both Q-T dispersion and Q-T interval returned to normal values (Q-Tmax − Q-Tmin = 28 msec; Q-T = 367 msec).

Patients in both groups presented comparable rates during escape rhythm, but the group with TdP had significantly longer Q-T intervals. After pacemaker implantation for treatment of the AV block, the pacing rate was varied between 50–100 beats/minute. The study confirmed that in the TdP group, the Q-T interval abnormally prolonged at slow rates. The investigators concluded that patients with complete AV block who develop TdP have a bradycardia-dependent repolarization abnormality that may account for the electrical vulnerability of their heart.

Because the development of EADs is one of the proposed mechanisms for TdP, and given that they are induced by slow heart rates, EADs may be responsible for the prolongation of Q-T interval in patients developing TdP in the presence of profound bradycardia. Indeed, in a recently reported study measuring monophasic action potentials in a patient with marked bradycardia, in the presence of hypokalemia, EADs developed with a marked prolongation of the Q-T-U interval.

A Genetic Marker for Torsade de Pointes?

According to some reports, individuals more prone to develop TdP as a consequence of pharmacologic treatment may present an abnormality of an essential component of drug metabolism. Cytochromes P-450 play a major role in oxidative drug metabolism. Their expression is genetically determined and shows considerable variability. For example, cytochrome P-450 CYP2D6 shows considerable polymorphism, with 5–10% of Caucasians not expressing this enzyme. These individuals are the poor metabolizers in which drug elimination may be defective, thus increasing the risk for the development of side effects.

This opens the way to genetic studies to ascertain whether or not the propensity to develop TdP, after administration of specific substances, might be a genetic trait. Accordingly, it is essential to study of the families of individuals with drug-induced TdP. To address this and related issues, a worldwide prospective registry/study has been initiated by a group of investigators in the United States and in Europe.

Therapy

Therapeutic decisions should be the logical extension of the degree of understanding of the underlying mechanisms. A rational approach to prevention and therapy of TdP has been recently described according to the principles put forward in the *Sicilian Gambit*.

The choice of therapy depends on the identification of a "vulnerable parameter," which represents the most critical concept proposed by the *Sicilian Gambit*. The assumption is that for each arrhythmogenic mechanism, a specific alteration in one or more of several electrophysiological properties will be sufficient to terminate the arrhythmia or to prevent its initiation. A second and related assumption is that among several potentially effective modifications in electrophysiological properties, it is possible to identify one that is at the same time most susceptible to alterations and minimally associated with undesirable effects on the heart. This property has been labeled the "vulnerable parameter."

Despite the alternate possibilities just listed, TdP is probably caused by triggered activity as a consequence of afterdepolarizations. The afterdepolarizations more directly related to TdP are those that interrupt the repolarization process, known as early afterdepolarizations, or EADs. EADs result from an excess of inward over outward currents during the plateau and phase 3 of the action potential, which delays or interrupts repolarization. Any intervention able to reduce plateau inward currents (e.g., I_{CaL}), or to increase outward currents (e.g., I_K), thus shortening action potential duration, will prevent EADs. EADs tend to arise after long pauses or at low heart rates, when action potential duration is maximal. Because all changes in ionic currents preventing EADs will also shorten repolarization, the prolonged action potential duration can be effectively considered as the vulnerable parameter for EAD-dependent triggered activity. Action potential duration may be shortened either by blocking inward or by enhancing outward currents. In the first case, Ca^{++} antagonists and magnesium would be the drugs of choice. Alternatively, the best current practical option to enhance outward currents is to increase heart rate by β-receptor agonists or vagolytic agents.

In the following section we briefly review the current consensus on TdP therapy in light of the vulnerable parameter on which a given intervention is based (Table 20.2).

HEART RATE INCREASE

Isoproterenol

Isoproterenol infusion adjusted to maintain a ventricular rate above 90 beats/minute has been shown to effectively suppress episodes of TdP. However, the isoproterenol infusion is not devoid of risks, as some of the electrophysiologic effects of catecholamines may favor the onset of ventricular tachyarrhythmias. Therefore, it is advisable to use alternative therapies to increase heart rate.

Atropine

Extreme bradycardia often associated with AV block is a condition in which TdP may develop. Atropine has the potential to enhance AV conduction and therefore to increase the ventricular rate. On the other hand, atropine may even enhance the block

Table 20.2
Therapeutic Approaches for Torsade de Pointes

Acquired prolonged Q-T syndromes
   Pharmacological therapy
      Isoproterenol
      Atropine
      Magnesium sulfate
      Amiodarone
   Nonpharmacological therapy
      Temporary atrial or ventricular pacing
      Permanent pacemaker
Idiopathic LQTS[a]
   Pharmacological therapy
      β-Blockers (propranolol, nadolol)
   Nonpharmacological therapy
      Left cardiac sympathetic denervation
      Antibradycardia pacemaker
      Implantable cardioverter-defibrillator

[a]LQ-TS, long Q-T syndrome

in the His-Purkinje network by increasing atrial rate. Accordingly, inconsistent results have been obtained when atropine has been given intravenously at doses of 0.03 mg/kg.

Temporary or Permanent Pacing

During the occurrence of TdP, temporary atrial or ventricular pacing with rates between 90–110 beats/minute may interrupt bradycardia-dependent TdP and also inhibit their recurrence, while washout of the offending agent is completed. This procedure is viewed by many as the first-choice treatment for TdP during the acute phase. Pacemaker implantation may be beneficial as well in patients affected by the idiopathic long Q-T syndrome. Indeed, although permanent pacing does not provide complete protection, it has been found to reduce the rate of recurrent syncopal events.

REDUCTION OF INWARD CURRENTS

Magnesium sulfate at intravenous (i.v.) doses of 2–3 g, is effective in suppressing drug-induced TdP, even in patients with normal plasma magnesium levels. The mechanism by which magnesium abolishes TdP is not known, and it remains intriguing that even when TdP is successfully terminated, the Q-T interval remains prolonged. It has been speculated that the calcium blocking properties of magnesium may inhibit the development of triggered activity, thus acting as a selective antiarrhythmic agent for this form of automaticity.

INCREASE OF OUTWARD CURRENTS

This approach has the potential to represent the most innovative therapeutic strategy for TdP. In fact, the availability of drugs that shorten the action potential duration and abolish EADs, such as nicorandil and pinacidil, has raised the possibility of their use in prolonged repolarization syndromes. Still, caution is necessary, and whether their use will provide progress in the management of TdP must await confirmation from carefully conducted clinical studies.

POLYMORPHIC VENTRICULAR TACHYCARDIA

Polymorphic Ventricular Tachycardia and Ischemic Heart Disease

Polymorphic VT in the course of acute myocardial infarction (MI) is uncommon. The appropriate management of this arrhythmia is not well defined. In a study of 11 patients with post-MI polymorphic VT, the arrhythmia was not consistently related to an abnormally long Q-T interval, sinus bradycardia, preceding sinus pauses, or electrolyte abnormalities but was often associated with signs or symptoms of recurrent myocardial ischemia. The arrhythmia had a variable response to class I antiarrhythmic agents but could be suppressed in some patients by i.v. amiodarone. Coronary revascularization appeared to be effective in preventing recurrence of polymorphic VT when associated with recurrent postinfarction angina. These findings are consistent with the observations of other investigators. For example, in a study of polymorphic VT and chronic ischemic heart disease, significant coronary artery stenosis was present in a majority of patients. The polymorphic VT was successfully treated with revascularization, including coronary angioplasty, and a few patients responded to amiodarone.

Polymorphic Ventricular Tachycardia without Significant Structural Heart Disease

Structural heart disease is absent in up to 5% of survivors of out-of-hospital cardiac arrest. There are few reports of polymorphic VT/ventricular fibrillation (VF) in patients with no significant structural heart disease. In one report, polymorphic VT occurred in 13 patients with no cardiac abnormality found on echocardiogram, cardiac catheterization, or autopsy. All patients had normal Q-T interval, no electrolyte abnormality, and were on no medications. In four patients, the arrhythmia was reproducibly initiated by isoprenaline infusion and/or exercise, and all four patients responded to chronic β-blockade. Two patients had the arrhythmia during coronary spasm and both responded to calcium blocking agents. In five of the remaining seven patients, the arrhythmia was pause-dependent. Those patients were treated by pacing, β-blockade, and calcium blocking agents alone or in combination. A short coupling interval in the patients with pause-dependent polymorphic VT formed a high-risk subgroup.

Patients with polymorphic VT and minimal or no structural heart disease seem to respond erratically to antiarrhythmic drugs. Because they are at high risk for sudden cardiac death, an implantable cardioverter-defibrillator may have to be considered in some cases.

There may be electrophysiologic similarities between fast polymorphic VT without significant structural heart disease and idiopathic VF. There are few reports of VF in the presence of minimal or no structural heart diseases. In a review of 54 cases of idiopathic VF, 50 patients required resuscitation, while four had nonsustained VF with syncope. Ventricular fibrillation was initiated by a ventricular premature beat with a very short coupling interval in many of the cases, and a short-long-short cardiac cycle preceded some of the tachyarrhythmia episodes. Induction of polymorphic VT and VF has been considered a nonspecific response to programmed stimulation in this group of patients, and its incidence varied from 39–69% in two large study groups. Sustained monomorphic VT was rarely induced. Thus, programmed stimulation may not be useful in guiding therapy in survivors of idiopathic VF.

Similar to polymorphic VT without significant structural heart disease, there is no recommended strategy for the management of idiopathic VF at present. Pharmacologic therapy has been tried often. Failure of amiodarone as a single drug therapy was seen in three of four cases in a recent report. Those investigators found class Ia drugs to be associated with better prognosis in the short term. However, the value of pharmacologic therapy in idiopathic VF has yet to be established.

In a recent report, a 10-center retrospective study provided information on 28 survivors of VF with minimal or no structural abnormalities who were treated with an implantable cardioverter-defibrillator. The 3-year survival rate with the device was excellent and superior to that reported in survivors of cardiac arrest with structural heart disease treated similarly. Only a small number of patients (four of 28) received shocks considered to be appropriate. However, the implanted device had no arrhythmia disclosure capability to provide an accurate estimate of the incidence of appropriate shocks. The report suggests than an implantable cardioverter-defibrillator may be a valid option in patients with idiopathic VF to avoid the potential risk of recurrent cardiac arrest.

Polymorphic Ventricular Tachycardia Induced by Programmed Stimulation

Polymorphic VT is frequently induced by programmed ventricular stimulation. The prognostic significance of induced polymorphic VT is controversial and seems to depend largely on the clinical presentation. It is customary to consider induced polymorphic VT a valid endpoint in patients with documented resuscitation from VF or with a high likelihood of having had such an arrhythmia. At present, such patients are more likely to be candidates for the implantable cardioverter-defibrillator than for serial antiarrhythmic drug trials.

Conversely, in patients with no such history, the induction of a polymorphic VT is considered a nonclinical response to programmed stimulation that lacks prognostic significance, particularly if the stimulation is carried out in the first few weeks after MI. The electrophysiologic rationale for this position is not clear, considering that induced polymorphic VT in the presence of ischemic heart disease is most likely due to reentry that may also underlie the spontaneous arrhythmia. This approach simply highlights our limited current understanding of the relationship between induced polymorphic tachyarrhythmia and its spontaneous occurrence.

A recent study demonstrated that conversion of inducible polymorphic VT into inducible monomorphic VT after procainamide can occur in approximately 30% of patients. This response occurred almost exclusively in patients with coronary artery disease and prior MI with significant ventricular dysfunction who had experienced spontaneous sustained ventricular tachyarrhythmias. In a few patients in this group, the conversion of polymorphic VT to monomorphic VT by procainamide permitted mapping of the ventricular activation pattern of the tachycardia. It also allowed successful application of surgical or catheter ablative therapeutic techniques that would otherwise not have been possible in these patients. In the same study, the prevention of induction of polymorphic VT by procainamide did seem to represent a favorable response. For this reason it is not advisable to extend the use of procainamide or other type Ia agents to all patients with induced polymorphic VT. This could be reserved for those patients with a high likelihood of having the substrate for monomorphic VT, such as those with previous MI, left ventricular aneurysm, and an abnormal signal-averaged ECG.

SUGGESTED READING

El-Sherif N. Clinical significance of polymorphic ventricular tachycardia induced by programmed stimulation. J Am Coll Cardiol 1993;21:99–101.

Jackman WM, Friday KJ, Anderson JL, et al. The long QT syndromes: a critical review, new clinical observations and a unifying hypothesis. Prog Cardiovasc Dis 1988;31:115–172.

Nguyen PT, Scheinman M, Seger J. Polymorphous ventricular tachycardia: clinical characterization, therapy and QT interval. Circulation 1986;74:340–346.

Schwartz PJ, Moss AJ, Vincent GM, Crampton RS. Diagnostic criteria for the long QT syndrome: an update. Circulation 1993;88:782–784.

Tzivoni D, Keren A, Cohen AM, et al. Magnesium therapy for torsades de pointes. Am J Cardiol 1984;53:528–530.

Wolfe CL, Nibley C, Bhandari A, Chaterjee K, Scheinmann MM. Polymorphous ventricular tachycardia associated with acute myocardial infarction. Circulation 1991;84:1543–1551.

21 Sudden Cardiac Death/Ventricular Fibrillation

POPULATION STUDIES AND RISK FACTOR IDENTIFICATION

Several large population-based epidemiologic studies have provided information on the incidence of sudden cardiac death (SCD) among various populations. In most of these studies, SCD was defined as death occurring within 1 hour from the onset of acute symptoms of a terminal episode in others, SCD was defined as death occurring within 2, 6, or 24 hours.

In the Framingham Study, during a 26-year follow-up of 5,209 men and women 30–59 years of age who were free of coronary heart disease at baseline, SCD (within 1 hour of onset of symptoms) accounted for 46% of all coronary disease deaths among men, while only 34% of such deaths in women were sudden. Women also had a three times lower incidence of SCD than men. The incidence of SCD increased with age, but the proportion of SCD among all coronary heart disease deaths was greater at younger ages. Sudden coronary death was significantly and positively associated with obesity, cigarette smoking, pulse rate, and strenuous physical activity.

Pooled data from two studies in the United States, in Albany, NY (1,838 men, aged 35–59) and in Framingham, MA (2,282 men, aged 30–59), indicated that SCD (1-hour definition) was the initial and terminal manifestation of coronary heart disease in more than half of all SCD victims. The incidence of SCD was four times greater among those who had known coronary heart disease at baseline compared with those who did not. The risk of SCD was equal among those with angina and those with previous myocardial infarction (MI). However, the proportion of coronary deaths that were sudden was not significantly different among those who had recognized coronary heart disease at baseline examination from those who did not.

In another U.S. study of 8,641 subjects in Tecumseh, Michigan, 46% of all coronary heart disease deaths occurred within 1 hour of the onset of acute symptoms. The vast majority of SCD cases had no prodromal symptoms, but a substantial proportion of them had known coronary heart disease prior to death. In 84% of those dying suddenly, electrocardiogram (ECG) evidence of cardiac arrhythmias or conduction disturbances were found. In a study of 269,755 U.S. men aged 20–65, 1,839 coronary heart disease deaths occurred during a 5-year follow-up period. A sample of 1,023 men aged 40–65 was selected at the beginning of the study and was followed for 5 years, including periodic, standardized examinations. About 60% of all coronary deaths in this group were classified as SCDs (within 2 hours). One-third of those who died suddenly did not have documented coronary heart disease prior to death. Major risk factors for arrhythmic cardiac death were hypertension, cigarette smoking, heavy alcohol consumption, and prior history of coronary heart disease. The most potent findings functioning as clinical risk factors

344

for sudden, arrhythmic death were chronic heart disease, left ventricular (LV) hypertrophy by ECG, enlarged heart as assessed by chest x-ray, congestive heart failure, and premature ventricular contractions.

In the Yugoslavia Cardiovascular Disease Study among 6,614 men, aged 35–62 years and free of coronary heart disease at baseline, 75% of all coronary heart disease deaths occurred suddenly. Two-thirds of SCD victims had no documented coronary disease prior to death, and about 45% of them died instantaneously. The proportion of all coronary deaths that were sudden and unexpected was significantly greater in men aged 45–54 than in the other age groups. The most significant and independent risk factors in the incidence of SCD among Yugoslav men were age, blood pressure, and cigarette smoking; significant although not independent SCD risk factors were pulse rate, LV hypertrophy on ECG, alcohol consumption, and hematocrit level.

In a follow-up of a cohort of 7,591 middle-aged Japanese men living in Hawaii, who were free of coronary heart disease at baseline examination, blood pressure, serum cholesterol, serum glucose, cigarette smoking, history of parental heart attack, and electrocardiographic evidence of LV hypertrophy were positively associated with the incidence of SCD in less than 1 hour. Alcohol consumption and social factors, such as number of years spent in Japan, were inversely related to SCD.

Several studies have reported data on the epidemiology of SCD among women. The Framingham study has shown that the incidence of SCD was significantly lower in women than in men, but 64% of all SCD in women occurred without prior clinically apparent coronary heart disease, indicating that SCD was often the first and last manifestation of coronary heart disease in women. In this study, the strongest predictors of SCD in women were an increased hematocrit level and a decreased vital capacity. It has been suggested that these associations could not be explained by the SCD-cigarette smoking association because smoking was not a significant and independent predictor of SCD in Framingham women. Among clinical characteristics, LV hypertrophy was found as the strongest predictor of SCD in this group of women. Another U.S. study also showed that at similar levels of major risk factors, the incidence of SCD was lower among women than among men. In this study, cigarette smoking was the strongest risk factor in the incidence of SCD among women: all of those 45 years old or younger who died suddenly were heavy smokers. From the study in the county of North Karelia, Finland, the proportion of SCD (within 1 hour) of all coronary heart disease deaths among persons aged 35–64 was 57% for men and 45% for women. The strongest SCD risk factor in this population was serum cholesterol. In a study of 300 cases of SCD among persons below the age of 70 years in Aukland, New Zealand, the incidence of SCD (defined as death within 24 hours after the onset of symptoms of terminal episode) was three times higher among men than among women and significantly higher among Maoris (who had the highest prevalence of cigarette smoking and the lowest high-density lipoprotein [HDL]-cholesterol levels) than among individuals of European or other ethnic origin.

Most but not all epidemiologic studies indicated that African Americans have a higher incidence of SCD than Caucasians. The reasons for this difference are not fully explained. It has been suggested that different levels of health care delivery provided for African Americans and Caucasians may be a strong contributor to the difference. Further epidemiologic studies are needed to provide better insights into risk factors and incidence of SCD in men and women of different race and ethnic origin.

Despite a large number of epidemiologic studies that have shown a strong relationship of major risk factors (blood pressure, serum cholesterol, cigarette smoking, body weight, physical activity) to the incidence of coronary heart disease in general, and SCD in particular, there is as yet not a single or a set of risk factors identified as being specific for SCD (Fig. 21.1). Although the strength of the relationship of various risk factors to the incidence of SCD does not hold equally in all populations, none of these risk factors can be used to distinguish individuals at risk for SCD from those whose deaths are more protracted. Therefore, until risk factors specific for SCD are found, prediction of SCD in the general population remains a matter of predicting SCD on the basis of standard risk factors, with continued difficulty in identifying the specific individuals at risk. This creates a problem regarding the limited efficiency of preventive interventions and the ability of such interventions to affect the large numbers of SCD candidates hidden within the general population.

MANAGEMENT OF THE SUDDEN CARDIAC DEATH VICTIM

The occurrence of ventricular fibrillation (VF) and SCD is a catastrophic event during which there is no active cardiac contraction and no cardiac output. VF in the human heart does not spontaneously terminate, and therefore survival is dependent upon prompt CPR and the reestablishment of organized electrical activity and a stable sinus or supraventricular rhythm. The only effective approach to terminating VF is defibrillation using 200–400 J of energy delivered transthoracically in a nonsynchronized fashion. The initial success of defibrillation depends upon the duration of the arrhythmia. When VF has been present for seconds to a few minutes and the fibrillatory waves are coarse, the success rate is high. However, as VF continues for a longer period of time, the fibrillatory waves become finer, the result of a depletion of myocardial epinephrine stores, and the ability to terminate the arrhythmia is decreased. Additionally, when VF continues for more than 4 minutes, there is irreversible damage to the central nervous system and other organs. This damage will affect survival, even if there is successful defibrillation.

The management of the patient who has survived an episode of SCD is complex and involves a complete and intensive evaluation of the precipitating event, underlying heart disease, and the degree of electrical instability (Table 21.1). Complete neurologic and psychologic evaluations are essential.

Provoking Factors

The evaluation of the patient who has had a cardiac arrest begins immediately after resuscitation. The physician needs to establish any obvious provoking factors

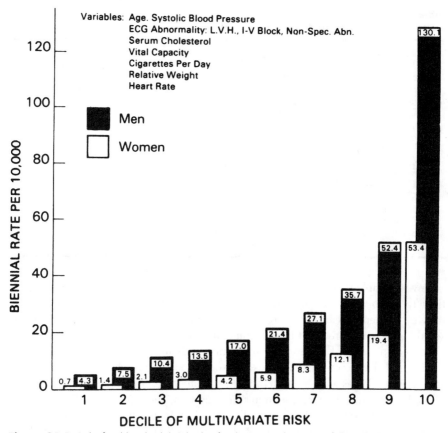

Figure 21.1. Risk of sudden death by decile of multivariate risk: 26-year follow-up, the Framingham Study. LVH, left ventricular hypertrophy; I-V, intraventricular; Non-Spec. Abn., nonspecific abnormality. (From Kannel WB, Schatzkin A. Sudden death: lessons from subsets in population studies. J Am Coll Cardiol 1985;5:141B–149B. Reprinted with permission from the American College of Cardiology.)

that may have led to the event and that need to be corrected so as to prevent an immediate recurrence. As soon as historical information can be obtained, the patient and family should be questioned about previous diagnoses of heart disease, the use of any medication, especially cardioactive drugs such as antiarrhythmics, diuretics, or digoxin, and antecedent symptoms, especially evidence of ischemia. Unfortunately, the cardiac arrest is often unwitnessed, or if there are observers, they are often unaware of any symptoms that may have preceded the event. More importantly, the patient resuscitated from VF often has retrograde amnesia and is unable to remember anything that occurred prior to the cardiac arrest. This retrograde amnesia may extend from several minutes to many hours or days before the collapse. Thus, a coherent history of chest pain or palpitations that heralded the event may not be ascertainable.

Table 21.1
Management of the Sudden Death Survivor

Diagnostic workup
- Establish the nature and extent of heart disease
- Evaluate left ventricular function
- Establish tthe type, frequency, and reproducibility of spontaneous ventricular arrhythmia in a drug-free state with ambulatory monitoring and exercise testing
- Document inducibility with electrophysiologic testing in drug-free state

Therapeutic
- Discontinue drugs, especially antiarrhythmic agents (if possible)
- Correct metabolic and electrolyte abnormalities
- Evaluate for precipating factors
- Optimize left ventricular function
- Control symptoms of active ischemia
- Evaluate neurologic state
- Attend to psychologic factors
- Systematic evaluation of antiarrhythmic drugs (noninvasive and invasive)
- Consider alternative therapy for drug-refractory patients

Any reversible metabolic abnormalities should be identified and corrected, particularly hypokalemia or low magnesium, as it is well established that such electrolyte imbalances can predispose to ventricular tachyarrhythmias. However, it should be remembered that hypokalemia may be present immediately after resuscitation as a result of the cardiac arrest rather than as a cause. It has been well established that a transient decrease in serum potassium occurs during VF and subsequent CPR as a result of an increase in catecholamine levels and stimulation of the β_2 receptors, an increase in insulin secretion, and acidosis-mediated hydrogen-potassium exchange. It is especially hazardous to ascribe a cardiac arrest to an electrolyte or metabolic derangement alone unless there is particularly compelling evidence of an association. Mistaken attribution of a major arrhythmia to an innocent laboratory abnormality places the patient at a high risk of recurrence.

Whenever possible, cardioactive drug therapy should be discontinued prior to any diagnostic studies. If clinically indicated, digoxin- and angiotensin-converting enzyme inhibitors can be continued for control of congestive heart failure and β-blockers, nitrates, or calcium channel-blocking agents for therapy of hypertension or ischemia. It is especially important that antiarrhythmic drugs be discontinued prior to an evaluation of baseline arrhythmia. These agents themselves can contribute to the likelihood of an event and can alter the electrophysiologic milieu at the time of testing. Of particular concern are patients who have had a cardiac arrest while receiving an antiarrhythmic drug. It is very difficult to be certain in many of these cases if the arrest was provoked by the drug or occurred despite its use. This dilemma is especially difficult in making decisions about chronic therapy for such patients.

Congestive Heart Failure and Ischemia

The majority of patients who experience SCD have LV dysfunction and a history of congestive heart failure. Prior to any baseline evaluation, overt congestive heart failure should be treated and LV function optimized. This includes therapy with digoxin, diuretics, and afterload reduction, as generally indicated. Active ischemia should be aggressively treated with aspirin, β-blockers, nitrates, and/or calcium channel blockers, or, if necessary, with revascularization utilizing angioplasty or bypass surgery, so as to render the patient free of symptoms. Infrequently, active overt or silent ischemia is the provoking factor for the sudden death episode, and revascularization is the only necessary therapy. However, for the majority of patients who survive an episode, an ischemic event cannot be regarded as the critical factor, even though the patient may have significant underlying coronary artery disease. For such patients, revascularization is an adjunctive but not primary therapy. A full arrhythmia evaluation is still essential.

Neurologic and Psychologic Assessment

Patients who have been resuscitated from SCD should have a complete neurologic examination to establish the nature and extent of impairment resulting from the arrest. It is also important to exclude conditions that could mimic an arrhythmic event, such as a seizure disorder. Equally important is an assessment of the patient's psychologic state, which often becomes a concern to the patient and the family, particularly after hospital discharge. Patients who have been resuscitated from SCD frequently have emotional problems and anxieties that prevent them from resuming a normal and active life and that can interfere with family interactions. Such potential problems should be identified and discussed with the patient and the family prior to discharge. Support groups that include individuals who have received an implantable device have become particularly popular and useful in making proper long-term adjustments.

Cardiac Evaluation

Once previous drug therapy has been discontinued and the drugs cleared from the body, and after metabolic derangements, ischemia, and hemodynamic abnormalities have been corrected, the patient should undergo a full cardiac examination. The first step is to establish the nature and extent of underlying heart disease and state of LV function by physical examination, echocardiography, inspection of the ECG, cardiac catheterization, and myocardial biopsy if indicated. Contemporary evaluations also include a signal-averaged ECG, done specifically to find a late potential. The presence of this abnormality suggests that there is an area of slow conduction within which a reentrant arrhythmia may propagate. The absence of a late potential does not exclude the possibility that a reentrant arrhythmia was responsible for the collapse, especially in patients with a nonischemic cardiomyopathy, although the chance of inducing such an arrhythmia in the laboratory is reduced.

Although the most frequent heart disease associated with VF is coronary artery disease, many other cardiac disease states can result in this arrhythmia. Determining the nature of the underlying heart disease is important for several reasons. It may expose a significant abnormality that contributed to the acute event and that requires therapy. Some examples of such abnormalities include critical aortic stenosis, a severe proximal coronary artery lesion, acute myocarditis, or hypertrophic cardiomyopathy. The nature of the cardiac abnormality and the severity of LV dysfunction may be helpful in deciding the best method for evaluating the patient (invasively vs. noninvasively), in the selection of an antiarrhythmic drug, or in a decision to treat the patient nonpharmacologically. For example, electrophysiologic testing may be less useful in patients with congestive cardiomyopathy compared to patients who have ischemic heart disease. Antiarrhythmic drugs are less effective and more likely to cause serious cardiac toxicity in patients with congestive heart failure and significant LV dysfunction.

When severe coronary artery disease is present, revascularization is an important part of therapy, although a complete arrhythmia evaluation is essential. In the presence of the Wolff-Parkinson-White syndrome, ablation of the accessory pathway could be the procedure of choice for preventing a recurrence of SCD.

Arrhythmia Evaluation

Once the underlying condition has been diagnosed and treated appropriately, a complete arrhythmia evaluation follows. The goal of this evaluation is to establish at baseline the type, frequency, and reproducibility of spontaneous ventricular ectopy and inducibility of a ventricular tachyarrhythmia. This involves the use of noninvasive extended ambulatory monitoring for 48 hours, an exercise test, and an invasive electrophysiologic study. Invasive and noninvasive techniques are both required, and they each provide important and complementary information. Electrophysiologic testing is necessary to evaluate the underlying myocardial substrate and the ability to generate and sustain reentry, the usual mechanism for ventricular tachyarrhythmias. Clinically, the reentrant circuit is activated by some trigger such as spontaneous ectopy or perhaps changes in heart rate. These triggers are best evaluated using ambulatory monitoring and exercise testing. Lastly, there are a number of modulating factors that may affect the stability of the substrate and the potential for reentry, and may also alter the triggers. These modulating factors include ischemia, pH changes, electrolyte abnormalities, sympathetic nervous system inputs, and circulating catecholamines, among others. Because these modulating factors are extremely changeable, they are best evaluated noninvasively with extended ambulatory monitoring and exercise testing. It is therefore preferable that both invasive and noninvasive methods be used in the evaluation and management of patients who have experienced SCD because the data derived from both methods are important. Indeed, each of these techniques has strengths and weaknesses that must be considered.

Noninvasive Testing

Ambulatory monitoring and exercise testing are widely available, easily performed, and are relatively inexpensive (Table 21.2). The data gathered about spon-

Table 21.2
Noninvasive Techniques

Strengths
    Widely available
    Easily performed
    Inexpensive (relatively)
    Can be repeated as often as necessary
    Results easy to interpret
    Normal physiologic changes evaluated
    Can follow patients over time as substrate changes

Weaknesses
    Requires high density of arrhythmia
    Frequent complex forms must be present
    Arrhythmia must be reproducibly present
    No unifrom criteria for drug efficacy
    Different criteria for drug effect (VPB suppression) vs. drug efficacy (prevention of sustained
      arrhythmia)

taneous arrhythmia and heart rate are fairly easy to interpret. Additional information, such as Q-T interval changes, ST segment changes, and heart rate variability can also be obtained. Noninvasive testing can be repeated as often as necessary, such as when the dose of the antiarrhythmic drug is changed, another drug is begun or discontinued, or the patient has a symptom suggesting arrhythmia recurrence or a drug-related conduction abnormality. It must be remembered that underlying heart disease itself is generally progressive, and therefore there are changes in the underlying substrate that occur over time. This can influence the presence of arrhythmia and the action of an antiarrhythmic drug, making it essential that evaluation of the drug effect be repeated on a regular basis. Importantly noninvasive methods are essential for evaluating the many modulating factors that can interact with and alter the substrate and the triggers. These factors are often transient and highly variable and can be assessed only by prolonged observation.

A noninvasive approach has a number of limitations. Its usefulness depends upon the presence of a high density of spontaneous ectopy, particularly runs of nonsustained ventricular tachycardia (NSVT), which are reproducibly present and stable in frequency and type from day to day. In many patients, spontaneously occurring arrhythmia manifests a great deal of daily variability. This variability makes it impossible to establish a baseline or to assess the effect of any intervention, especially antiarrhythmic drugs, because it is difficult to distinguish between drug effect and random changes. A number of investigators have reported considerable random variability of arrhythmia in patients with and without heart disease. The spontaneous ventricular arrhythmias seen in patients who have experienced a sustained arrhythmic event are often reproducibly present each day and tend not to vary. A large percentage of patients who have been resuscitated from SCD do not demonstrate spontaneous ventricular arrhythmia, and in them noninvasive methods cannot be utilized. Whether or not ambient arrhythmia is itself a trigger for a sustained event or is merely a marker of underlying electrical instability still remains uncertain. In addition, endpoints of therapy have not been established. For example, it has been reported that NSVT is an arrhythmia of concern and its suppression should be the major goal of therapy, but this is highly controversial. It must be remembered that while suppression of spontaneous arrhythmia by an antiarrhythmic agent defines a drug's activity, it does not necessarily establish drug efficacy for preventing a sustained ventricular tachyarrhythmia and SCD.

In a number of trials in which new antiarrhythmic agents have been evaluated, drug efficacy has been defined by a certain percentage of VPB suppression; however, these studies generally involved patients with a high density of spontaneous arrhythmia and not those who had an episode of SCD. The purpose of these studies was to establish the activity of the agent in certain circumstances rather than its effect on the patients' long-term survival. There have been a few studies in which patients who had a history of sustained VT or VF were managed noninvasively and followed over the long term. Criteria for efficacy in these studies were based not only on a percent reduction in the amount of arrhythmia but also on the elimination of certain forms. Most often used is total elimination of runs of NSVT, >90% reduction in the number of couplets, and >50% reduction in VPBs.

Regardless of whether ambulatory monitoring or electrophysiologic testing is used, exercise testing is an important adjunctive technique. Exercise testing is not only important as an additional way of provoking arrhythmia, but it has a more major role in the evaluation of the beneficial or potentially harmful effect of an antiarrhythmic drug (arrhythmia aggravation, conduction abnormalities). A number of physiologic changes that occur during exercise may interact with antiarrhythmic drug action and may in some cases negate the effect of the drug or perhaps even result in a drug-induced toxic effect, particularly arrhythmia aggravation or a significant conduction abnormality. With exercise there is activation of the sympathetic nervous system and an increase in circulating catecholamines. As a result, there are a number of metabolic changes, including ischemia, electrolyte shifts, and pH changes that can alter the activity of the antiarrhythmic drugs. Membrane-active drugs typically cause slowing of impulse conduction, reduction in membrane excitability, and a decrease in automaticity. In contrast, catecholamines enhance conduction velocity, excitability, and automaticity. Hypokalemia may produce similar changes that can negate the antiarrhythmic drug effect, while hyperkalemia (often a result of ischemia) may intensify the drug effect.

Invasive Testing

Because invasive electrophysiology evaluates the stability of the substrate and the ability to activate a reentrant circuit and induce a sustained ventricular tachycardia, spontaneous ectopy and its variability are less important (Table 21.3). Indeed, electrophysiologic testing is helpful and necessary when spontaneous arrhythmia is absent, often the case in patients who have had SCD. Electrophysiologic testing is also important for a complete evaluation of the conduction system, including the sinus node, atrioventricular node, and His-Purkinje

Table 21.3
Invasive Techniques

Strengths
    Arrhythmia variability unimportant
    Can document and expose clinical arrhythmia as necessary
    Useful for localizing arrhythmogenic area
    May expose certain groups of patients at risk for sudden death

Weaknesses
    Morbidity and mortality
    Costly
    Requires special training and equipment
    Definition of drug efficacy uncertain
    Many patients not inducible
    Meaning of nonclinical arrhythmia uncertain
    Normal physiologic changes not accounted for
    Nonreproducibility
    Studies not routinely repeated
    Changes in substrate occurring over time not evaluated

---

system, as conduction abnormalities may be present in patients who have significant underlying heart disease. In some patients, severe conduction problems may have contributed to the sudden death episode. Electrophysiologic studies are also useful for exposing supraventricular tachycardia, especially important in young patients in whom an accessory pathway may be present, and may have been the cause of SCD. In older patients with coronary artery disease, a rapid supraventricular tachycardia may precipitate a serious sustained ventricular tachyarrhythmia. Electrophysiologic testing is essential if nonpharmacologic therapy (surgery, ablation, or implantable device) is considered as a mode of therapy. Electrophysiologic testing is more sensitive and perhaps more accurate for establishing drug efficacy. Noninducibility of a previously induced arrhythmia likely indicates stability of the reentrant circuit and its inability to generate and sustain a reentrant arrhythmia, regardless of the presence of spontaneous ectopy or other "triggers."

Electrophysiologic testing has a number of important limitations. It is costly, especially when repeated several times in a hospitalization. There is also a risk of morbidity and mortality. A single center reported one death in 1000 studies, which has become the commonly quoted statistic for risk of death during diagnostic electrophysiology studies. The other complications were similarly uncommon and were comprised mostly of the morbidity implicit in right heart catheterization. Electrophysiologic testing is generally not repeated during long-term follow-up unless recurrent arrhythmia is documented or suspected because of symptoms. This is an important factor if one considers that the underlying heart disease is itself progressive. Variability of arrhythmia induction in a baseline, drug-free state as well as during drug therapy has been reported and is an important concern. This may be because electrophysiologic testing is performed at one point in time under artificial conditions and does not account for the physiologic changes (modulating factors) that can alter the stability of the substrate. For example, there are a substantial number of SCD victims who do not have inducible arrhythmia, ostensibly because of an alteration in the substrate that gives rise to a reentrant arrhythmia. Variations in inducibility appear to be related to the type of heart disease and/or the presenting arrhythmia.

Although more than 90% of patients with coronary artery disease who present with sustained monomorphic VT have this arrhythmia induced in the laboratory, the rate of induction is substantially less in patients with a nonischemic cardiomyopathy in whom reentrant arrhythmia may not be present and in whom other mechanisms may be responsible. Likewise, when the patient presents with VF or SCD in which the initiating arrhythmia is not documented, as many as 30–40% of patients do not have an arrhythmia induced, even with an aggressive protocol. This is especially the case in those patients who have a nonischemic cardiomyopathy, and is of particular concern in those who undergo drug therapy. In these cases, the inability to induce an arrhythmia in a drug-free state completely obviates the use of the serial drug testing procedure. Inducibility may also be viewed with a jaundiced eye inasmuch as day-to-day variability in this cohort is substantial.

Additionally, a number of patients have nonclinical arrhythmia induced, and its meaning remains uncertain. The only reported reliable endpoint of electrophysiologic testing is a sustained monomorphic VT; thus, the meaning of polymorphic VT or VF induced in the laboratory in a patient who has had syncope or SCD due to VF is uncertain. Of particular concern is the meaning of nonclinical arrhythmia that is induced during drug therapy, because it is uncertain whether this represents an artifact or drug-induced arrhythmia aggravation.

Lastly, the definition of drug efficacy based on electrophysiologic testing remains controversial. Although it is widely accepted that noninducibility of a previously induced VT represents drug efficacy and a good outcome, this endpoint is only infrequently achieved. Indeed, it is not certain what defines noninducibility, specifically, whether induction of <3, <5, or <15 repetitive complexes is the most optimal result. It is possible, although not established, that other endpoints may represent an adequate drug effect, correlating with improved survival, although not predicting freedom from all recurrences of arrhythmia (Fig. 21.2). These include a significant slowing of the rate of the induced VT (by a certain percentage or an increase in the R-R cycle length by >100 msec), greater difficulty in induction, or conversion of a sustained VT to a nonsustained arrhythmia.

Outcome of Guided Pharmacologic Therapy

Generally the first approach to therapy of patients who have had SCD is pharmacologic, guided by objective criteria based upon either an invasive or noninvasive approach. A number of studies have reported that an effective drug, identified by either technique, prevents recurrent arrhythmia and improves survival. It has been observed, however, that an effective drug is more often identified when ambulatory monitoring is used compared to electrophysiology testing. The response rate for individual agents based on the noninvasive approach typically is 50–80%,

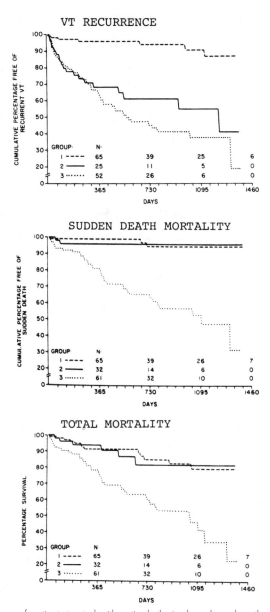

Figure 21.2. Outcome of patients treated with antiarrhythmic drugs based on the results of electrophysiologic testing. Group 1 are patients who were drug responders and were without induced VT. Group 2 patients had VT induced, which was hemodynamically tolerated because of rate slowing, while group 3 patients had no benefit from drugs, and the VT remained rapid and hemodynamically unstable. Although group 2 had a higher frequency of VT recurrence in follow-up, compared with group 1, sudden death and total mortalities were equivalent to the group 1 patients. (From Waller TJ, Kay HR, Spielman SR, Kutalek SP, Greenspan AM, Horowitz LN. Reduction in sudden death and total mortality by antiarrhythmic therapy evaluated by electrophysiologic drug testing: criteria of efficacy in patients with sustained ventricular tachyarrhythmia. J Am Coll Cardiol 1987;10:83–89.)

compared with a 10–25% response rate by invasive criteria (Table 21.4). The lower response rate quoted in the literature may be an artifact of demanding the most rigorous result, that is, complete noninducibility. Nevertheless, the long-term outlook for responders in either group is encouraging. One study of 123 patients referred for management of a sustained ventricular tachyarrhythmia, used monitoring and exercise testing to select an effective antiarrhythmic drug. Effective therapy was responsible for an annual SCD rate of 2.3%, while it was 43.6% in the patients for whom no drug was found to suppress spontaneous arrhythmia (Fig. 21.3).

Table 21.4
Drug Efficacy in the Electrophysiology (EP) Study Versus Electrocardiographic Monitoring Trial

Drug	N Tested	N (%) with Adverse Effects	Efficacy (%) Holter	Efficacy (%) EP
Imipramine	71	43	45	10
Mexiletine	162	27	67	12
Pirmenol	84	23	55	19
Procainamide	116	24	50	26
Propafenone	160	26	48	14
Quinidine	116	24	59	16
Sotalol	196	16	56	35
P value			0.347	<0.001 (Sotalol compared to other drugs)

From Mason JW for the ESVEM Investigators. A comparison of seven antiarrhythmic drugs in patients with ventricular tachyarrhythmias. N Engl J Med 1993;329:452–458.

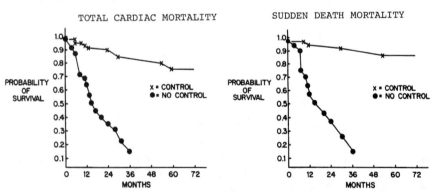

Figure 21.3. Total cardiac and sudden death mortality among 123 SCD patients undergoing a noninvasive method for drug selection. There were 98 patients in whom an antiarrhythmic drug suppressed arrhythmia, based on both ambulatory monitoring and exercise testing (*control*), and 25 patients who failed to respond to any antiarrhythmic agent (*no control*) but who were treated with the most effective agent. (From Graboys TB, Lown B, Podrid PJ, De Silva R. Long-term survival of patients with malignant ventricular arrhythmia treated with antiarrhythmic drugs. Am J Cardiol 1982;50:437–443.)

In a follow-up study of 161 patients with coronary artery disease and a history of sustained VT or VF, suppression of NSVT as assessed by ambulatory monitoring and exercise testing obtained at the time of discharge was a significant predictor of a favorable outcome. At 1 year, the SCD rate was 5% among patients without NSVT, and it was 19% among those with persistent NSVT. At 5 years the SCD rate was 29 and 48%, respectively (P<.02). Similar results were reported in a group of 59 patients. After a follow-up of 700 days, 82% of those who responded to a drug (NSVT was absent on a discharge ambulatory monitor) were free of recurrence in contrast to a 42% event-free survival among those patients with persistent runs of NSVT (P<.002). The sensitivity and specificity of ambulatory monitoring were 100 and 68%, respectively, with a predictive accuracy of 73%. Several other studies in which therapy with amiodarone was evaluated with ambulatory monitoring have also reported that suppression of NSVT by drug correlates with freedom from recurrence.

There have been numerous reports of improved survival in patients with SCD in whom electrophysiologic testing was used for the selection of an effective antiarrhythmic drug. In a group of 131 patients with out-of-hospital SCD, during a 15-month follow-up there were no recurrences among 91 patients who responded to a drug based upon electrophysiologic testing, while there was a 50% recurrence rate in the group with arrhythmia that remained inducible. In a report involving 239 patients followed for 14.8 months, the recurrence rate was 12% when arrhythmia was noninducible on drug therapy compared with 31% when arrhythmia was still induced (Fig. 21.4). Many other studies of similar design have reported comparable results. Overall, electrophysiologic testing has a predictive accuracy of approximately 90%; that is, noninducibility predicts a good outcome and freedom from recurrence in the majority of patients. Although the recurrence rate is higher when an arrhythmia remains inducible by electrophysiologic techniques, as many as 50% of such patients will not have a clinical event during follow-up. The reliability of such statistics is questionable because patients whose arrhythmias remain inducible frequently undergo therapy with a drug deemed "partially effective."

Apparently, both ambulatory monitoring and electrophysiologic testing are useful methods for selecting an effective antiarrhythmic drug. If an effective and well-tolerated drug is identified, recurrent arrhythmia can be prevented. However, it must be emphasized that none of the studies to date involving patients with serious arrhythmia have been placebo-controlled. Therefore, it is uncertain whether antiarrythmic drugs are effective, as has been suggested, or whether a positive response to these agents selects patients who will have a better outcome, irrespective of therapy.

Nonpharmacologic Therapy

Pharmacologic therapy with antiarrhythmic drugs is often the first approach used for the management of the SCD patient, but there are many patients for whom alternative approaches are necessary. This includes patients who do not respond to antiarrhythmic drugs or those who have significant side effects from

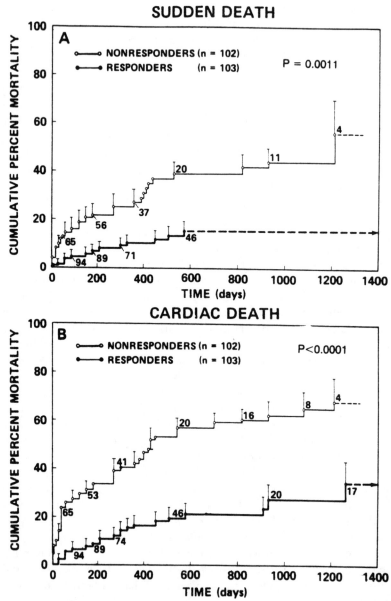

Figure 21.4. Actuarial curves for sudden death and cardiac death in patients responding or not responding to antiarrhythmic drugs as assessed by electrophysiologic testing. (From Swerdlow CD, Winkle RA, Mason JW. Determinants of survival in patients with ventricular tachyarrhythmias. N Engl J Med 1983;308:1436–1439.)

these agents, those who have a recurrence of a serious tachyarrhythmia, despite treatment with what was predicted to be effective therapy, or patients who have no objective way to judge the effect of an antiarrhythmic drug; that is, they have no spontaneous arrhythmia on monitoring and have no arrhythmia induced in the electrophysiology laboratory.

Another factor to consider is that the risk of a cardiac toxic effect from antiarrhythmic drugs is greatest in those patients who often have severe disease, poor LV function, and significant congestive heart failure. For these patients, nonpharmacologic approaches are necessary, including surgery or an implantable defibrillator. In fact, given the dramatic improvements in device technology and concerns about the reliability of drug testing, nonpharmacologic therapy is now considered by some to be the preferred approach in most SCD victims. Ongoing clinical trials hopefully will be able to confirm or refute this notion definitively. An NIH study, Antiarrhythmic Drugs Versus Implantable Devices (AVID), will address this issue in patients with VT or VF who will be randomized to therapy with implantable defibrillators or antiarrhythmic drugs (amiodarone or sotalol).

PROGNOSIS

Using the most sophisticated forms of therapy, including antiarrhythmic drugs, surgery, and a device, the expected survival of the victim resuscitated from SCD is only fair. Much depends on whether the patient has suffered major morbidity from the event itself, especially a neurologic complication. Survival of these patients is very much dependent upon the degree of LV dysfunction, regardless of the form of therapy selected. The survival of those with poor LV function and reduced ejection fraction is significantly less than that of patients with better LV function (Fig. 21.5), regardless of response to drug evaluated invasively or noninvasively. In addition, these patients may be protected from recurrence of arrhythmia and sudden arrhythmic death, but overall survival may not be influenced. This is because these patients generally have far advanced heart disease and often die from progression of the underlying disease state and worsening of LV function. As has been already pointed out, there are as yet no controlled trials proving that survival is enhanced with device or pharmacologic therapy. Likewise, there are no data comparing the outcome of these therapies in patients with preserved versus those with poor ventricular function. Unfortunately, current data are limited by a relatively short period of follow-up, by failing to analyze the adverse effects of device complications and repeated generator changes, and by failing to account for the progression of disease over the observation period. This is especially important in those patients with coronary artery disease who do not have adequate risk factor modification. These patients may be susceptible to new coronary events that may manifest as an arrhythmia that is unrelated to the index event.

Extended life in a patient surviving a sudden death episode has important lifestyle implications. There may be a prolonged and difficult adjustment phase associated with significant psychologic upheaval. Once the patient is discharged from the hospital and returns home, there is a prolonged period of adjustment to an

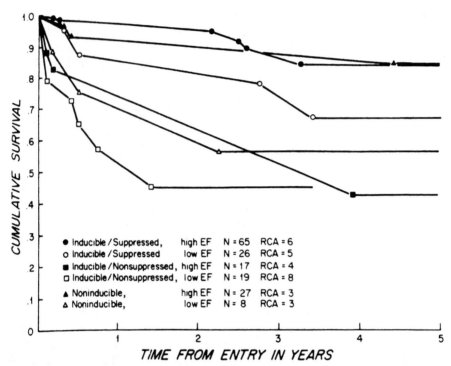

Figure 21.5. Outcome of patients with malignant ventricular tachyarrhythmia based upon drug response evaluated by electrophysiologic testing and ejection fraction (EF): high EF, >30%; low EF, <30% (inducible or noninducible in control, suppressed or nonsuppressed by drug); RCA, recurrent cardiac arrest. (From Wilber DJ, Garan H, Finklestein D, et al. Out-of-hospital cardiac arrest. Use of electrophysiologic testing in the prediction of long-term outcome. N Engl J Med 1988;318:19–24.)

unmonitored and unprotected environment. Those patients who have neurologic deficits as a result of cerebral anoxia from the arrest itself may find it difficult to cope with new mental and physical impairments. The fear of recurrence and the absence of trained personnel who can intervene immediately create worry and panic. Nighttime is especially difficult for the patient. As a result, the patient may experience a number of psychologically mediated symptoms such as dizziness, lightheadedness, and chest discomfort that mimic and may suggest arrhythmia recurrence or even a device discharge. For those patients receiving an implantable defibrillator, the arrhythmia is not prevented, and therefore the patient may still experience loss of consciousness. The very anticipation of such an occurrence itself may cause many psychologic problems for the patient. Also, certain daily activities may be interdicted, for example, driving an automobile. Decisions about these activities should be made on an individual basis.

The occurrence of "inappropriate" discharges for asymptomatic arrhythmias is another source of concern for the patient. Many come to dread device discharges that can cause a significant amount of discomfort if the patient has not lost consciousness. Patients who are treated pharmacologically may magnify their complaints about the side effects from the drugs and require close attention and often careful management. Continued contact with and input from their physician is important, especially during the initial posthospital period, but it is also important that the patient be encouraged to be as active as possible and to avoid chronic dependency which may develop in many of these patients. As mentioned earlier, support groups may be very helpful in allaying fears simply by providing a sympathetic environment wherein the patient's problems can be discussed.

PRIMARY PREVENTION

Although most of the focus of this chapter has been on the management of the patient resuscitated from SCD, it is more rational—but more difficult—to concentrate efforts on primary prevention by identifying those patients at risk and by intervening to prevent the first episode. Given the large number of patients at risk, the difficulties of resuscitation, and the poor survival rates for the majority of victims, the public health impact of effective primary prevention has enormous potential.

The first step in this effort is risk stratification. A fairly simple set of tests may be applied to exclude the lowest risk individuals so that an intervention of low complexity and cost can be applied to the remaining majority of potential victims. An epidemiologic profile is most helpful to identify a subgroup who may be approached, such as patients with coronary artery disease who have had a recent MI. In such patients, a battery of low-risk tests, such as exercise testing, signal-averaged ECG, ambulatory monitoring, and a measurement of global LV function may be advisable. Once this risk assessment has been completed, and the highest risk individuals have been segregated out for the most intensive therapy, it is common practice to prescribe drugs such as β-adrenergic blocking agents and aspirin, interventions with proven benefit. It should be emphasized that the intention of this approach may not be specifically to prevent SCD, but rather to reduce overall mortality, as the interventions used may not be antiarrhythmic. For example, it is possible that the β-blockers reduce mortality unassociated with any effect on ventricular arrhythmia.

Risk stratification may be more aggressive. Here the intention is to identify a smaller population at particularly high risk to target therapy which itself may be harmful. The data to support this approach are much less definitive. There are a number of parameters reported to be of use in post-MI patients for the purpose of risk stratification (Table 21.5). Invasive testing to delineate coronary anatomy

Table 21.5
Risk Stratifiers Postmyocardial Infarction

1. Left ventricular ejection fraction
2. Nonsustained ventricular tachycardia on ambulatory monitoring
3. Late potentials on signal-averaged ECG
4. Inducible VT during electrophysiologic testing (?)
5. Prolonged Q-Tc on surface ECG, a Q-T dispersion
6. Absence of heart rate variability on 24 hr of ambulatory monitoring
7. Abnormal baroreceptor response

may be important in some subgroups, and intervention in these patients may be applied with a realistic expectation of improving outcome, although well-done clinical trials in this area are rare. Similarly, the use of programmed electrical stimulation to define an arrhythmogenic substrate and identify patients at risk for SCD is intuitively appealing but unproven, and itself is the subject of active clinical research. Electrophysiologic studies performed on patients after an acute MI have reported conflicting results (Table 21.6). In patients with a cardiomyopathy, electrophysiologic studies appear to be unhelpful, although there have been several trials that have addressed this issue (Table 21.7). In the future, it may be feasible to apply such testing to individuals with a high pretest probability of having a positive test, such as those with a reduced LV ejection fraction, NSVT on ambulatory monitoring, or a late potential on signal-averaged ECG. Because the interventions that could be employed as a result of these tests themselves carry a significant chance of harm, we will require definite evidence of benefit before recommending that they be applied to the large population at risk.

Most of the information available regarding primary prevention comes from studies of patients with ischemic heart disease. We have much less information to guide the evaluation and management of patients with other forms of heart disease. Nevertheless, patients with all forms of heart disease have an increased susceptibility to SCD, and the magnitude can be defined epidemiologically. Unfortunately, when the event rates are low, as in patients with intact LV function, studies of methods that could further define risk are problematic. Without a high event rate, these studies require recruitment of such large number of patients that valid conclusions can almost never be reached within the constraints of a modern clinical trial. Similar problems exist for intervention analyses.

Redefining epidemiologic principles remains one of the most important tasks in future research. Likewise, techniques of risk assessment must be better understood and defined. Once these methods are more exacting, it may be possible to apply more sophisticated methods to protect patients, such as the use of simpler, cheaper, more plentiful antitachycardia devices, implanted prophylactically in the highest-risk individuals. Other options will include drugs designed to be mechanism-specific so that they may protect against arrhythmic events without exposing the patient to the potential toxicity of conventional antiarrhythmic agents. These efforts will be the challenge of the next decade of research in the field of SCD.

Table 21.6
Electrophysiologic Studies in Patients after Myocardial Infarction

Study	No. of Patients	Follow-up (Mo)	Inducible (%)	No. with Arrhythmia (%)	Non-inducible (%)	No. with Arrhythmia (%)	EP Prognostic
Hamer et al. (1982)	70	12	12 (17)	5 (33)	58 (83)	5 (9)	Yes
Richards et al. (1983)	165	12	38 (23)	13 (21)	127 (77)	3 (2)	Yes
Marchlinski et al. (1983)	46	18	10 (22)	1 (6)	36 (78)	5 (14)	No
Waspe et al. (1985)	50	23	17 (34)	7 (41)	33 (61)	0 (0)	Yes
Roy et al. (1985)	150	10	35 (23)	2 (6)	115 (72)	2 (2)	No
Santarelli et al. (1985)	50	11	33 (46)	0 (0)	27 (54)	0 (0)	No
Breithardt et al. (1982)	132	15	61 (46)	10 (16)	71 (54)	3 (4)	Yes
Bhandari et al. (1985)	45	12	20 (44)	2 (10)	35 (56)	1 (3)	No
Gonzales et al. (1984)	84	20	19 (23)	0 (0)	65 (77)	4 (6)	No
Kowey et al. (1990)	187	18	119 (64)	25 (21)	68 (36)	20 (29)	No
	979		364 (36)	65 (18)	615 (65)	43 (7)	

Table 21.7
Role of Electrophysiologic Studies in Patients with Cardiomyopathy and NSVT

Study	No. with Cardiomyopathy	No. Inducible (%)	Follow-up (mo)	Prediction
Veltri et al. (1985)	6	3 (50)	23	No
Sulpizi et al. (1987)	9	5 (56)	29	No
Das et al. (1986)	24	8 (33)	12	No
Poll et al. (1986)	20	1 (5)	18	No
Gomes et al. (1984)	10		30	Yes
Zheutlin et al. (1986)	13	7 (54)	22	Yes
Buxton et al. (1984)	18	9)50)	33	No
		14 (50) CAD		
Hammill et al. (1990)	53		50	No
		1 (4) idio		

SUGGESTED READING

Kowey PR, Marinchak RA, Rials SJ. Sudden death prevention after myocardial infarction: what are the choices? J Cardiovasc Electrophysiol 1991;2(suppl S):S192–S201.

Lown B, Wolf M. Approaches to sudden death from coronary heart disease. Circulation 1971; 44:130–142.

Myerburg RJ, Castellanos A. Cardiac arrest and sudden cardiac death. In: Braunwald E, ed. Heart disease. A textbook of cardiovascular medicine. 4th ed. Philadelphia: WB Saunders, 1992:756–789.

Myerburg RJ, Kessler KM, Castellanos A. Sudden cardiac death: epidemiology, transient risk, and intervention assessment. Ann Intern Med 1993;119:1187–1197.

Myerburg RJ, Kessler KM, Zaman L, et al. Factors leading to decreasing mortality among patients resuscitated from out-of-hospital cardiac arrest. In: Brugada P, Wellens HJJ, eds. Cardiac arrhythmias: where do we go from here? Mount Kisco, NY: Futura, 1987:505–525.

Ward DE, Camm AJ. Dangerous ventricular arrhythmias—can we predict drug efficacy [Editorial]. N Engl J Med 1993;329:498–499.

22 Supraventricular Tachycardia: Diagnosis and Etiology

ROLE OF 12-LEAD ELECTROCARDIOGRAM IN THE DIAGNOSIS OF NARROW COMPLEX QRS TACHYCARDIAS

Narrow QRS tachycardias fall into two broad categories: atrial and atrioventricular (AV) junctional (Table 22.1). Of the latter, most are either due to AV nodal reentry or AV reentry involving an accessory AV connection. Fig. 22.1 provides a simple algorithm for the differentiation of these arrhythmias..

Table 22.1
Classification of SVT Based on Site of Origin with Usual Electrocardiographic features

	ECG Appearance
Atrial	
Atrial fibrillation	P waves substituted by multiple "F" waves of variable amplitude and morphology. Ventricular rate irregularly irregular.
Atrial flutter Type I Type II	Organized, regular, and rapid atrial rhythm (usually around 300/min) with a characteristic morphology in leads II, III, and aVF. Ventricular rate may be regular or irregular.
Multifocal atrial tachycardia	Presence of at least three different P-wave morphologies. Varying P-P, P-R, and R-R intervals.
Unifocal atrial tachycardia Paroxysmal Sinoatrial reentry Intraatrial reentry Nonparoxysmal Automatic atrial	P waves usually identified and frequently precede the QRS. AV dissociation may be present or demonstrable. P-wave morphology similar to sinus rhythm. P wave morphology depends on site of origin of tachycardia. Spontaneous onset and rate may vary depending on autonomic tone.
AV junctional	
AVNRT Common (slow:fast) Uncommon (fast:slow) Others (slow:slow)	Pwave usually not identified (85%) or may deform end of QRS (10–15%). Inverted P waves in II, III, and aVF with long R-P and short P-R. P wave location intermediate with R-P:P-R ratio close to 1.
Automatic junctional tachycardia	AV dissociation common. Rate may be irregular because of occasional sinus capture.
AVRT (Circus movement tachycardia) Paroxysmal Permanent	AV dissociation never seen. P wave following QRS may be identified in 70–80% of cases. Spontaneous onset with long R-P and short P-R. P wave inverted in II, III, and aVF.

AVNRT, AV nodal reentrant tachycardia; AVRT, AV reentrant tachycardia (accessory pathway)

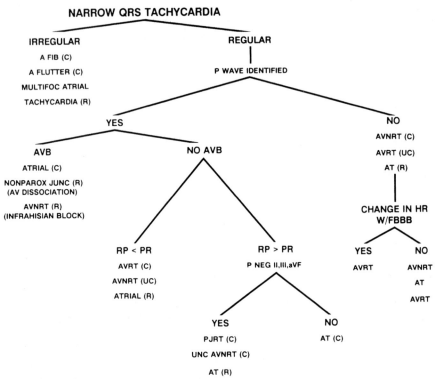

Figure 22.1. A simple algorithm for the differential diagnosis of narrow QRS tachycardia by surface electrocardiography. The frequency with which a specific feature is seen is indicated in parentheses. AT, atrial tachycardia; AVNRT, atrioventricular nodal reentrant tachycardia; AVRT, atrioventricular reentrant tachycardia; C, common; FBBB, functional bundle branch block; PJRT, permanent form of junctional reciprocating tachycardia; R, rare; UC, or UNC uncommon.

Regularity of Tachycardia

An irregular ventricular rate during tachycardia suggests the presence of either a continually changing tachycardia cycle length or variable AV block or both. The former is usually seen in atrial fibrillation (AF) when no organized atrial activity is seen on the surface electrocardiogram (ECG) or during multifocal atrial tachycardia in which the P wave activity is identifiable but is irregular and has multiple morphologies. In other types of atrial tachycardia or atrial flutter, although the atrial activity is regular, variable AV block results in an irregular ventricular rate. In AV junctional tachycardias, on the other hand, except for minor beat-to-beat variability, the heart rate is regular. A characteristic, albeit uncommon finding in patients with accessory pathway-mediated tachycardia is an abrupt decrease in heart rate with the development of ipsilateral functional bundle branch block, although the rhythm is still regular.

PRESENCE OF AV BLOCK DURING TACHYCARDIA

Demonstration of AV block during tachycardia is strong presumptive evidence for an atrial origin of the tachycardia (Fig. 22.2). When 1-1 AV conduction is seen, it may be useful to produce transient AV block either by vagal maneuvers, such as carotid sinus massage, or by the use of AV nodal blocking agents. Perpetuation of tachycardia, despite AV block, occurs primarily with atrial tachycardia (Fig. 22.3). Participation of the AV node in the tachycardia circuit can be presumed if tachy-

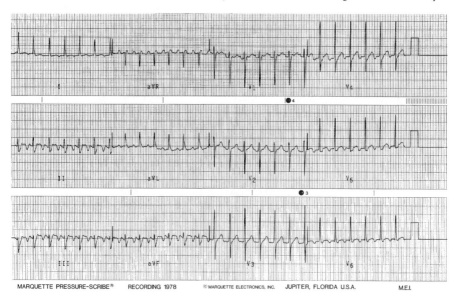

Figure 22.2. 2:1 Block during SVT. A 12-lead ECG of atrial flutter with 2:1 AV block is shown. With the aid of multiple electrocardiographic lead recordings (best seen in lead aVR in this example), atrial flutter with 2:1 AV conduction is noted.

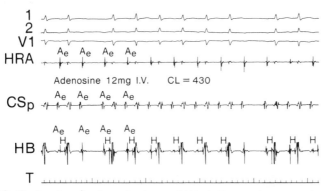

Figure 22.3. Continuation of tachycardia despite AV block. Tracings from top to bottom are ECG leads (1, 2, and V₁), high right atrial (HRA) electrogram, proximal coronary sinus (CSp) electrogram, His bundle (HB) electrogram, and time lines (T). Recordings obtained following administration of adenosine reveal a continuation of tachycardia, cycle length (CL), 430 msec, despite the presence of AV nodal block.

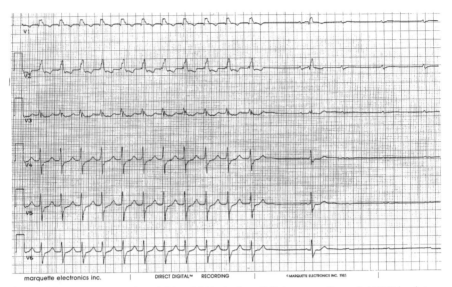

Figure 22.4. Diagnostic value of AV nodal blockade in SVT diagnosis. Precordial ECG leads in a patient with orthodromic reciprocating tachycardia with right bundle branch aberration is shown. Following administration of adenosine, termination of tachycardia is seen with a P wave not followed by a QRS, suggesting that the tachycardia circuit involves the AV node in the antegrade direction.

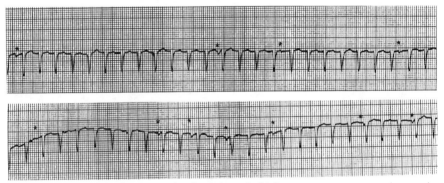

Figure 22.5. Example of a junctional tachycardia with AV dissociation in a patient with an underlying cardiomyopathy. Seen is a narrow complex junctional tachycardia at a rate of 180. Intermittently seen are P waves (asterisks).

cardia terminates with antegrade block, i.e., with a P wave that is not followed by a QRS, because the site of block with vagal maneuvers or adenosine is usually the AV node (Fig. 22.4). Occasionally AV block may be seen during AV junctional tachycardias as well. When AV block is seen during AVNRT, the site of block is usually infra-Hisian and functional in nature (except in patients with prior His-Purkinje disease).

Another AV junctional tachycardia in which AV dissociation may be present is the nonparoxysmal form of AV junctional tachycardia (Fig. 22.5). This arrhythmia is often seen in the postoperative population and at times after acute myocardial infarction (MI) and is due to increased automaticity in the AV node. Frequently, the ventricular rate exceeds the atrial rate during the tachycardia. Because of occasional sinus capture, this rhythm at times may be irregular. In an accessory pathway-mediated tachycardia, AV dissociation is never seen, as the atrium is a necessary part of the circuit.

P-QRS RELATIONSHIP

In the diagnosis of tachycardias with 1-1 AV conduction, the location of the P wave in relation to the QRS is helpful (Fig. 22.6). Part of the reason for this is the fact that most of these arrhythmias are of AV junctional origin, and continuation of tachycardia requires intact conduction in the antegrade and retrograde directions. It is useful to classify these tachycardias on the basis of the P wave location into those with short R-P-long P-R intervals and long R-P-short P-R intervals. A third not uncommon category are tachycardias in which the P waves cannot be recognized on the surface ECG.

SHORT R-P-LONG P-R TACHYCARDIAS

In these tachycardias the P-R interval is longer than the R-P interval. This electrocardiographic appearance may be seen in the orthodromic type of AV reentrant tachycardia, as the conduction time in the antegrade direction via the AV node is

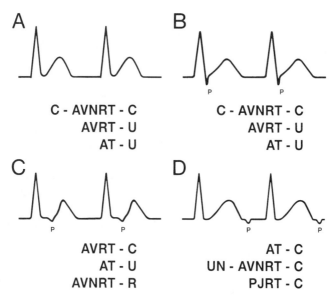

Figure 22.6. Relationship of P to QRS in SVTs. AVNRT, AV node reentrant tachycardia; AVRT, AV reentrant tachycardia; AT, atrial tachycardia; PJRT, permanent junctional reciprocating tachycardia; C, common; U, uncommon; R, rare.F

frequently longer than the retrograde conduction time through the accessory pathway. This results in a short R-P and a long P-R interval. Occasionally in left-sided pathways, the R-P interval—which is a reflection of intramyocardial and accessory pathway conduction—is sufficiently long enough for the R-P:P-R ratio to approach 1 and may even exceed it. A short R-P-long P-R electrocardiographic appearance may also be seen in the common form of AV node reentrant tachycardia, where the slow pathway of the AV node is used antegradely and the fast pathway retrogradely. A similar type of electrocardiographic appearance is less frequent with atrial tachycardia, unless there is concomitant AV conduction delay. The latter is usually physiologic and secondary to the atrial tachycardia rate encroaching on AV nodal refractoriness.

LONG R-P-SHORT P-R TACHYCARDIAS

This type of electrocardiographic appearance would require a reversal of conduction characteristics mentioned earlier, i.e., fast antegrade conduction and slow retrograde conduction, and is seen in both the uncommon type of AVNRT and the permanent form of junctional reciprocating tachycardia. A long R-P-short P-R relationship is also common in atrial tachycardias. Because the presence or absence of ventriculoatrial conduction is incidental in atrial tachycardias, the P wave location is determined by the degree of AV conduction delay. Therefore, in the absence of significant AV conduction delay, the P-R interval is usually shorter than the R-P interval.

NO IDENTIFIABLE P WAVES

A P wave distinct from the QRS may not be appreciable in nearly half of the patients with sustained ventricular tachycardias (SVTs). In common AVNRT, as the P wave occurs simultaneously with the QRS, it is frequently obscured by the latter. Inscription of the P wave in the terminal part of the QRS during AVNRT sometimes results in the so-called pseudo-R deflection in V_1 or an S wave in 2, 3, and AVF. However, appreciation of this change requires comparison with the ECG after tachycardia termination. Less commonly, in the orthodromic type of AV reentry and atrial tachycardia, the timing, magnitude, or polarity of the P wave may prevent its recognition. Hence, although the recognition of a P wave on the surface ECG is suggestive of either an AV reentrant or atrial tachycardia, these diagnoses cannot be excluded if P waves cannot be identified. Absence of a visible P wave on the surface ECG does, however, usually reflect 1:1 AV relationship, where the P wave has a fixed timing relative to the QRS. If the P wave has an inconsistent relationship with the QRS (such as AV dissociation), the presence of the P wave may be suspected because it is likely to alter the appearance of the ST-T segment.

INITIATION AND TERMINATION

Onset of SVTs, when observed, may offer clues to possible mechanisms. Initiation of SVT during sinus rhythm is often seen in the incessant types of SVT, such as a permanent form of junctional reciprocating tachycardia and atrial ectopic tachycardia. AV reentrant tachycardia and AV nodal reentrant tachycardia are frequently initiated by a premature atrial contraction. The P-R interval of these premature beats is frequently prolonged because of antegrade conduction via the slow pathway, which has a short refractory period. At the same time there is antegrade block in the fast pathway, which has a longer refractory period. This slow AV conduction facilitates recovery of retrograde conduction in the fast pathway, which is usually required for initiation of tachycardia. Although premature ventricular contractions can also induce all types of SVT, they are more likely to induce tachycardias associated with accessory AV connections.

Termination of tachycardia with AV nodal block, i.e., with a P wave not followed by a QRS, usually implies that the AV node is part of the reentrant circuit. This may occur spontaneously or be induced by vagal maneuvers or intravenous (i.v.) adenosine. Atrial tachycardia usually terminates with a QRS not followed by a P wave, except in an unusual situation, such as when accompanied by concomitant AV block as may be seen occasionally with adenosine administration. AV junctional tachycardia may also terminate with a QRS not followed by a P wave when tachycardia termination occurs with block in the retrograde limb of the tachycardia circuit (fast pathway of the AV node or accessory pathway in AVNRT and AV reentrant tachycardia, respectively).

Other electrocardiographic features that have been used in the differential diagnosis of SVTs include the heart rate and the presence of QRS alternans. Both of these findings are relatively insensitive and nonspecific, although the latter if noted during slower tachycardias is suggestive of AV reentry. Vagal maneuvers, e.g., carotid sinus massage or AV nodal blocking agents such as verapamil or adenosine, may be used both from a therapeutic as well as a diagnostic viewpoint and are primarily helpful in differentiating atrial from AV junctional tachycardias (Figs. 22.3 and 22.4).

ELECTROPHYSIOLOGIC BASIS OF SUPRAVENTRICULAR TACHYCARDIAS

AV NODE REENTRANT TACHYCARDIA

The electrophysiologic basis of AV node reentrant tachycardia is the presence of a reentry circuit in the AV node. It consists of two or more AV nodal pathways with different conduction times and refractory period properties. This is best demonstrated by the atrial extrastimulus technique. In patients with dual AV nodal physiology, at a critical coupling interval, the effective refractory period of the fast pathway is reached, and conduction proceeds through the slower conducting pathway that has a shorter refractory period. Thus, rather than a gradual prolongation, a sudden prolongation in the A-H intervals is seen. Depending on the conduction time of the slow pathway and the site of block in the fast pathway, the impulse traveling down the slow pathway may be able to turn around and conduct up the fast pathway, resulting in an AV nodal echo beat. Continuation of this phenomenon results in sustained AV nodal reentrant tachycardia of the common type. The retrograde His to atrial interval is <50 msec.

In the uncommon variety of AV nodal reentry, the direction of impulse propagation is reversed, with antegrade conduction occurring over the fast pathway and retrograde over the slow pathway. Tachycardia can be initiated either by atrial or ventricular pacing. During the atrial extrastimulus method, the tachycardia starts with relatively minor prolongation of the A-H interval as the tachycardia circuit employs the fast pathway for antegrade conduction.

It can be appreciated that the common type of AVNRT has a long A-H and short H-A interval and in the uncommon variety this relationship is reversed. The atrial activation sequence in these two varieties of AVNRT are also frequently different with the earliest atrial activation occurring in the region of the His bundle recording site in common AVNRT, and around the coronary sinus ostium in the uncommon variety.

ORTHODROMIC RECIPROCATING TACHYCARDIA

Perhaps the most common tachycardia associated with AV connections and the only tachycardia in which the concealed accessory pathways participate is orthodromic tachycardia. This tachycardia circuit involves antegrade conduction from the atrium to the ventricle via the AV node-His-Purkinje system (AVN-HPS) and retrograde conduction back to the atrium through the accessory pathway.

The electrophysiologic differentiation of this arrhythmia from AVNRT and atrial tachycardia is usually straightforward. The V-A interval during tachycardia is usually constant and exceeds 60 msec, and the introduction of premature ventricular complexes during tachycardia timed when the His bundle is refractory from antegrade conduction is able to advance atrial activation. This finding is diagnostic of the presence of an accessory pathway, as atrial advancement can only occur if an alternate conduit to ventriculoatrial (V-A) conduction is present. However, inability to preexcite the atrium does not exclude the presence of an accessory pathway.

PREEXCITED TACHYCARDIAS

In the presence of accessory pathways capable of rapid antegrade conduction, several mechanisms may result in preexcited tachycardias. In true antidromic tachycardia, the accessory pathway functions as the antegrade limb and the HPS-AVN as the retrograde limb of the tachycardia circuit. All types of atrial rhythms may result in preexcited tachycardias. Identification of the nature of the underlying atrial activity and the demonstration of AV dissociation are the keys to characterization of these arrhythmias.

UNUSUAL ACCESSORY PATHWAY-MEDIATED TACHYCARDIAS

In permanent junctional reciprocating tachycardias, the antegrade limb is the AVN-HPS, and the retrograde limb is a concealed accessory pathway with a long conduction time and decremental properties reminiscent of the AV node. Because antegrade conduction via the AV node is faster than retrograde conduction through the accessory pathway, this tachycardia bears a strong resemblance to the uncommon type of AVNRT. In fact, this pathway may represent an accessory AV node.

Recent observations suggest that pathways formerly considered to be nodoventricular Mahaim (AV node to ventricular myocardium) are more likely atriofascicular in nature, arising from the right atrium and inserting into the right bundle. During right atrial pacing, increasing preexcitation with a typical left bundle branch block pattern is seen. Tachycardia initiation requires antegrade AV nodal block, conduction down the accessory pathway, and return to the atrium via the right bundle to the His and AV node. Therefore, the typical electrophysiologic appearance is that of a preexcited tachycardia with a typical left bundle branch block morphology, right bundle recording preceding His bundle recording, and atrial activation via the normal pathway.

ATRIAL TACHYCARDIAS

These tachycardias are a heterogeneous group of tachyarrhythmias that arise above the AV junction. The electrophysiologic hallmark of this group of tachycardias is the demonstration that AV conduction is not required for initiation or perpetuation of the tachycardia. This may be readily apparent on the surface ECG or may require vagal or pharmacologic maneuvers or electrophysiologic testing.

Type 1 or common atrial flutter generally has a rate of around 300 beats/minute, with a sawtooth appearance on the surface ECG. It also has an excitable gap, and is therefore amenable to overdrive pacing. The reentrant circuit in this tachycardia appears to be confined to the right atrium.

Sinus node reentry and atrial reentrant tachycardia share many similarities electrophysiologically and, as the name implies, have features that during programmed electrical stimulation suggest a reentrant mechanism, such as initiation and termination with programmed stimulation and entrainment. The atrial activation pattern in sinus node reentry shows an atrial activation sequence similar to sinus beats (Fig. 22.7), and, in atrial tachycardia, it is dependent upon the site of origin of the tachycardia.

An incessant form of atrial tachycardia occurring predominantly in the pediatric age group is the so-called "automatic atrial ectopic tachycardia." Unlike the tachycardia discussed previously, these tachycardias are not initiated or terminated by incremental atrial pacing or programmed atrial stimulation, although they may be temporarily suppressed by the former.

PRACTICAL APPROACH TO THE DIAGNOSIS OF A TACHYCARDIA WITH A WIDE QRS COMPLEX

Causes of a Wide QRS Tachycardia

Tachycardias with a wide QRS complex (QRS width ≥ 0.12 seconds) can originate in supraventricular or ventricular structures (Table 22.2). During SVT, widening of the QRS complex occurs when the supraventricular impulse is conducted

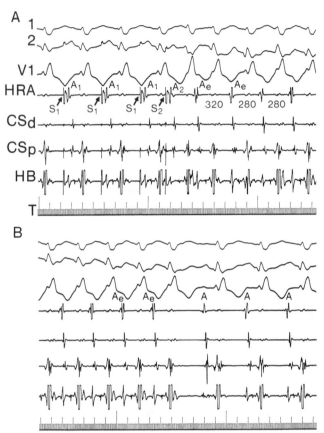

Figure 22.7. Electrophysiologic features of sinoatrial reentrant tachycardia. Tracings from top to bottom are surface ECG leads (1, 2, V₁), high right atrial (HRA) electrogram, proximal (CSp), and distal (CSd) coronary sinus electrograms, His bundle (HB) electrogram and time lines (T). At a drive cycle length of 350 msec, an atrial premature beat (A2) initiates a tachycardia. Several features suggest sinoatrial reentry as the mechanism of the tachycardia. The sequence of atrial activation is similar to that during sinus rhythm; no consistent V-A relationship is seen, especially at the initiation of the tachycardia, and the tachycardia terminates with an A followed by a V. This latter finding is less likely to be seen in AVNRT and orthodromic tachycardia where tachycardia usually terminates with AV nodal block (A not followed by a V). Ae, atrial echo; A, atrial; S, sinus.

antegradely over an accessory pathway or when conduction over the normal intraventricular conduction system is blocked in either the right or the left bundle. When aberrant intraventricular conduction is already present during sinus rhythm and before the onset of the tachycardia, it is called preexistent. When intraventricular conduction is normal during sinus rhythm but aberrant during tachycardia, two main mechanisms have to be considered. Functional or physiologic phase 3 aberration may occur in normal fibers and is rate related. Patients receiving antiarrhythmic drugs, especially the Ic agents, may have a rate-related aberration as a result of the drug's depressant effect in intraventricular conduction. These

Table 22.2
Causes of a Wide QRS Complex Tachycardia

1. VT
2. Any type of SVT
   + bundle branch block, preexistent
     Rate (phase 3)-dependent
     Concealed retrograde conduction
   + Antegrade conduction over AP

agents have "use-dependent" effects, i.e., the slowing of conduction is more pronounced at higher heart rates. Hence, they may cause a rate-related aberrancy.

In a preexcitation syndrome, if antegrade conduction occurs over an accessory pathway and retrograde conduction occurs either over the AV node or another accessory pathway (antidromic tachycardia), a wide QRS complex tachycardia results. This presentation is very difficult to differentiate from VT, because in both forms, ventricular activation starts outside the normal intraventricular conduction system.

Finally, it should be stressed that widening of the QRS complex can occur in any type of supraventricular arrhythmia (atrial tachycardia, atrial flutter, AF, AV nodal reentrant, and AV reentrant tachycardias) and may also be seen with sinus tachycardia.

General Clinical Approach to Diagnosis of a Wide Complex Tachycardia

The approach to establishing the etiology of a wide complex tachycardia involves evaluation of information obtained from the history, physical examination, response to certain maneuvers, as well as careful inspection of the ECG, including a rhythm strip and a 12-lead tracing (Table 22.3). Comparison of the ECG during the tachycardia with that recorded during sinus rhythm is of great importance.

HISTORY

Patients with VT tend to be older than those with an SVT, but there is a great deal of overlap, making this assumption unreliable. The presence of structural heart disease, especially coronary artery disease and a previous MI, is of particular importance and strongly suggests VT as an etiology. The length of time during which the tachycardia has occurred is of some help, and when it has been present for >3 years, an SVT is more likely. The first occurrence of the tachycardia after a MI strongly suggests VT as the etiology. Therapy with antiarrhythmic drugs is important, as it might result in rate-related aberration during any supraventricular arrhythmia (sinus tachycardia, atrial flutter or AF, and SVT).

PRESENTING SYMPTOMS

The symptoms associated with a tachycardia may be mild, such as palpitations, lightheadedness, weakness, diaphoresis, a chest sensation, or polyuria. Symptoms reflecting hemodynamic instability, include dizziness, angina, presyncope or syn-

Table 22.3
Wide Complex Tachycardia: VT versus SVT with Aberrancy

Diagnostic Aids	Usefulness
Presenting symptom	Unhelpful
History	
CAD[a] and previous MI	VT
First arrhythmia after MI	VT
Physical exam	
Evidence of AV dissociation	VT
Blood pressure	Unhelpful
Heart rate	Unhelpful
ECG	
Rate	Unhelpful
QRS width >0.16	VT
QRS width <0.16	Unhelpful
Axis shift	VT
Left axis	Suggests VT
Right or normal axis	Unhelpful
QRS morphology	Usually helpful
Positive QRS concordance	VT
Negative QRS concordance	Unhelpful
AV dissociation	Unhelpful
No AV dissociation	
Response to lidocaine	Suggests VT
Response to verapamil	Suggests SVT

[a]CAD, coronary artery disease; MI, myocardial infarction.

cope, and cardiogenic shock or seizures. Hemodynamic effects and symptoms are not related to the mechanism but are the result of the elevated heart rate, associated heart disease, and left ventricular function. They are also related to the presence of AV asynchrony and the location of the VT focus and hence sequence pattern of the left ventricular activation.

PHYSICAL EXAMINATION

Blood pressure and heart rate are not helpful. However, evidence of AV dissociation is of great importance. In approximately 60–75% of patients with VT, AV dissociation is present (although not always evident), while it is rarely seen in SVT. The presence of AV dissociation may be established with the ECG or physical examination (Table 22.4).

AV dissociation results in AV asynchrony and hence variability in the relationship between atrial and ventricular contraction. Examination of the jugular pulsation in the neck reveals cannon "A" waves, which are intermittent and irregular pulsations of greater amplitude, reflecting simultaneous atrial and ventricular contraction. The contraction of the atria against a closed AV valve produces a transient increase in atrial and venous pressure. There is fluctuation in the blood pressure, which may be highly variable because of the variability in the degree of atrial contribution to left ventricular filling, stroke volume, and cardiac output. As a result of AV asynchrony, there is variability in the occurrence and intensity of heart sounds, especially S1.

RESPONSE TO INTERVENTIONS

Carotid sinus pressure results in an enhancement of vagal tone and hence depresses sinus and AV nodal activity. The heart rate during sinus tachycardia will gradually slow with carotid sinus pressure and then accelerate upon release. The ventricular rate of atrial tachycardia and atrial flutter will also transiently slow, the result of increased AV nodal blockade. The arrhythmia itself, which is generated within the atria, is unaffected. An SVT will either terminate or remain unaltered. In general, VT is unaffected, although carotid sinus pressure will slow the atrial rate and in some cases will expose the presence of AV dissociation not otherwise obvious, establishing the diagnosis of VT. In rare cases, a VT may terminate with carotid sinus pressure. Response to lidocaine suggests, but does not prove, that VT is the mechanism, while a response to digoxin, verapamil, or adenosine strongly suggests SVT, although very infrequently VT may terminate. However, unless the etiology for the wide complex tachycardia is definitely established, verapamil and even adenosine should not be given, as they have been reported to cause hemodynamic collapse in patients with VT.

Table 22.4
Establishing AV Dissociation

1. Physical examination
   a. Cannon "A" waves
   b. "Cacophony" of heart sounds
   c. Variability of first heart sound
   d. Variability of blood pressure

2. ECG
   a. Dissociated P waves with rate slower than ventricular rate
   b. Irregular changes in S-T waves
   c. Non-rate-related changes in QRS width and morphology
   d. Fusion betats
   e. Dressler beats (intermittent capture)

3. Esophageal lead (or NG tube or central i.v. line)
   a. P wave and QRS complexes at different rates

4. EP techniques
   a. Dissociated atrial electrograms with cycle length greater than ventricular electrograms
   b. No His electrogram before the ventricular electrogram (none present or follows the ventricular electrogram)
   c. His potential preceding ventricular electrogram with short H-V interval

NG, nasogastric.

ELECTROCARDIOGRAM

Careful inspection of the ECG (12-lead and rhythm strip) is of great importance. Additionally, comparison of the ECG obtained during the tachycardia with an ECG recorded during sinus rhythm is very helpful (Fig. 22.8). A significant shift in axis and marked change in QRS morphology are of great diagnostic help in establishing VT, while their similarity suggests SVT. VT is often associated with slight irregularity of R-R intervals, subtle or more marked variation of QRS morphology, and variability in ST-T waves (Figs. 22.8 and 22.9). Occasionally seen is evidence of AV dissociation, manifest as obviously dissociated P waves (Fig. 22.10), fusion beats, and intermittent captured (Dressler) beats (Figs. 22.11 and 22.12). In some cases marked changes in the QRS morphology and ST- and T-waves are manifestations of AV dissociation (Figs. 22.8A and 22.12). With SVT there is uniformity of the R-R intervals, QRS morphology, and ST and T waves. This occurs because the activation of the ventricular myocardium always follows the same pathway, which involves the AV node and His-Purkinje system or an accessory bypass tract. Usually there is 1:1 atrial and ventricular activity.

ESTABLISHING AV DISSOCIATION

The most diagnostic ECG finding associated with VT is the presence of AV dissociation. AV dissociation results from the absence of retrograde atrial activation (i.e., no V-A conduction) due to retrograde AV nodal block. Hence, atrial activity or the P wave is independent of the ventricular activity or QRS complex and is usually at a rate slower than the ventricular rate. Dissociated P waves may be obvious on the ECG or rhythm strip or may be superimposed on the ST segment or T-wave, altering their morphology. If P waves are not obvious nor suggested on the ECG, alternative methods for their identification are the use of a modified chest lead placement (Lewis leads), carotid sinus pressure, an esophageal lead (using an electrode wire or nasogastric tube), or a right atrial recording obtained by an electrode catheter in the right atrium or from a central i.v. line. Certainly invasive electrophysiologic (EP) studies will expose AV dissociation if present, establishing the diagnosis (Fig. 22.13).

The presence of a fusion beat that has a morphology intermediate between the sinus beat and ventricular complex results from simultaneous activation of the ventricular myocardium via the atrium and AV node and from the ventricular focus (Fig. 22.12). An intermittent captured or a Dressler beat is a QRS complex that is normalized and is identical to the sinus QRS complex (Fig. 22.11). It results from ventricular activation, which is entirely the result of impulse conduction from the atrium via the AV node and His-Purkinje system. Fusion and Dressler beats are features of AV dissociation and are more commonly seen when the tachycardia rate is slower. Fusion and capture do not alter the rate of the VT, although they may produce a change in R-R intervals. However, a narrower beat during a wide QRS tachycardia is not always a marker for VT. It may occur in SVT with bundle branch block and PVCs arising in the ventricle near to or within the bundle branch

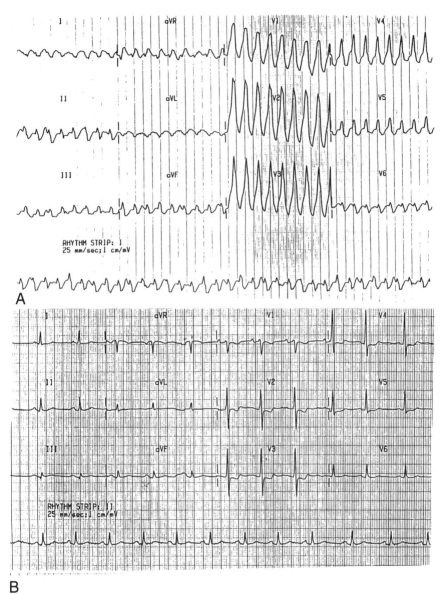

Figure 22.8. A. Example of a wide complex tachycardia. The axis is rightward (negative QRS complexes in leads I and aVL), and there are tall, monophasic R waves in leads V_1–V_5 and a deep S wave in V_6. These ECG findings favor VT. Most importantly, there is evidence of AV dissociation, best seen in leads II, III, and aVF. The II rhythm strip shows obviously dissociated P waves as well as marked changes in QRS morphology and of the ST segments and T waves. B was recorded after sinus rhythm was restored. The ECG shows a normal axis and normal QRS morphology in the limb and precordial leads.

LEAD II CONTINUOUS TRACING

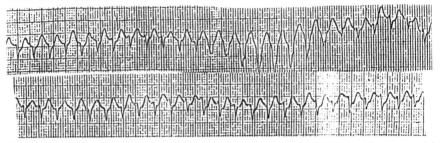

Figure 22.9. Continous lead II rhythm strip of VT. Seen are subtle changes in the ST segments and T waves. Importantly, there is a sudden change of QRS morphology, becoming widened, which is not rate-related but occurs spontaneously.

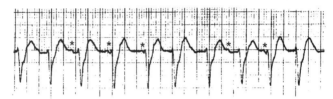

Figure 22.10. Example of VT with obvious AV dissociation. P waves (*asterisks*) are dissociated from the QRS complexes and occur at a rate slower than the ventricular rate.

that has the block. Furthermore, in Wolff-Parkinson-White syndrome, AF occasionally can conduct over the AV nodal-His axis, resulting in narrower beats, although in this case the R-R intervals are very irregular.

Classic ECG Criteria for the Differential Diagnosis Between Ventricular Tachycardia and Supraventricular Tachycardia with Aberrant Conduction

Classic criteria suggestive of VT or SVT are summarized in Figure 22.14.

QRS MORPHOLOGY PATTERN IN THE PRECORDIAL LEADS

V1-Positive Wide QRS Tachycardias

RBBB aberrancy can be identified in lead V_1 from a triphasic rSR' pattern and in lead V_6 from a triphasic qRS pattern with the R:S ratio greater than 1.

The small initial waves (rV_1 and qV_6) reflect normal septal activation that is preserved in RBBB, whereas the tall terminal forces ($R'V_1$ and SV_6) indicate late activation of the right ventricle, due to conduction delay in the right bundle.

In VT, intraventricular conduction is bizarre and does not follow the rules that apply to functional or structural interruption of the normal conduction system. A monophasic R or a biphasic qR pattern in lead V_1 and a deep S-wave (R:S ratio <1) in lead V_6 suggest a ventricular origin of the tachycardia.

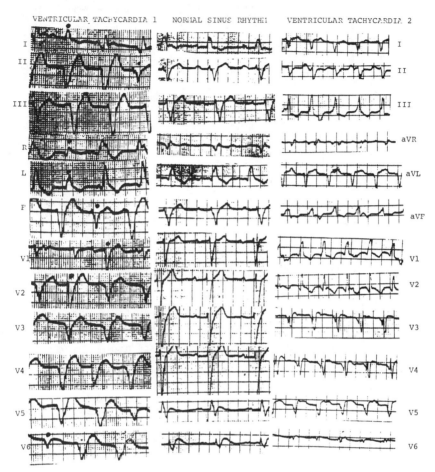

Figure 22.11. Patient with VT of two different morphologies. Ventricular tachycardia 1 has a QRS morphology that resembles that seen in sinus rhythm in all leads. However, the complexes are wider. Noted are occasional QRS complexes (black circles) that are different in morphology from the others but that are identical to the QRS morphology recorded during sinus rhythm. A P wave and constant P-R interval can be seen prior to these "normal" QRS complexes, and the P-R interval is the same as measured during sinus rhythm. These are Dressler beats, i.e., QRS complexes that are normalized due to intermittent capture. Ventricular tachycardia 2 has a QRS morphology different from sinus rhythm and VT 1. Although the QRS is narrowed, there has been a marked shift in axis, there is a tall monophasic R wave in V_1, and most importantly, there is AV dissociation, best seen in the limb leads. Noted are marked changes in the ST segments and T waves and occasional distinct P waves.

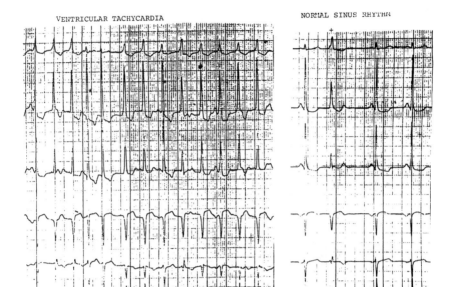

Figure 22.12. Example of VT. Seen are the six limb leads recorded simultaneously. During VT there are marked changes in QRS morphology best seen in leads I (1st line) and aVL (5th line). In lead II (2nd line) there are distinct P waves that are dissociated from the QRS complexes. Some of the P waves can be seen within the ST segment or T wave. Occasionally there is a P wave that is followed by a normalized QRS complex (for example, the 4th and 8th QRS [*asterisk*]). These are Dressler beats. Also occasionally seen are fusion complexes (*circle*). When compared to sinus rhythm, the captured beats are identical to the sinus QRS complexes. Additionally, the QRS complexes during VT are identical in morphology to a spontaneous ventricular premature beat (+) seen during sinus rhythm.

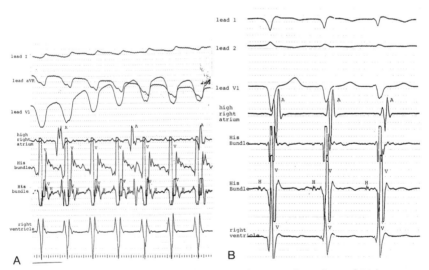

Figure 22.13. A. Example of an EP study of a patient with VT. Noted is evidence of AV dissociation, i.e., the atrial activity (A) is at a slower rate compared to the ventricular activity (V), and there is no relationship between A and V. Additionally, His bundle activation (H spike on the His-bundle electrogram) follows ventricular activity, indicating retrograde activation of the bundle of His. B. Example of an EP study during SVT with aberration. Noted is 1:1 atrial (A) and ventricular (V) activation, which occur simultaneously, although the retrograde A electrogram occurs slightly after ventricular activity. Prior to each V wave is a bundle of His spike (H), with a fixed H-V interval, indicating a supraventricular origin for the tachycardia.

When a double-peaked R wave is recorded in V_1, with a left peak taller than the right one (the so-called rabbit ear sign), ventricular ectopy is likely. However, a taller right rabbit ear does not help in distinguishing a ventricular from a supraventricular site of origin.

V_1-Negative Wide QRS Tachycardia

A ventricular origin of a V_1-negative (LBBB-like) wide QRS tachycardia is highly suspected in the presence of the following ECG findings:

1. A broad initial R wave of 30 msec or more in lead V_1 or V_2 (this initial R wave in V_1 is often taller during tachycardia than during sinus rhythm);
2. A slurred or notched downstroke of the S wave in lead V_1 or V_2;
3. A duration of 70 msec or more from the onset of the ventricular complex to the nadir of the QS or S wave in lead V_1 and V_2; and
4. The presence of any Q wave in lead V_6.

In LBBB the electrical activation of the septum, which normally occurs from left to right, is reversed. This results in a small right to left vector, which is the normal right septal vector. In LBBB this vector is unopposed by the left to right force of the left septal mass. The unopposed but small right septal vector causes a small narrow R wave in V_2 and often absence of any initial positive deflection in V_1. Furthermore, the right-to-left septal vector is directed towards V_6, causing initial positivity and absence of any Q wave in this lead. Finally, during LBBB aberrancy, the downstroke of the S wave is clean, without any slurring or notch and has a swift inscription.

QRS WIDTH AND QRS AXIS

Other currently used diagnostic criteria are related to the width of the QRS complex and the QRS axis in the frontal plane. A QRS duration of 0.14 seconds or more and a superior axis, especially in the "northwest" quadrant, favor the diagnosis of VT. A marked rightward or leftward shift in axis, primarily of the initial portion of the QRS complex, when compared with the axis during sinus rhythm, is strongly suggestive of VT.

A New Stepwise Approach to Wide QRS Tachycardias

ALGORITHM 1: DIFFERENTIAL DIAGNOSIS BETWEEN VT AND SVT WITH ABERRANT CONDUCTION

This algorithm is based on observations that the prolongation of the R-S interval in LBBB-like wide QRS complex tachycardias strongly favors the diagnosis of VT. It is hypothesized that prolongation of the intrinsic deflection in any precordial lead showing a clear-cut R-S complex could be a marker of VT, irrespective of the morphology pattern in V_1, RBBB, or LBBB-like wide QRS complex tachycardias.

In the first step all precordial leads are inspected to detect the presence or absence of an R-S complex. If an R-S complex cannot be identified in any precordial lead, the diagnosis of VT can be made with 100% specificity. If this is the case, further analysis is not needed. If an RS complex is clearly distinguished in one or

1. QRS width > 0.14 sec

2. Superior QRS axis

3. Morphology In precordial leads

RBBB like pattern	LBBB like pattern

V1:
 V6 : R/S < 1
	V1: r tachy > r sinus
	 V2 1 : 30 msec
	       2 : notch
	       3 : 70 msec
	 V6 : qR

4. AV. Dissociation, Fusion, Captures present

Figure 22.14. Criteria used in the differential diagnosis between SVT with intraventricular aberrant conduction and VT which favor VT.

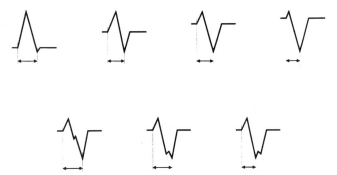

Figure 22.15. R-S complexes and how to measure the R-S interval.

more precordial leads, one has to proceed to the second step. This step consists of carefully measuring the interval between the onset of the R wave and the deepest part of the S wave (R-S interval). The onset of ventricular activation can be more accurately measured if all precordial leads are recorded simultaneously (Fig. 22.15).

If the R-S interval exceeds 100 msec, the diagnosis of VT can be made with a specificity of 98%. If RS complexes are present in multiple precordial leads, the one with the largest R-S interval is considered (Fig. 22.16).

If the R-S interval is less than 100 msec, either a ventricular or supraventricular site of origin of the tachycardia is possible, and the third step follows, namely, determining the presence or absence of AV dissociation. Clear-cut demonstration of AV dissociation is 100% specific for the diagnosis of VT.

The fourth step of the algorithm is the classic morphology criteria for V_1-positive and V_1-negative wide QRS complex tachycardias. When diagnosing VT it is essential that the classic morphology criteria be present, both in lead V_1 (V_2) and lead V_6. In the presence of a discordant morphology pattern, suggesting VT in one lead and SVT in the other, a supraventricular site of origin of the tachycardia is assumed.

ALGORITHM 2: DIFFERENTIAL DIAGNOSIS BETWEEN VT AND ANTIDROMIC
TACHYCARDIA

Important arrhythmias that present difficulty in differential diagnosis are VT, SVT with aberrant conduction resulting from an antidromic tachycardia, and SVT with aberration due to treatment with antiarrhythmic drugs (classes Ia and Ic). In

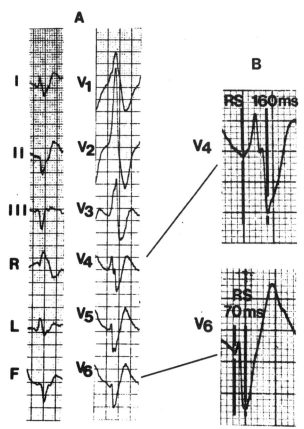

Figure 22.16. Tracings from the 12-lead ECG illustrating the measurements of the R-S interval. A VT with an RBBB-like QRS complex is shown. An R-S complex is observed in the precordial leads V_3–V_6. S wave is, however, not sharp enough in lead V_3 to measure confidently an R-S interval. R-S interval (enlarged in the right panel) measures 160 msec in lead V_4 and 70 msec in lead V_6. Thus, the longest R-S interval is more than 100 msec and diagnostic of VT. Paper speed was 25 mm/second.

fact, in antidromic tachycardia as in VT, ventricular activation starts outside the normal intraventricular conduction system. To differentiate VT from antidromic tachycardia, algorithm 2 was developed based on the following information:

1. Accessory pathways (APs) are located in the AV ring. Hence they activate the ventricles from the base to the apex, resulting in predominantly positive QRS complexes in the precordial leads V_4–V_6. Therefore, predominantly negative complexes in these leads cannot be observed during a preexcited tachycardia and will favor the diagnosis of VT.
2. In the absence of structural heart disease, qR complexes in leads V_2–V_6 cannot be observed in antidromic tachycardia.
3. AV relation different from 1:1 with more QRS complexes than P waves excludes antidromic tachycardia and is 100% specific for VT.

In the first step the polarity of the QRS complex in leads V_4–V_6 is defined either as predominantly positive or predominantly negative. If predominantly negative the diagnosis of VT can be made with 100% specificity, and further analysis is unnecessary. If the polarity of the QRS complex is predominantly positive in V_4–V_6, one should proceed to the second step, being the presence of a qR complex in one or more of precordial leads V_2–V_6. If a qR complex can be identified, VT can be diagnosed with an equal specificity of 100% and further analysis is omitted. If a qR wave in leads V_2–V_6 is absent, the third step has to be considered. The AV relationship has to be evaluated. More specifically the question has to be answered whether the AV relationship is different from 1:1 and whether there are more QRS complexes than P waves present. If this is the case, a third diagnostic criterion for VT, also having a specificity of 100%, is available. If all these steps are answered negatively, the diagnosis of preexcited (antidromic) tachycardia has to be considered.

SUGGESTED READING

Akhtar M, Shenasa M, Jazayeri M, Caceres J, Tchou PJ. Wide complex tachycardia. Reappraisal of a common clinical problem. Ann Intern Med 1988;109:905–912.

Brugada P, Brugada J, Mont L, et al. A new approach to the differential diagnosis of a regular tachycardia with a wide QRS complex. Circulation 1991;83:1649–1659.

Dancy M, Camm AJ, Ward D. Misdiagnosis of chronic recurrent ventricular tachycardia. Lancet 1985;2:320–323.

Morady F, Baerman JM, DiCarlo LA, DiButleir M, Krol RB, Wahr DW. A prevalent misconception regarding wide-complex tachycardias. JAMA 1985;254:2790–2792.

Stewart RB, Bardy GH, Greene HL. Wide complex tachycardia: misdiagnosis and outcome after emergency therapy. Ann Intern Med 1986;104: 766–771.

Tchou P, Young P, Mahmud R, Dinker S, Jazayeri M, Akhtar M. Useful clinical criteria for the diagnosis of ventricular tachycardia. Am J Med 1988;84:53–56.

Wellens HJJ, Bär FW, Lie KI. The value of the electrocardiogram in the differential diagnosis of a tachycardia with a widened QRS complex. Am J Med 1978;64:27–33.

Wellens HJJ, Bär FW, Vanagt EJ, et al. The differentiation between ventricular tachycardia and supraventricular tachycardia with aberrant conduction: the value of the 12-lead electrocardiogram. In: Wellens HJJ, Kulbertus HE, eds. What's new in electrocardiography. Boston: Martinus Nijhoff, 1981:184–192.

23 Conduction Abnormalities

ATRIOVENTRICULAR NODAL BLOCK

Atrioventricular (AV) block is a delay in transmission of the cardiac impulse from atrium to ventricle or actual failure of transmission of one or more such impulses.

Traditionally, AV block is divided into three categories. First-degree AV block refers to prolongation of the P-R interval beyond that seen in a normal population, i.e., >0.2 seconds. Second-degree block refers to failure of one or more P waves but not all P waves to be conducted. Second-degree AV block is further subdivided into type I, in which there is progressive delay in AV transmission prior to the blocked P wave type II, in which the P wave is suddenly blocked without a preceding progressive delay in AV transmission; and high-grade second-degree block, in which there is a fixed ratio of conduction, e.g., 2:1, 3:1, 4:1. Third-degree AV block is complete absence of AV conduction.

AV block can result from delay or blockade of impulse transmission between the sinoatrial and AV nodes, i.e., intraatrial block, delay or blockade of impulse transmission within the AV node itself, i.e., AV nodal block, or delay or blockade of impulse transmission in the distal conducting system, i.e., subnodal or intranodal block. It often is not possible to determine with certainty which part of the conduction system is responsible for AV block based on the electrocardiogram (ECG) pattern of block alone.

Etiology

A variety of conditions or disease processes may lead to impaired AV nodal conduction, and the degree of impairment of AV nodal conduction in each of these circumstances may range in severity from first-degree AV block to third-degree or complete AV nodal block (Table 23.1). In general the prognosis in such situations is determined by the nature of the condition or disease process leading to AV nodal block rather than by the severity of the AV block itself.

Prevalence and Prognosis of AV Nodal Block

Many conditions or disease states that affect AV nodal conduction also affect conduction in other segments of the conduction system. Because sites of block usually cannot be determined precisely from electrocardiographic criteria alone and because most clinical studies of AV block are based on electrocardiographic criteria alone, it is virtually impossible to describe accurately the prevalence and significance of AV nodal block per se for each of the conditions or disease states in which it is seen. Nevertheless, some general statements are possible.

Table 23.1
Causes of AV Block

Congenital block
  Associated with other anomalies (ostium primum defect, corrected transposition of great arteries)
  Not associated with other congenital anomalies

Primary causes
  Cardiomyopathy
  Lev's disease
  Lenègre's disease

Secondary causes
  Atherosclerotic heart disease
    Acute myocardial infarction
      Anterior
      Inferoposterior
    Myocardial infarction healed
  Calcific interruption of AV conduction system
    Calcified mitral or aortic valve or combination
  Inflammatory diseases
    Acute infective endocarditis ("ring abscess")
    Myocarditis
      Bacterial
        Acute rheumatic fever
        Diphtheria, syphillis, pertussis, Lyme disease, tuberculosis
      Parasitic
        Chagas' disease
      Viral
        Mumps, measles

Drugs
Collagen disease
  Dermatomyositis, scleroderma, systemic lupus erythematosus, rheumatoid arthritis, ankylosing
  spondylitis, Wegener's granulomatosis
Infiltrative diseases
  Hemachromatosis, primary oxalosis, sarcoidosis
Trauma
  Surgical trauma, radiation therapy, catheter ablation
Tumors
  Rhabdomyoma, rhabdomyosarcoma, mesothelioma

Functional block
  Vagally induced

Several large studies have indicated that the incidence of unexplained P-R prolongation of >0.2 seconds in a healthy population ranges between 0.5–1.5%. Importantly, the morbidity and mortality in the group with first-degree AV block were the same as expected in a normal population without first-degree AV block. First-degree AV block occurring in a young, otherwise healthy individual with no obvious cause for impairment of AV conduction usually is simply a manifestation of enhanced vagal tone with resultant slowing of conduction in the AV node.

Complete AV block is rarely asymptomatic and may affect prognosis adversely. The most common cause of acquired complete AV block is acute myocardial infarction (MI) (Table 23.2). Complete AV nodal block during an inferior wall MI may be encountered in 10–15% of such patients. Complete AV block in this setting is rarely sudden in onset and usually is preceded by a period of second-degree type I block. The site of AV block in such patients is typically the AV node and is caused by a combination of factors, including ischemia of the AV node, local release of adenosine, and activation of autonomic reflexes, particularly enhanced vagal tone. This type of AV block often responds readily to treatment with atropine or isoproterenol and seems not to have an adverse impact on the overall prognosis of affected patients. Complete AV block in the setting of acute anterior MI is less common, occurring in only 5% of patients. The site of block in such patients is usually the bundle of His rather than the AV node. Such patients have a much more grave prognosis than do individuals with complete AV block in the setting of inferior infarction, but this is probably because of the greater extent of necrosis usually seen in anterior infarction rather than as the result of the accompanying AV block per se.

In rare patients complete AV block is congenital; the site of block in such patients is typically the AV node. Congenital complete AV block may occur as an isolated abnormality or it may be seen in association with other cardiac defects. The prognosis of patients with congenital complete AV block is good and is largely determined by the nature and severity of accompanying anatomic lesions, if any are present. Most infants with complete AV block as their sole cardiac abnormality will develop and grow normally. Studies and case reports in children and young adults with congenital complete AV block indicate that the heart rate in such patients, which is usually determined by automaticity in the His bundle, responds well to a variety of hemodynamic and pharmacologic stimuli. The patients can engage in active sports and can even carry normal pregnancies to term. However, this benign prognosis has been questioned recently. Patients with resting heart

Table 23.2
AV Block in Acute Myocardial Infarction

	Anterior MI	Inferoposterior MI
Pathology	Extensive infarction Injury to His-Purkinje system, intranodal block	Less extensive infarction Nodal block
Hemodynamic compromise	Often present	Often absent
QRS width	Wide	Narrow
Treatment	Pacing	No therapy Atropine Infrequent pacing
Prognosis	80% mortality	30% mortality

rates less than 50 beats/minute may be prone to syncope and may require permanent pacing to relieve symptoms.

Associated Symptoms and Hemodynamic Effects

First-degree AV nodal block almost never leads to symptoms. When AV nodal block causes symptoms, these are usually the result of second or third-degree block. Second-degree block can give rise to the symptoms of palpitation in individuals who sense the irregular cadence due to block of P waves. Other symptoms that are the consequence of slow heart rate with an attendant decline in cardiac output and impaired oxygen delivery to peripheral tissues are dizziness, lightheadedness, and syncope. These symptoms are usually seen in patients with complete AV nodal block, but they may also be reported by patients with second-degree AV nodal block in association with marked sinus bradycardia. Syncope is a particularly ominous symptom. It may result from bradycardia itself or may be the result of bradycardia-dependent torsade de pointes ventricular tachycardia. Severe bradycardia or torsade de pointes may even be a cause of sudden death.

Physical Examination

The most salient features of AV nodal block on physical examination are abnormalities of the jugular venous pulse and the intensity of the first heart sound. A prolongation of the interval between "a" and "c" waves in the jugular venous pulse is typical of first-degree AV nodal block. If this interval prolongs progressively until a c wave is suddenly absent or if there is sudden absence of a c wave, second-degree AV block may be suspected. Dissociation of a and c waves in the jugular venous pulse with "cannon a" waves due to atrial contraction against a closed tricuspid valve are hallmarks of complete AV block.

The intensity of the first heart sound, which represents closure of the mitral and tricuspid valves, is a function of the position of these valves at the onset of ventricular systole. If ventricular systole occurs after a short P-R interval, when the valves are still widely open, S1 will be loud as the valve snaps back. With marked prolongation of the P-R interval, as occurs in first-degree AV block, the valves have time to float back to their closed position before onset of ventricular systole, resulting in a soft S1. If the P-R interval is constantly changing, as occurs in type I second-degree AV, the intensity of S1 will vary.

The diagnosis of complete AV block may be suspected on the basis of physical examination. The pulse is typically slow (<40 beats/minute) and strong. Simultaneous examination of the venous and arterial pulses may reveal jugular a waves occurring independently of the carotid upstroke. Cannon a waves can be appreciated as the atrium contracts against the closed tricuspid valve. The systemic arterial pulse pressure is wide. The first heart sound varies in intensity, with an increase in intensity as the atrial systole moves closer in time to ventricular systole, until eventually a booming first sound can be appreciated. This has been termed as "bruit the cannon" and results from opening of the AV valves by atrial contraction immediately prior to ventricular systole.

ECG Manifestations

The ECG manifestations of first-degree AV nodal block are a 1:1 relationship between P waves and QRS complexes but with a P-R interval of >0.20 seconds, up to 0.60 seconds (Fig. 23.1). Even in the same patient, the P-R interval may vary over a wide range, depending upon the interplay among factors like heart rate, autonomic tone, drug levels, and metabolic state.

The cardinal ECG manifestation of second-degree AV nodal block is the failure of some but not all P waves to be conducted to the ventricles. Type I second-degree AV nodal block is characterized by Wenckebach periodicity in which the P-R interval gradually prolongs until a P wave fails to conduct to the ventricles. After the blocked P wave conduction then resumes, the P-R interval of this next conducted beat shortens. In its "typical" form, the largest increment in R-R interval occurs between the first and second beat of the Wenckebach cycle (Fig. 23.2). Although the

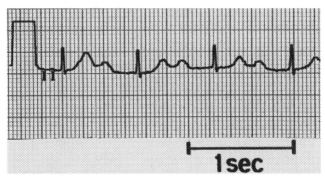

Figure 23.1. Marked first-degree AV block. The normal QRS suggests that the site of block is in the AV node.

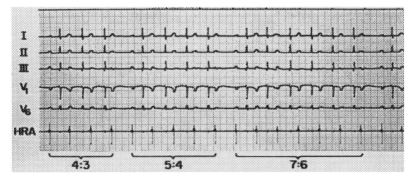

Figure 23.2. Multiple surface ECG leads recorded simultaneously with a high right atrial electrogram (HRA) during type I second-degree AV block. The HRA electrograms are coincident with regularly occurring P waves. During the cycle labeled 5:4 there is typical Wenckebach periodicity, the R-R intervals progressively decreasing with a progressively increasing P-R interval. The cycle labeled 7:6 is atypical.

P-R interval continues to lengthen during subsequent beats, it does so by progressively smaller increments. Thus, during such "typical Wenckebach" cycles (about 50% of cases) the R-R intervals actually decrease progressively, even though the P-R intervals are progressively increasing. It is quite common, however, to observe R-R intervals that do not decrease progressively or P-R intervals that may actually stabilize or shorten for several beats during the Wenckebach cycle (Fig. 23.2).

Type II second-degree AV nodal block is characterized by sudden failure of one or several consecutive P waves to conduct to the ventricles without progressive lengthening of the P-R interval prior to the blocked P wave (Fig. 23.3). In some patients apparent type II second-degree block may actually be the same electrophysiologic phenomenon as type I block, but with increments in the P-R interval too small, i.e., <50 msec, to be detected at the usual ECG recording paper speed of 25 mm/second. Another explanation for apparent type II AV nodal block is the sporadic occurrence of concealed junctional extrasystoles. The third ECG pattern of second-degree AV nodal block is characterized by a fixed ratio of P waves to QRS complexes, e.g., 2:1, 3:1, 4:1. This type of block cannot be classified as type I or type II. Instead, it is usually referred to as "advanced" or "high-grade" second-degree block.

Third-degree or complete AV nodal block is total absence of conduction between atria and ventricles. In the presence of sinus rhythm or some other organized atrial rhythm like atrial tachycardia, there is AV dissociation, the ventricular rate being slower than the atrial rate and being governed by a subsidiary sub-AV nodal pacemaker (Fig. 23.4). In the presence of second- or third-degree heart block, ventriculophasic arrhythmia may be observed, i.e., the P-P interval surrounding a QRS complex is shorter than the P-P interval without a QRS complex in between. The reason for this is not clear, but a proposed mechanism is ventricular contraction resulting in atrial stretch or pulsatile flow to the sinus node artery, resulting in enhanced sinus node automaticity. Complete AV nodal block in the presence of atrial fibrillation may be easily overlooked with only casual inspection of the ECG. A regular ventricular rate in the presence of atrial fibrillation should heighten one's suspicion of complete AV block.

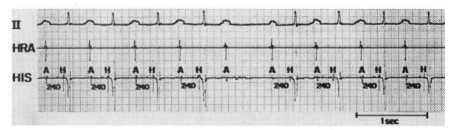

Figure 23.3. Surface ECG lead II recorded simultaneously with high right atrial (HRA) and His bundle (HIS) bipolar electrograms. The ECG shows type II second degree AV block. The fifth P wave fails to conduct through the AV node, despite constant P-R and A-H intervals before and after the blocked P wave. This may reflect momentary increase in vagal tone.

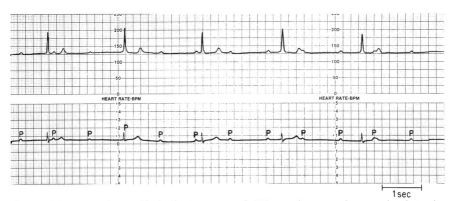

Figure 23.4. Complete AV block. The P waves and QRS complexes are dissociated with regular R-R intervals that are slower than the P-P intervals. Note that P-P intervals that span a QRS complex (6th and 7th P waves, 8th and 9th P waves) are shorter than other P-P intervals (5th and 6th P waves). This is referred to as ventriculophasic sinus arrhythmia.

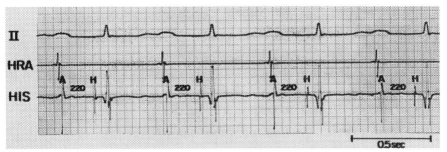

Figure 23.5. Same organization of tracings as in Fig. 23.3. The prolonged P-R interval is due to prolongation of the A-H interval. This localizes the site of AV conduction delay to the AV node.

Clinical Electrophysiology

The P-R interval in the surface ECG represents the total time required for transmission of the cardiac impulse from its point of origin in the sinus node to the ventricular myocardium. This interval is the sum of conduction times over each different segment of the AV conducting system, namely, conduction time between the sinus and AV nodes, conduction time through the AV node itself, and conduction time from the His bundle to ventricular myocardium. Although specific information about conduction over each of these segments is not apparent from the surface ECG, it is available from simultaneous recordings of the surface ECG and a His bundle electrogram.

The interval between the onset of a normal sinus P wave in the surface ECG and depolarization of the right atrial myocardium (A in the His bundle electrogram) represents intraatrial conduction time from the sinus node to the AV node.

Most of the normal delay during AV transition occurs within the AV node. AV nodal conduction time, therefore, accounts for the majority of the P-R interval. Because the atrial deflection recorded by a His bundle electrode catheter represents depolarization of atrial muscle near the cranial border of the AV node, the A-H interval provides an accurate measure of AV nodal conduction time. AV nodal conduction times in normal persons span a wide range, usually between 50–140 msec, due largely to variations in sympathetic and parasympathetic tone within the richly innervated AV node (Fig. 23.5).

The terminal portion of the P-R interval in the surface ECG represents conduction through all segments of the AV conduction system distal to the AV node. This includes conduction over the His bundle, down to right and left bundle branches and through the subendocardial ramifications of the Purkinje network to ventricular myocardium. Total conduction time in this subnodal portion of the AV conduction system is reflected in the H-V interval, measured from the H spike in the His bundle electrogram to the earliest point of ventricular depolarization in any intracardiac or surface lead. The H-V interval normally ranges between 35–55 msec.

Guidelines for Treatment

Decisions about treatment of AV nodal block are influenced by whether the block is related to some transient active problem or occurs as a chronic condition. Acute AV nodal block, such as that encountered in the setting of digitalis toxicity or acute inferior MI, usually subsides with resolution of the underlying problem. The need for intervention in such patients should be determined by the symptomatic state of the patient. First-degree AV nodal block is not an indication for treatment. However, acute second- and third-degree block that results in symptomatic bradycardia are indications for therapy. Intravenous atropine 0.5–1.0 mg administered as a bolus is often helpful at reducing the degree of block or eliminating block altogether in patients with acute block. Intravenous infusion of isoproterenol may also be used in emergency situations, but is not recommended in patients with digitalis intoxication or acute MI because of the likelihood of precipitating ventricular arrhythmias or exacerbating myocardial ischemia. If symptomatic bradycardia persists despite atropine, a temporary pacemaker should be utilized.

In chronic AV nodal block, prognosis is determined predominantly by the nature and severity of the associated underlying heart disease. The major contribution of permanent pacemaker implantation is relief of symptoms related to bradycardia rather than having a marked impact on prognosis. Guidelines have been published by the joint American Heart Association/American College of Cardiology task force for implantation of permanent pacemakers (see chapters on pacing and bradyarrhythmias).

HIS-PURKINJE DISEASE

The His-Purkinje system is composed of specialized cardiac tissue that extends from the AV node to the terminal Purkinje fibers with their insertion into the ventricular myocardium. It is an "electronic highway" that transmits and distributes the depolarizing impulses to the ventricular working myocardium so that contraction can proceed in a synchronized and effective manner.

Etiology and Mechanism of His-Purkinje Disease

His-Purkinje block presents in various forms of heart disease, including:

1. Valvular lesions (rheumatic, degenerative, calcific, aging);
2. Hypertension;
3. Ischemic;
4. Cardiomyopathy;
5. Inflammatory diseases;
6. Infectious diseases;
7. Infiltrative diseases;
8. Neuromuscular disorders;
9. Neoplastic disease;
10. Idiopathic (Lev's disease, Lenègre's disease);
11. Congenital heart disease; and
12. Reversible conditions (antiarrhythmic drugs, hyperkalemia, hypoxia, acidosis, mechanical, trauma).

Electrocardiographic Manifestations and Diagnosis

The concept of the trifascicular nature of the intraventricular conduction system has become accepted. It has been proposed that the system consists of the right bundle branch and a left bundle branch that subdivide into anterior and posterior fascicles. Although more recently the existence of a fourth septal fascicle has been proposed, its origin and constancy has not been well defined.

The electrocardiographic presence of bundle branch block or fascicular block indicates a delay in ventricular activation. This delay may represent a complete block in the bundle branch or fascicle or a partial block with delayed conduction. It is the effect of the delay in depolarization that is observed on the surface ECG. Occasionally, this delay is due to slow conduction within a localized portion of the myocardium, not necessarily including the bundle branch or fascicles. In this case the block has been termed a "parietal block."

Right bundle branch block is characterized by a prolonged QRS duration of 0.12 seconds or more, associated with abnormal terminal QRS forces directed anteriorly and to the right, indicating delayed activation of the right ventricle. These terminal forces will produce an R, rSR', or qR wave in V1; wide, slurred S waves in leads I, aVL, V5, and V6; and a wide terminal r wave in aVR.

Left bundle branch block is characterized by prolonged QRS duration of 0.12 seconds or more and delays in both initial and mid QRS forces, which are directed leftward and posteriorly indicating delayed left ventricular activation. This results in a broad, notched R wave without q waves in leads I, aVL, and V6, and an rS pattern in lead V1 (Fig. 23.6).

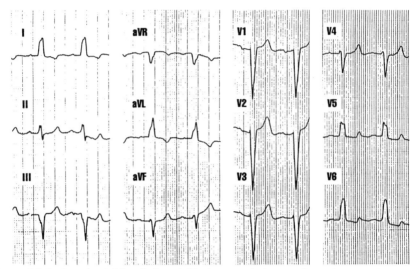

Figure 23.6. Complete left bundle branch block. 12-lead electrocardiographic recording (paper speed 25 mm/second) showing a wide QRS with M-shaped morphology in lead I and aVL.

Left anterior fascicular block is characterized by minimally prolonged QRS duration of 0.09–1.0 seconds and a leftward axis of –45° or more. The initial QRS activation is directed rightward and inferiorly, resulting in a qR in leads I and aVL and an rS pattern in leads II, III, and aVF (Fig. 23.7).

Nonspecific intraventricular conduction delay is characterized by prolonged QRS duration in the absence of a specific bundle branch or fascicular block pattern. This type of widened QRS complex probably represents additional intramyocardial conduction delay and not an isolated lesion of the conduction system.

Left posterior fascicular block is characterized by a minimally prolonged QRS of 0.9–1.0 second duration with a right axis deviation of >90°. The initial QRS forces are directed superiorly, resulting in a qR in leads II, III, and aVF and an rS in I and aVL. Other causes of right axis deviation, such as right ventricular hypertrophy, must be excluded prior to making this diagnosis.

Combinations of right bundle branch block and left anterior fascicular block or right bundle branch block and left posterior fascicular block are defined as bifascicular blocks (Figs. 23.8 and 23.9). Most authors will classify complete left bundle branch block as bifascicular, although some argue that lesions prior to the division of the left bundle (predivisional block) are not truly bifascicular.

Alternating bundle branch block is an electrocardiographic pattern where both left and right bundle branch block conduction patterns are present either on the same or different tracings of the same patient. Intermittent bundle branch block is present when normal intraventricular conduction alternates with bundle branch block or fascicular block patterns (Fig. 23.10).

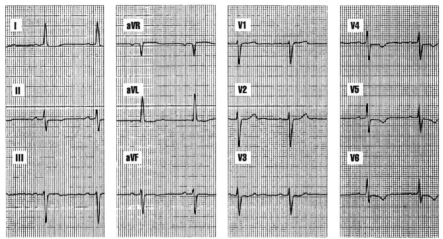

Figure 23.7. Left anterior fascicular block. Note that there is left axis deviation (–45°) in frontal plane with a small q in aVL.

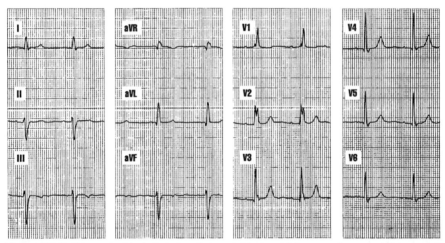

Figure 23.8. Bifascicular block. Right bundle branch block and left anterior fascicular block. Frontal plane QRS axis of –60°.

CHRONIC INTRAVENTRICULAR BLOCKS

The clinical significance of the presence of bundle branch block on the ECG depends on the population under investigation. Epidemiologic studies report that bundle branch block develops in 2.4% with an annual incidence of 0.13%. Right bundle branch block is the most common, and its appearance is not associated with any overt acute clinical event. Most of the patients who develop this conduction defect are hypertensive. Compared with a matched control group without

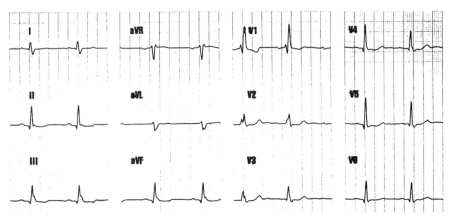

Figure 23.9. Bifascicular block. Right bundle branch block and left posterior fascicular block. Note wide QRS complexes with rSR' in V1 and small q waves in II, III, and aVF and frontal plane QRS axis of +100°.

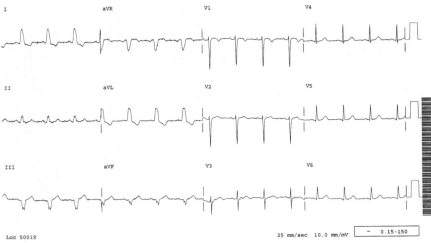

Figure 23.10. Example of an intermittent left bundle branch block. The QRS complexes in the limb leads have a left bundle branch morphology while the complexes in the precordial leads show normal conduction. The P-R and R-R intervals are identical throughout.

right bundle branch block, the incidence of coronary artery disease is 2.5 times greater, the incidence of congestive heart failure is four times greater, and cardiovascular mortality is three times greater in the group with right bundle branch block. Less common is left bundle branch block. In contrast to right bundle branch block, 48% of the cases have a clinically diagnosable vascular event at the time of developing the left bundle branch block. There is also a strong association between the presence of left bundle branch block and the occurrence of hypertension, cardiomegaly, and coronary artery disease in these patients. The cumulative mortality is 50% within 10 years, which is five times greater than the population at large without left bundle branch block.

Left anterior fascicular block is the most common intraventricular conduction defect (prevalence—4.5%). Isolated left posterior fascicular block is a rare electrocardiographic finding. The prevalence of right bundle branch block is 1.15–3.19% and 1% for left bundle branch block. Retrospective electrocardiographic studies examining the prognosis of patients with chronic isolated bundle branch or bifascicular block report a 9–14% progression to complete heart block over an unspecified period of time.

The natural history and management of patients with chronic intraventricular conduction disease and the risk of advanced heart block during noncardiac surgery has revealed that transient complete heart block is only rarely seen. Thus, temporary pacing is rarely required in patients with chronic bifascicular block who undergo noncardiac surgery and should not be routinely used.

ACUTE INTRAVENTRICULAR BLOCKS

The overall incidence of acute intraventricular conduction block occurring with an MI varies between 10–35%, with an average of 19%. The mortality of patients with intraventricular conduction defects is twice that of patients without intraventricular conduction block. Left anterior fascicular block is the most common type of intraventricular conduction defect (7%) and left posterior fascicular block is the rarest. Isolated fascicular blocks do not appear to worsen the course of acute MI.

Left bundle branch block is the second most common form of an acute intraventricular conduction defect, with an average incidence of 4% and the progression to third-degree heart block is 9%, and there is a high in-hospital mortality (41%) associated with this conduction defect. Isolated right bundle branch block has a frequency of 2%. The progression to complete AV block is 19%. The associated mortality is 50%. In the presence of nonadjacent bifascicular blocks, i.e., right bundle branch block and left anterior fascicular block, right bundle branch block and left posterior fascicular block, and alternating bundle branch block, pathological examination reveals extensive necrosis of the intraventricular septum. The progression to complete heart block in these patients is markedly increased. Mortality associated with bilateral bundle branch block is very high (50–70%). Transient intraventricular blocks during an acute MI appear to have a more favorable clinical course and prognosis.

The presence of an old versus new intraventricular block also seems to influence outcome. The progression to third-degree (AV) block is twice as frequent in patients with new intraventricular blocks than in patients with old intraventricular blocks (22% vs. 13%). The mortality rate for patients with new intraventricular block is slightly higher than that in those with existing block (43% vs. 36%), although both carry a high in-hospital mortality. ECG variables define groups at low, intermediate, and high risk for progression to advanced or complete AV block. These variables are first-degree AV block, "new" bundle branch block, and bilateral bundle branch block. The lowest risk group, defined by having only one of the three variables present, has a 10–13% incidence of progression. The intermediate risk group, defined as having any two of the variables present, except for new bilateral bundle branch block, has a progression rate of 19–20%. The highest risk group, having either all three variables present or a new bilateral bundle branch block, has a progression rate of 31–38%.

The long-term prognosis of patients who have permanent or transient complete heart block in association with an intraventricular block during an acute MI is ominous but is related to the extent of disease. The use of permanent pacemakers is uncertain and is further complicated by the fact that not all of the sudden death in this population are clearly the result of recurrent heart block and asystole. Furthermore, most of the longitudinal studies were carried out before thrombolytics were used, limiting their reliability in the modern era of coronary intervention.

Clinical Electrophysiologic Manifestations and Diagnosis

RECORDING OF HIS BUNDLE ELECTROGRAM, CONDUCTION TIMES, REFRACTORY PERIOD, AND ABERRANCY

The H-V interval, measured from the onset of His potential to the onset of ventricular activation, as determined from the earliest deflection of the surface QRS, is a measure of conduction time through the His bundle (distal to the recording site) and bundle branches. In patients with bundle branch block, the H-V interval reflects conduction time in the functioning bundle branch.

There is an increase in H-V interval with increasing age. The H-V interval, recorded from the proximal His bundle, for infants varies from 13–27 msec, while for those of 15 years of age and older the normal interval is 35–55 msec. Atrial pacing can be used to stress the conduction system and uncover abnormalities not apparent during sinus rhythm. Atrial pacing at rapid rates does not affect the His bundle potential or the H-V interval under normal conditions. The development of block distal to His during rapid atrial pacing is definitely an abnormal finding and indicates His-Purkinje disease (Fig. 23.11).

The refractory period of the His-Purkinje system is rate dependent, and as the rate increases, the refractory period of the His-Purkinje system and the ventricular muscle decreases. The cycle length dependency of the refractory period of the His-Purkinje system accounts for a number of electrocardiographic and electrophysiological observations. Aberrant conduction of premature supraventricular impulses mostly exhibits right bundle branch block pattern (80–90%), although some may have left bundle branch block aberration or both patterns may be observed. Occasionally, axis shifts are seen without the appearance of bundle branch block. Most of these axis shifts are leftward, indicating a delay in the left anterior fascicle. The presence of aberrancy, conduction delays, and blocks is dependent on multiple factors, including the preceding cycle, conduction time over the AV node, refractoriness of the His-Purkinje system, and presence of catecholamines.

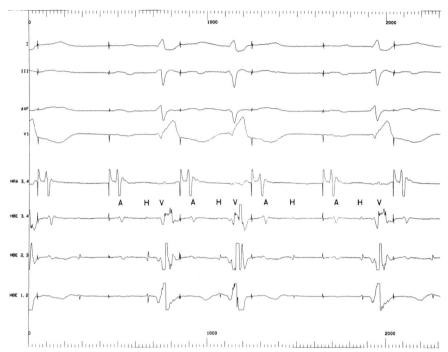

Figure 23.11. Infra-Hisian block during atrial pacing in a patient with a right bundle branch block and left anterior fascicular block. The first and fourth atrial paced beats are conducted to the His bundle but not to the ventricle (the His spike is seen, but there is no ventricular electrogram following it). Loss of distal conduction is sudden, not decremental. AV nodal conduction times (A-H interval) are constant. HBE, His bundle electrograms recorded from proximal (3, 4) and distal (1, 2) poles. HRA, high right atrial signals recorded from proximal poles (3, 4).

CHRONIC AV BLOCKS

During first-degree AV block (PR >0.20 seconds), the delay most commonly occurs in the atrioventricular node. However, occasionally in the presence of a narrow QRS, P-R prolongation is related to delay in the His bundle, with recording of split His potentials (H-H'). Prolongation of the H-V interval in the presence of a wide QRS denotes disease in the His bundle or the bundle branches. Prolongation of the H-V interval accounting by itself for first-degree AV block is quite rare. Most commonly, first-degree AV block represents a combination of prolongation of intraatrial, AV nodal, and His-Purkinje conduction times.

During second-degree AV block, the His bundle recording can delineate three sites of block, including (*a*) block proximal to the His potential (AV nodal); (*b*) block within the His potential (intra-Hisian); and (*c*) block distal to the His potential (intra-Hisian or trifascicular block), in which the blocked P wave is followed by a His potential. The clinical significance of second-degree AV block is related to the site of block rather than to the electrocardiographic type of block.

Type I block usually represents AV nodal block (72%) and less commonly intra-His block (8%) or infra-His block (20%). Type II AV block most commonly represents infra-His block (71%) and less commonly intra-His block (29%). In the presence of 2:1 and 3:1 block, the site of block is infra-His in 51% of cases, intra-His in 20%, and in the AV node in 29%.

The prognosis of second-degree intra-Hisian block is controversial. Chronic second-degree block distal to His has a poor prognosis with most patients becoming symptomatic with syncope.

In complete heart block, the use of His bundle recording allows the delineation of three sites of block, including (a) proximal to His (AV node); (b) intra-Hisian (split His potential); and (c) distal to the His bundle (complete trifascicular block). The site of complete heart block cannot be predicted with accuracy from the surface ECG. In patients with AV nodal or intra-Hisian block, the escape rhythm may have narrow or wide QRS complexes. In patients with block distal to His, the escape rhythm always has wide QRS complexes. The distribution of the site of block in complete heart block varies with different series. It is AV nodal in 14–35%, intra-Hisian in 14–18%, and distal to the His bundle in 49–72% of cases. Patients with complete heart block are frequently symptomatic with dizziness, syncope, or congestive heart failure. A distal site of block is frequently correlated with syncopal manifestations. The incidence of syncope is 29% in AV nodal block, 25% in intra-Hisian block, and 71% in distal to His block.

CHRONIC INTRAVENTRICULAR BLOCKS

Prognostic Significance of H-V Interval in Patients with Bundle Branch Block and Heart Disease

In patients with bifascicular block, the H-V interval reflects the function of the remaining fascicle, and the prolongation of the H-V interval suggests the presence of trifascicular disease. Prospective studies of patients with organic heart disease and bundle branch block demonstrate that there is a high prevalence of H-V prolongation. However, in spite of the high prevalence of trifascicular disease, the overall progression to complete heart block is uncommon and is approximately 2–4% per year. The progression to heart block is higher in those patients with H-V prolongation. There is a high total mortality associated with intraventricular conduction defect, and half of the mortality is related to sudden death. The available evidence to date suggests that the sudden death is more likely related to ventricular tachyarrhythmias and not to the development of heart block.

To improve the accuracy of electrophysiologic studies in patients with chronic bundle branch block, investigators have used various means to stress the conduction system. The development of block distal to His during incremental atrial pacing has been shown to predict the occurrence of spontaneous atrioventricular block (Fig. 23.11).

Prognostic Significance of H-V Interval in Primary Conduction Disease

Progression to AV block occurs in 3% of patients with primary conduction disease and in 7% of patients with organic heart disease. The cumulative incidence of sudden death over a 3-year period is 6% in the patients with primary conduction disease and 17% in patients with organic heart disease (P <.001). Thus, patients with bifascicular block in the presence of primary conduction disease have a significantly lower incidence of electrophysiologic abnormalities, subsequent AV block, as well as sudden death mortality than do patients with organic heart disease.

INTERMITTENT BUNDLE BRANCH BLOCK

Intermittent bundle branch block may be heart rate dependent, in which case it is defined as rate-dependent bundle branch block or unrelated to changes in heart rate. Most of the electrophysiologic observations in humans have been made in rate-dependent bundle branch block. Rate-dependent bundle branch block is diagnosed when the bundle branch block appears at a critical heart rate. This should be differentiated from functional bundle branch block, in which the block is dependent on a preceding long cycle length. Functional bundle branch block (aberrancy) may be a physiologic response, while rate-dependent bundle branch block is most commonly seen in patients with heart disease.

Indications for Electrophysiologic Studies and Pacing

INDICATIONS FOR ELECTROPHYSIOLOGIC STUDIES

The following recommendations are from the latest reports of the Task Force on Assessment of Diagnostic and Therapeutic Cardiovascular Procedures of the ACC and AHA.
Recommendations are categorized into three classes:

1. For Class I, general agreement that electrophysiologic study provides information that is very useful and important in the clinical management of the patient and should be done;
2. For Class II, conditions for which electrophysiologic studies are frequently performed but there is less certainty about the clinical usefulness of the information that is obtained (Experts are divided in their opinion of whether electrophysiologic studies for these conditions should be done.);
3. For Class III, conditions for which there is general agreement that electrophysiologic studies do not provide useful information and should not be done.

Recommendation for Electrophysiologic Study in the Presence of Acquired AV Block

1. Class I:
   (*a*) Symptomatic patients (syncope or near syncope) in whom His-Purkinje block, not established with electrocardiographic recordings, is suspected

as a cause of symptoms; (*b*) patients with second- or third-degree AV block treated with a pacemaker who remain symptomatic and in whom ventricular tachyarrhythmia is suspected as a cause of symptoms;

2. Class II:

(*a*) Patients with second- or third-degree AV block in whom knowledge of the site or mechanism of block or both may help to direct therapy or assess prognosis; (*b*) patients with suspected concealed junctional extrasystoles as a cause of second- or third-degree AV block (pseudo-AV block);

3. Class III:

(*a*) Patients in whom the symptoms and presence of AV block are correlated with electrocardiography; (*b*) asymptomatic patients with transient AV block associated with sinus slowing or increased vagal tone (nocturnal type I second-degree AV block).

Recommendation for Electrophysiologic Studies in Patients with Chronic Intraventricular Conduction Delay

Class I:

Symptomatic patients with bundle branch block in whom ventricular arrhythmias are suspected to cause the symptoms. The study is not designed to evaluated intraventricular conduction delay itself but the inducibility of sustained ventricular tachyarrhythmias;

Class II:

Symptomatic patients with bundle branch block in whom the knowledge of the site, severity of conduction delay, or response to drugs may help to direct therapy or assess prognosis;

Class III:

(*a*) Asymptomatic patients with intraventricular conduction delay; (*b*) Symptomatic patients with intraventricular conduction delay whose symptoms can be casually related to electrocardiographically documented events.

INDICATIONS FOR PACING

The recommendations from the Committee on Pacemaker Implantation of the same Task Force are categorized into three classes: class I, conditions for which there is general agreement that a permanent pacemaker should be implanted; class II, conditions for which permanent pacemakers are frequently used but there is a divergence of opinions with respect to the necessity of the use; class III, conditions for which there is an agreement that implantation of permanent pacing is unnecessary.

Indications for Pacing in Acquired AV Block In Adults (see chapter on pacing and bradyarrhythmias)

Indications for Pacing Following an Acute MI

Class I: Category *A*, persistent advanced second-degree or complete heart block after acute MI with block in the His-Purkinje system; Category *B*, patients with transient advanced AV block and associated bundle branch block;

Class II: Patients with persistent advanced block at the AV node;

Class III: Category *A*, transient AV conduction disturbances in the absence of intraventricular conduction defect; Category *B*, transient AV block in the presence of isolated left anterior or posterior fascicular block; Category *C*, acquired left anterior or posterior fascicular block in the absence of AV block; Category *D*, patients with persistent first-degree AV block in the presence of bundle branch block.

SUGGESTED READING

Alpert MA, Flaker GC. Chronic fascicular block. Recognition, natural history and therapeutic implications. Arch Intern Med 1984;144:799–809.

Amat y Leon F, Dhingra R, Denes P, Wu D, Wyndham C, Chuquimia R, Rosen K. The clinical spectrum of chronic His bundle block. Chest 1976;70:747–756.

Brown RW, Hunt D, Sloman JG. The natural history of atrioventricular conduction defects in acute myocardial infarction. Am Heart J 1969;78:460–472.

Dhingra RC, Amat y Leon F, Pouget M, Rosen KM. Infranodal block. Diagnosis clinical significance and management. Med Clin North Am 1976;60:175–187.

Dhingra RC, Palileo E, Strasberg B, et al. Significance of HV interval in 517 patients with chronic bifascicular block. Circulation 1981; 64:1265–1272.

Dreifus LS, Fisch C, Griffin JC, Gillette PC, Mason JW, Parsonnet V. Guidelines for implantation of cardiac pacemakers and antiarrhythmia

devices. A report of the American College of Cardiology/American Heart Association Task Force on Assessment of Diagnostic and Therapeutic Cardiovascular Procedures. Circulation 1991;84:455.

Karpavich PP, Gillette, PC, Garson A Jr, et al. Congenital complete atrioventricular block: clinical and electrophysiologic predictors of need for pacemaker insertion. Am J Cardiol 1981; 48:1098–1104.

Lenegre J. Etiology of bilateral bundle branch fibrosis in relation to complete heart block. Prog Cardiovasc Dis 1964;6:409–412.

Lev M, Bharati S. Atrioventricular and intraventricular conduction disease. Arch Intern Med 1975;135:405–411.

McAnulty J, Rahimtoola SH, Murphy E, et al. Natural history of "high risk" bundle branch block. Final report of a prospective study. N Engl J Med 1982;307:137–143.

24   Syncope

EPIDEMIOLOGY

Syncope is an important cause of morbidity in almost all age groups. Framingham study data, based on 26 years of follow-up in over 5000 individuals (2336 men and 2873 women), suggest that approximately 3% of the population experience a syncopal episode during their lifetime. The incidence may even be higher, reportedly up to 37%, if a young population of individuals is examined. Furthermore, given an initial syncopal event, recurrence of syncopal symptoms can be expected in about 30% of cases.

Syncope is reported to account for an estimated 3% of emergency room visits, and from 1–6% of general hospital admissions in the United States. In many of these cases, underlying structural cardiovascular disease may be present. However, in a broader population of individuals in the community, that is not the case. For example, in the Framingham study, "isolated" syncope (i.e., absence of cardiac or neurologic findings) accounted for 79% and 88% of syncopal episodes in men and women, respectively. Among these individuals, the initial syncopal event occurred at an average age of 52 years (range 17–78 years) for men and 50 years (range 13–87 years) for women. In addition, the prevalence of isolated syncopal episodes increased with advancing age, ranging from 8 per 1000 person-exams in the 35–44-year-old age group to approximately 40 per 1000 person-exams in the ≥75-year-old age group (Fig. 24.1). Indeed, among elderly patients confined to long-term care institutions, the annual incidence may be as high as 6%, with 30% recurrence rates.

DIFFERENTIAL DIAGNOSTIC CONSIDERATIONS IN THE SYNCOPE PATIENT

Although a number of studies have delineated the causes of syncope in various settings, application of such findings to general medical practice is limited by the nature of the environment in which patients were enrolled and the variable manner in which symptoms were evaluated. Recent reexamination of an ongoing study of syncope patients have provided important insights into the origins and assessment of syncope. Findings were reported in 433 syncope patients initially enrolled between April 1981 and February 1984. Evaluation of these patients included history, physical, and neurologic examination, hematologic and biochemical studies, 12-lead electrocardiogram (ECG), and a minimum of 24 hours of ambulatory electrocardiographic monitoring. Further studies, including angiography, electroencephalogram (EEG), and computer tomography scans, were obtained when clinically warranted. Electrophysiologic testing was available for only a portion of the time period encompassed by this report and was performed in relatively few patients. Head-up tilt testing was not available.

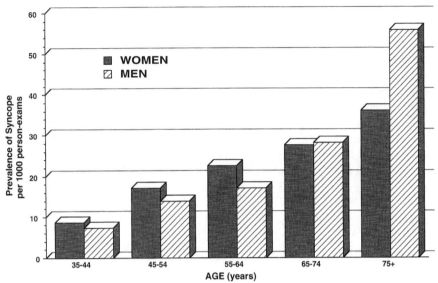

Figure 24.1. Graph depicting the age-specific prevalence of isolated syncopal events. These findings, obtained after 26 years of follow-up in the Framingham Study, illustrate that syncope in the absence of overt structural or neurologic disease occurs in all age groups, although there is a particular predilection in older individuals. (Modified from Savage DD, Corwin L, McGee DL, et al. Epidemiologic features of isolated syncope: the Framingham Study. Stroke 1985;16:626–629.)

Among the patients evaluated, a cause of syncope was assigned in 254 of 433 patients, with a cardiovascular cause being responsible in the vast majority of cases. The most common causes of syncope were neurally mediated (vasodepressor) syncopal syndromes (71 patients), ventricular tachycardia (VT) (49 patients), orthostatic hypotension (43 patients), and drug-induced syncope (nine patients). Carotid sinus syncope was identified in only five patients and seizure disorders in only seven patients. Vascular disease compromising cerebral blood flow accounted for 10 cases of 254 (4%).

History and physical examination were apparently the most useful means for assessing a "cause" of syncope, while the ECG and EEG monitoring were the next most valuable tools. Of importance, neurologic studies were of diagnostic utility in only four patients, while computed tomography (CT) scans were not reported to be of diagnostic utility in any patient.

The findings are consistent with what should be expected in general patient populations. These observations are important for physicians in emergency rooms and general medical and cardiological practice. By contrast, syncope patients described from electrophysiology laboratory studies are more highly selected and usually comprise a high proportion of older patients with structural cardiovascular disease, who in turn tend to exhibit a higher incidence of conduction system disease and ventricular and supraventricular arrhythmias as the cause of syncope.

This selection bias is particularly relevant to the interpretation of reports in which electrophysiologic testing was conducted without benefit of tilt-table study.

In the older patient who has traditionally comprised the predominant referral for conventional electrophysiologic testing (and consequent reports), VT has been the most commonly identified etiology of symptoms, although supraventricular tachyarrhythmias, conduction system disease, and sinoatrial dysfunction are also reported. Nonetheless, more recent studies suggest that within this patient population, as well as in the younger patient, neurally mediated syncopal syndromes represent an important diagnostic consideration. As a rule, then, the syncope patient with evident structural cardiac disease should undergo a conventional electrophysiological study first, and if that is nondiagnostic, then a tilt-table test is warranted. The reverse strategy would be appropriate in the individual with no evidence of structural cardiovascular disease. The sequence of the evaluation of a syncope patient will be discussed later in this chapter.

CLASSIFICATION OF THE CAUSES OF SYNCOPE

Neurally Mediated Reflex Disturbances of Blood Pressure Control

The neurally mediated (often referred to as "vasovagal") syncopal syndromes are probably the most common causes of syncope (Table 24.1). Current analysis suggests that the various conditions within this group exhibit a number of common pathophysiologic elements. Differences among the syndromes are primarily the result of "trigger factors" associated with each and possibly the manner in which the central nervous system (CNS) receives and processes incoming neural signals generated by these "triggers" (Fig. 24.2). In general, the afferent neural signals that initiate these forms of syncope may originate from the CNS directly or from any of a variety of peripheral "receptors" that respond to mechanical or chemical stimuli, pain, or possibly even temperature change. Noxious smells, unpleasant sights, unanticipated pain, venipuncture, prolonged exposure to upright posture, heat, dehydration, and physical exercise are among the most well known trigger factors. However, carotid sinus stimulation, drug effects, gastrointestinal or genitourinary stimulation, coughing, sneezing, and airway stimulation are also known to cause similar bradycardic-hypotensive episodes. In addition, emotional state may play an important contributory role in initiating or facilitating events.

In the case of carotid sinus syndrome, carotid artery mechanoreceptors (baroreceptors) are presumed to be the principal origin of the afferent neural signals triggering the event. In other neurally mediated syncopal episodes, other receptors located in any of a variety of organ systems are believed to be contributory. For example, mechanoreceptors and to some extent chemoreceptors located in atrial and ventricular myocardium have been implicated in triggering certain neurally mediated syncopal events by initiating afferent neural signals when subjected to increased wall tension (e.g., aortic stenosis, "empty" ventricle syndrome) or changes in the chemical environment (e.g., myocardial ischemia). However, in

Table 24.1
Diagnostic Classification

1. Neurally mediated reflex disturbances of blood pressure control
   Emotional (vasovagal) faint
   Carotid sinus syncope
   Cough syncope and related disorders
   Gastrointestinal, pelvic, or urologic origin (swallowing, defecation, postmicturition)
   Airway stimulation

2. Orthostatic and dysautonomic vascular control
   Idiopathic orthostatic hypotension
   Shy-Drager syndrome
   Diabetic neuropathy
   Drug-induced orthostatis

3. Primary cardiac arrhythmias
   Sinus node dysfunction (including bradycardia/tachycardia syndrome)
   AV conduction system disease
   Paroxysmal supraventricular tachycardias
   Paroxysmal ventricular tachycardia (including torsade de pointes)
   Implanted pacing system malfunction, pulse generator/lead failure, pacemaker-mediated
      tachycardia, "pacemaker syndrome"

4. Structural cardiovascular or cardiopulmonary disease
   Cardiac valvular disease
   Myocardial infarction
   Obstructive cardiomyopathy
   Subclavian steal syndrome
   Pericardial disease/tamponade
   Pulmonary embolus
   Primary pulmonary hypertension

5. Cerebrovascular disturbances
   Vertebrobasilar disease
   Carotid vascular disease
   Extrinsic vascular disturbances

6. Central nervous system substrates
   Seizure disorders
   Subarachoid hemorrhage
   Narcolepsy
   Hydrocephalus

7. Noncardiovascular origin metabolic/endocrine disturbances
   Hypoglycemia
   Volume depletion (Addison's disease, pheochromocytoma)
   Hypoxemia
   Hyperventilation (hypocapnia)

8. Psychiatric disorders
   Panic attacks
   Hysteria

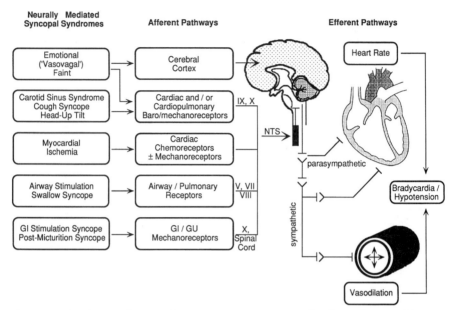

Figure 24.2. Schematic illustration depicting present concepts regarding the mechanisms of the neurally-mediated syncopal syndromes. The principal neurally-mediated syncopal syndromes are indicated at left. Currently suspected peripheral receptors ("triggers") and afferent neural pathways are also depicted. Efferent neural pathways are at the right. NTS, nucleus tractus solitarius. See text for discussion.

these cases CNS factors are often crucial. Furthermore, cardiac receptor sites are not the sole sources of afferent signals capable of provoking vasodepressor syncope in subjects susceptible to the "emotional" or vasovagal faint, as evidenced by the reported occurrence of vasovagal syncope in a heart transplant patient in whom ventricular and atrial mechanoreceptors were presumably decentralized. Clearly, peripheral receptors of multiple types in various organ systems may participate in initiating symptomatic episodes.

The ultimate cause of syncope in the neurally mediated syncopal syndromes is a transient disturbance of what is usually a well-regulated cerebrovascular perfusion pressure. Nonetheless, the electrophysiologic and hemodynamic picture may be quite heterogeneous. Certain patients exhibit a predominantly "cardioinhibitory" picture, with an extended period of bradycardia (or asystole) being the proximate cause of the faint. Most, however, present a mixed "vasodepressor" and cardioinhibitory response (Table 24.2). On rare occasions a pure vasodepressor syndrome may be observed. In all cases the bradycardia is primarily parasympathetically mediated via the vagus nerve. The mechanism of the vasodepressor element, on the other hand, is believed to be predominantly the result of abrupt peripheral sympathetic neural "withdrawal," with consequent inappropriate peripheral vascular dilation.

Table 24.2
Classification of Heart Rate and Hemodynamic Responses to Head-Up Tilt-Table Testing[a]

Type 1: Mixed
Heart rate rises initially then falls but the ventricular rate does not fall to less than 40 beats/min or falls to 40 beats/min for less than 10 seconds with or without asystole for less than 3 seconds. Blood pressure rises initially then falls before heart rate falls.
Type 2A: Cardioinhibitory
Heart rate rises initially then falls to a ventricular rate less than 40 beats/min for more than 10 seconds or asystole occurs for more than 3 seconds. Blood pressure rises initially then falls before heart rate falls.
Type 2B: Cardioinhibitory
Heart rate rises initially then falls to a ventricular rate less than 40 beats/min for more than 10 seconds or asystole occurs for more than 3 seconds. Blood pressure rises initially and falls to hypotensive levels less than 80 mm Hg systolic only at or after onset of rapid and severe heart rate fall.
Type 3: Pure vasodepressor
Heart rate rises progressively and does not fall more than 10% from peak at time of syncope. Blood pressure falls to cause syncope.

[a]Based on initial proposal of a recently formed international study group (VASIS, Vasovagal International Study) published in Sutton R, Petersen, M, Brignole M, et al. Proposed classification for tilt induced vasovagal syncope. Eur J Cardiac Pacing Electrophysiol 1992;3:180–183. Exceptions proposed by the study group are not incorporated into this table. Future modifications to this classification should be expected.

Excess β-adrenergic tone remains an additional potential contributor to the hypotension in vasodepressor episodes. Markedly elevated circulating epinephrine levels are known to occur in this circumstance, and conceivably an altered epinephrine/norepinephrine balance may undermine vascular control.

As suggested previously, the cerebral hypoperfusion associated with vasovagal episodes is believed to be principally secondary to marked central vascular hypotension. However, a recent study utilizing transcranial Doppler ultrasonic techniques raised the interesting possibility that paradoxic cerebrovascular arterial vasoconstriction may also participate. Further study of this phenomenon is needed to determine whether it is indeed unique to vasovagal syncope or whether it occurs in other hypotensive states as well.

Until quite recently, a diagnosis of neurally mediated syncope could not be obtained directly. For the most part, it was largely a diagnosis by exclusion, with the medical history being an extremely critical determinant. Over the last several years, however, head-up tilt testing has evolved into a valuable diagnostic tool for eliciting susceptibility to these syncopal syndromes and will be discussed later in this chapter.

Orthostatic and Dysautonomic Disturbances of Vascular Control

Presyncopal or syncopal symptoms associated with abrupt assumption of upright posture are extremely common. All age groups appear to exhibit susceptibility to this phenomenon. However, the elderly, less physically fit, or otherwise dehydrated/volume-depleted individuals are at greatest risk for frank syncope in this setting. Iatrogenic factors such as excessive diuresis or overly aggressive use of certain antihypertensive agents are important contributors.

In the older or infirm patient, environmental factors (e.g., excessive heat), impaired mobility, and/or a reduced appetite may aggravate susceptibility to orthostatic hypotension by both reducing circulating fluid volume and diminishing "fitness" level. The latter, in particular, adversely affects ability to vasoconstrict and venoconstrict promptly. Additionally, chronotropic incompetence may contribute to the problem by preventing appropriate compensatory heart rate changes with upright posture. Furthermore, in some cases, abrupt diminution of central volume with upright posture may trigger neural reflexes comparable to those described earlier for the neurally mediated syncope. The consequent vasodilation and relative bradycardia may then additionally complicate the pathophysiology of the "orthostatic" syncopal event. In certain cases, the coincidence of neurally mediated as well as intrinsic electrophysiologic disturbances appear to have been implicated in syncopal disturbances.

Primary autonomic nervous system dysfunction (such as Shy-Drager syndrome) leading to disturbances of vascular control is rare. More commonly, disturbances of autonomic vascular control are secondary in nature (e.g., neuropathies of alcohol or diabetic origin, spinal cord lesions, or paraneoplastic syndromes). Additionally, a wide range of commonly used vasoactive drugs or sedatives may impair normal neural reflex compensation and increase susceptibility to symptomatic orthostasis. For example, angiotensin-converting enzyme inhibitors and other vasodilators may prevent adequate vasoconstriction in the setting of movement to upright posture. β-Adrenergic blocking drugs or other sympatholytic antihypertensive agents may preclude appropriate heart rate response to gravitational stress.

Primary Cardiac Arrhythmias

Primary cardiac arrhythmias encompass those rhythm disturbances associated with intrinsic cardiac disease, accessory conduction pathways, or other structural abnormalities (e.g., postoperative disturbances). Intrinsic sinus node dysfunction (bradyarrhythmias and tachyarrhythmias), atrioventricular (AV) conduction system disturbances, and both supraventricular and ventricular tachycardias are included. In general, among patients with structural heart disease, primary cardiac arrhythmias are probably the most common cause of syncope. Thus, a careful physical examination and use of selected studies (particularly echocardiography and occasionally radionuclide scanning) is an important first step in determining the likelihood of a primary arrhythmic use for syncope. Subsequently, other studies may be appropriately selected in an attempt to ascertain a basis for symptoms. These studies may include ambulatory electrocardiography, exercise testing, signal-averaged electrocardiogram (SAECG), electrophysiology testing, and tilt-table testing.

Structural Cardiovascular or Cardiopulmonary Disease

Syncopal episodes resulting directly from structural abnormalities of the heart or blood vessels (excluding arrhythmias) are less frequent than the conditions discussed earlier. Probably the most common cause of syncope attributable to left ventricular disease is that which occurs in conjunction with acute myocardial ischemia or infarction. On the other hand, because coronary artery disease alone is ubiquitous, its mere presence should not be construed as providing adequate explanation for syncope. In such cases the causes of syncope are probably more often than not unrelated to coronary artery disease. However, when ischemia is at fault, it must be kept in mind that the proximate causes of syncope may be multiple, including not only transient reduction of cardiac output but also important neural reflex effects and cardiac arrhythmias.

Syncope associated with aortic stenosis or hypertrophic obstructive cardiomyopathy is relatively rare but important to recognize because of the reportedly poor prognosis (particularly in valvular aortic stenosis) if untreated. The basis for the fainting is often attributed to inadequate blood flow due to mechanical obstruction (often occurring with exercise, a result of peripheral vasodilation and inability to compensate because of the fixed obstruction), cardiac arrhythmias (tachyarrhythmia or bradyarrhythmia resulting from AV block), or both. However, ventricular mechanoreceptor-mediated bradycardia and vasodilation is thought to play an important role. In the case of hypertrophic obstructive cardiomyopathy, neural reflex mechanisms may also play a role, but syncope may be more often related to occurrence of atrial tachyarrhythmias or VT. In one study, syncope was reported to be an important predictor of sudden death in these patients, a finding yet to be confirmed by others. It is now recognized that asymmetric septal hypertrophy is common in the elderly patient, and that about one-third of patients with hypertrophic obstructive cardiomyopathy are over the age of 60.

Subclavian "steal" syndrome or severe carotid artery disease (e.g., atherosclerotic disease, Takayasu's disease) are also relatively rare causes of syncopal episodes. In the former, narrowing of the subclavian artery at its origin results in syncope or dizziness in conjunction with ipsilateral upper extremity exercise as blood is shunted from the brain to the exercising limb via the vertebral artery system. Usually a bruit can be detected over the affected subclavian artery, along with diminution of brachial artery pressure on the affected side.

Other even less common conditions that may be associated with syncope include left ventricular inflow obstruction such as in patients with mitral stenosis or atrial myxoma, right ventricular outflow obstruction, right-to-left shunting secondary to pulmonic stenosis, or pulmonary hypertension. In the latter case (i.e., pulmonary hypertension), neural-reflex effects may contribute to symptoms.

Syncope Caused by Cerebrovascular or Neurologic Disturbances

It has been estimated that 3% of the U.S. population are susceptible to seizures. For many of these cases, epilepsy is the etiologic diagnosis, and differentiation from true syncope may be made based upon careful history and appropriate neurologic assessment. On the other hand, seizure-like activity may occur in conjunction with cerebral hypoperfusion of any etiology. Susceptibility to neurally mediated hypotension-bradycardia may be present in a subset of patients in whom loss of consciousness with tonic-clonic reactions are unresponsive to antiseizure medication. These individuals are best assessed by head-up tilt-table testing and may prove to be better controlled by agents more typically used for treatment of the vasovagal fainter.

In some patients temporal lobe seizures may mimic (or induce) neurally mediated reflex bradycardia and hypotension. Differentiation of such events from true syncope may be difficult. However, occurrence of seizures tends to be independent of position, is usually associated with immediate convulsive activity and loss of bowel or urinary continence, and is typically followed by a confusional state. On the other hand, apparent seizure-like motor activity may also accompany transient cerebral hypoperfusion of any etiology (including neurally mediated reflex syncope). However, in the latter case, the abnormal motor activity tends to be relatively brief and unassociated with either bladder or bowel incontinence.

Cerebrovascular disease is not a common cause of true syncope. However, transient ischemic attacks due to vertebrobasilar disease may mimic syncope. (Only rarely is carotid vessel mediated ischemia associated with syncope, such as in the patient with an extremely compromised cerebral circulation.) In such cases, there are usually associated neurologic findings to lead the physician toward the correct diagnosis. Thus, vertebrobasilar disease is usually accompanied by at least some of the following symptoms: vertiginous complaints, ocular disturbances, or speech problems. On rare occasions, extrinsic disturbances of the cerebrovascular supply may be at fault. Syncope or dizziness may therefore be associated with neck extension or rotation resulting from vertebral artery compression by cervical spondylosis, cervical osteoarthritis, or a cervical rib.

Syncope of Noncardiovascular Origin

Metabolic/endocrine disturbances rarely cause true syncope. More often they result in confusional states or behavioral disturbances. Hyperventilation episodes with marked reductions of pCO_2, presumably leading to reduced cerebral blood flow, may be one of the more frequent causes of transient loss of consciousness in this category.

Finally, syncope may be mimicked by anxiety attacks, hysteria, or other psychiatric disturbances. In this regard, panic disorder and major depression are common findings in syncope patients and approximately 25–30% of events are attributed to such causes. Similarly, others report a psychiatric diagnosis in 24% (major depression 12%, others 12%). However, except in cases where loss of consciousness is witnessed and demonstrated to be associated with a normotensive state, such a diagnosis should be considered only once other causes have been clearly excluded.

The problem of persistent dizziness is often lumped with that of syncope. It has been estimated that dizziness accounts for about 8 million outpatient medical visits per year and is probably one of the most common and refractory of all medical complaints. In a recent evaluation of the problem, vertigo of various forms was the most common primary or contributory cause (54%), with psychiatric disturbances being second in frequency (16%). Others have observed a similar breakdown of diagnoses (Table 24.3). In perhaps more than 50% of instances, however, dizziness is multifactoral, and the establishment of an etiologic diagnosis requires substantial persistence on the part of the physician.

DIAGNOSTIC WORKUP

The approach to the diagnosis of the causes of syncope is present in Figure 24.3 and is discussed in the following sections.

History

Questions surrounding the event of the syncopal spell are invaluable for diagnosis. It is important to establish if the patient truly lost consciousness. A description of any warning or premonitory symptoms can be extremely useful (Table 24.4). A history of syncope on movement of the neck laterally or during shaving of the neck or wearing a tight necktie is suggestive of carotid sinus hypersensitivity. Drugs like digitalis, verapamil, and propranolol can aggravate carotid sinus hypersensitivity. Provoking events include neck pressure, sneezing, shaving, and tight collar. Potential triggers for vasovagal or situational syncope include cough, defecation, micturition, deglutition, pain, fear, or the postprandial state. A history of positional change preceding the episode suggests orthostasis. Vasovagal syncope is often precipitated by emotionally distressing circumstances such as venipuncture, prolonged standing, excessive heat, dental surgery, or physical injury or threat.

Table 24.3
Causes of Persistent Dizziness[a]

Cause	% of Total Cases
Vertigo	45–54
Benign positional	12–17
Ménière's disease	1–10
Nonspecific vertigo	≈10
Psychiatric disorder	9–21
Presyncope	4–14
Disequilibrium	1–16
Hyperventilation	1–23
Multicausal[b]	12–13
Unknown	8–19

Modified from Kroenke K, Lucas, CA, Rosenberg ML, et al. Causes of persistent dizziness. A prospective study of 100 patients in ambulatory care. Ann Intern Med 1992;117:889–904.

[a]Note that the principal subcategories under "vertigo" are noted, but these do not add up to the total due to omission of less frequent categories.

[b]Multicausal means one or more primary causes as listed above were identified, but no single one predominated. Six of these patients had 2 causes, and 7 patients had 3 causes.

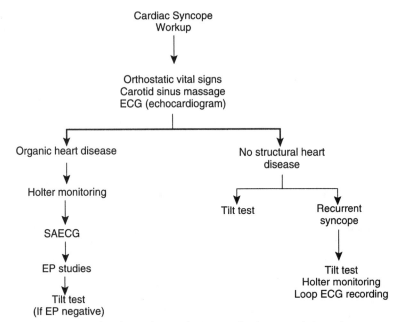

Figure 24.3. An approach to the evaluation of patients with a history and physical examination suggestive of cardiac syncope.

Table 24.4
History of Syncope

Situational syncope
    Relationship to meals, alcohol, drugs, cough, swallowing, micturition, defecation, posture, pain, movement of head and neck

Cardiac syncope
    Abrupt onset, effort or exertion, major injury
Vasovagal syncope
    Premonotory symptoms—yawning, pallor, diaphoresis, stress, pain, crowding, standing a long time; procedure, instrumentation

Iatrogenic syncope
    First-dose syncope (prazosin, captopril nitroglycerine)
    Arrhythmias precipitated by antiarrhythmics, phenothiazines, tricyclics, β-blockers, digoxin, diuretics-induced hypokalemia

Cardiac syncope due to tachyarrhythmias is of sudden onset, preceded by palpitations, dyspnea, chest tightness or diaphoresis and resolves promptly. If cardiac arrest occurs, seizure activity or other signs of cerebral hypoxia may be evident. Syncope in aortic stenosis tends to occur during activity, whereas in patients with hypertrophic obstructive cardiomyopathy, it tends to occur after exercise.

The patient or witnesses may provide information regarding the events, especially the posture, activities, and sensation immediately prior to the attacks. If there is a history of repeated attacks with identical aggravating factors and epiphe-nomena, then one can with certainty make the diagnosis of a reflex-mediated form of syncope. The onset, frequency, and duration of premonitory symptoms, pres-ence of predisposing disorders such as diabetes mellitus, prolonged bed rest, blood loss, hypovolemic states, circumstances surrounding the attack, associated symptoms, and the medications used will assist in the diagnosis and direct the physician in the evaluation of patients.

The elderly are prone to develop syncope or presyncope. They take three times as many drugs as younger patients, and some of these medications aggravate or precipitate syncope. The commonly used diuretics, vasodilators, psychoactive drugs, β-blockers, and antiarrhythmic drugs potentiate the tendency for syncope. The proarrhythmic effect of antiarrhythmias in the elderly, who often have severe heart disease and left ventricular dysfunction, is a recognized problem. Over-the-counter medications such as sedatives, antidiarrheal preparations, and antihista-mines may have anticholinergic properties that can exacerbate the already impaired multiple sensory and physiologic reflexes that contribute to syncope. In the elderly the compensatory mechanisms for maintaining cerebral blood flow and cardiac output are blunted. Hence, the elderly are more sensitive to antihyper-tensive drugs and diuretics. Changes in intravascular volume and blood pressure make the elderly very vulnerable to syncope.

A history of the patient's dietary habits may be useful in cases of fad dieting and bulimia, which can lead to electrolyte deficiencies. A psychiatric history may reveal panic disorders, major depression, and hysterical personality disorder.

PHYSICAL EXAMINATION

Accurate recording of blood pressure in upright and recumbent positions can establish the diagnosis of orthostatic hypotension. If there is orthostatic hypoten-sion, the systolic blood pressure falls 30–70 mm Hg with the development of symptoms in 1–2 minutes.

In evaluating for vascular lesions, one should evaluate blood pressure in both arms and legs. Differences of >20 mm Hg in the arms is indicative of subclavian steal syndrome or aortic dissection. One should also look for cardiovascular clues by examining for cyanosis, clubbing, and other signs of congenital heart disease. Auscultation of bruits in the carotid, subclavian, and temporal vessels should be routinely performed. Careful auscultation of the heart to uncover aortic stenosis, hypertrophic cardiomyopathy, mitral valve prolapse, and pulmonary hypertension should be performed with standard maneuvers. Head flexion and extension and arm exercises may provoke vertebrobasilar insufficiency of subclavian steal syn-drome. Bedside carotid sinus massage should be performed with ECG monitor-ing, blood pressure monitoring, and intravenous access. The duration of the massage should be limited to 3–5 seconds. Hypersensitivity of the carotid sinus may be either (a) cardioinhibitory, in which there is bradycardia with sinus arrest or advanced AV block; or (b) vasodepressor, in which there is a significant drop in blood pressure with heart rate unchanged. The cardioinhibitory response can be abolished with atropine or AV sequential pacing.

ELECTROCARDIOGRAPHY

The ECG is a routine screening test for patients with syncope and is helpful in identifying a cardiac cause of syncope, which might include prolongation of the Q-T interval, ventricular preexcitation, high-degree AV block, premature ventricular or atrial beats or runs, myocardial infarction (MI), and right or left ventricular hypertrophy, which might suggest pulmonary hypertension, aortic stenosis, or hypertrophic cardiomyopathy. Patients with a normal ECG and no clinical cardiac findings have a low likelihood of arrhythmias and are at low risk of sudden cardiac death and arrhythmogenic cardiac syncope.

ECHOCARDIOGRAPHY

In the absence of clinical, historical, or physical findings of cardiac abnormality, the diagnostic yield from echocardiography is low. Therefore, echocardiography in the absence of cardiac findings is not routinely indicated for the diagnostic workup of syncope. Echocardiography may be very useful in the presence of large pericardial effusion, hypertrophic cardiomyopathy, aortic valve disease, atrial myxoma, and abnormal left ventricular function. Cardiac catheterization and other diagnostic tests may be necessary in patients with echocardiographic findings.

EXERCISE STRESS TESTING

In any patient who has cardiac symptoms or findings, a stress test should be performed to evaluate for myocardial ischemia and exercise-induced arrhythmias. Exercise stress testing can provoke ventricular arrhythmias and paroxysmal VT induced by exertion in patients without clinical evidence of organic heart disease. The significance of exercise-induced arrhythmias has been controversial, but it may identify patients at high risk for sudden death. In a patient with severe aortic stenosis, exercise testing should not be performed. In mild to moderate stenosis, it can be done with extra caution.

AMBULATORY ELECTROCARDIOGRAPHIC MONITORING

In patients with a known cardiac condition, ambulatory ECG monitoring is frequently used as the initial screening test for syncope. The yield from ambulatory monitoring is low. In one study of 1500 patients who underwent ambulatory monitoring, only 1% of patients had syncope during the monitoring period. In this study many asymptomatic arrhythmias, which can compound the diagnostic problem, were recorded. Incidental findings such as sinus pauses, AV Wenckebach block, or bursts of VT may not be related to syncope, but they could be used to direct further diagnostic workup. If symptoms are absent, the data obtained by ambulatory ECG monitoring must be interpreted with the understanding that such arrhythmias and conduction disturbances can be detected during monitoring in an asymptomatic general population. As many as 33% of patients may have symptoms with normal sinus rhythm, implying that the ambulatory ECG can be a useful screen to rule out an arrhythmic cause for syncope.

Prolonged ambulatory ECG monitoring for durations of 48 and 72 hours does not help to establish the causal relation between arrhythmias and syncope. One group performed three 24-hour periods of ambulatory ECG monitoring. For the first 24 hours, the findings showed arrhythmias in 14.7% during the first day, an additional 11.1% the second day, and an additional 4.3% the third day. But only one of 95 patients had symptom-related arrhythmias that occurred during the first 24 hours.

In patients who have recurrent syncope, patient-activated intermittent loop recorders may capture the rhythm disturbance during syncope after the patient regains consciousness, as retrograde ECG recording for several minutes can be obtained. Loop recording may be useful in a small group of patients, especially if they have recurrent syncopal episodes. The loop recorder devices have up to 4 minutes of replay capacity and can be worn for weeks at a time, continuously recording and erasing the heart rhythm. The rhythm is stored into memory when the patient depresses the record button, and the stored rhythm can be transmitted via telephone to a monitoring service. According to one study, the diagnostic yield of loop ECG recording was 25% in patients with unexplained syncope. In the next few years, more experience with an implantable event recorder will be available.

SIGNAL-AVERAGED ECG

Signal-averaged ECG (SAECG) has become a valuable tool for the detection of patients at risk for ventricular tachyarrythmias. SAECG allows the detection of late potentials, which are low-amplitude, high-frequency signals occurring at the end of a filtered QRS complex that persist for tens of milliseconds into the ST segment. Signal averaging is used to reduce noise produced by the skeletal muscle activity frequency, which is close to the high-frequency cardiac potentials. After signal averaging by a computer, time domain analysis by high-pass bidirectional filtering is then performed to reduce high-amplitude low-frequency signal content. A filtered QRS complex using a 40-Hz filter of longer than 114 msec with voltage in the last 40 msec of the QRS of less than 20 µV or duration under 40 µV longer than 38 msec is considered abnormal.

Detection of late potentials has a sensitivity of 80% and a specificity of >90% for prediction of inducible sustained VT in patients with syncope. This technique can be used as a screening test in selecting patients for electrophysiological studies (EPS). Late potentials in the terminal portion of the QRS complex may identify heterogenous myocardial activation in areas of infarction that possibly provide anatomic substrate for sustained ventricular tachyarrhythmias. A negative SAECG suggests that VT will not be inducible by EPS.

UPRIGHT TILT TESTING

The upright tilt test has been very helpful in identifying vasovagal or neurocardiogenic syncope in up to 70% of patients with so-called recurrent unexplained syncope. Individuals susceptible to vasovagal syncope, on assumption of the upright posture, can develop bradycardia and hypotension leading to syncope. This is neurally mediated syncope. In these individuals there is accentuated adrenergic activity with intense activation of cardiopulmonary mechanoreceptors resulting in bradycardia and hypotension.

The test is performed after hydration and an overnight fast. Baseline ECG, blood pressure, and heart rate are recorded. The patient is supported by a belt across the torso and foot support. In this test the patient is kept in an upright posture with head-up position for a period of 20–60 minutes at 60–80°. In normal individuals in this upright posture there is central venous pooling and this activates the renin-angiotensin system, which leads to vasoconstriction and compensatory mechanisms, leading to tachycardia and increase in cardiac output and normotension. A normal response includes an increase in heart rate of >10 beats/minute and >5 mm Hg increase in diastolic blood pressure, with no change in systolic blood pressure.

However, in patients with neurocardiogenic syncope, there is a marked decrease in blood pressure and heart rate. In patients who have a negative upright tilt test, a graded infusion of isoproterenol is started, initiating with a 1 µg/minute dose to a maximum of 5 µg/minute. Upright tilt testing using isoproterenol provocation can identify neurocardiogenic syncope in many patients. With this test, 75% of patients develop symptomatic hypotension or bradycardia or both. With the combination of isoproterenol infusion and tilt testing, the sensitivity is increased to 87%, with a specificity of 85%. However, in other studies, the specificity was much lower, i.e., 65%. Hypotension and bradycardia may be nonspecific responses to tilt testing since they can be provoked in normal persons without a history of syncope or presyncope (false-positive rate of 31%). Still, tilt testing is very useful for identifying neurocardiogenic syncope with recurrences, especially in young patients without heart disease and in those with negative EPS. Isoproterenol infusion is best avoided but can be used if neurocardiogenic syncope is strongly suspected.

ELECTROPHYSIOLOGICAL STUDIES

Electrophysiological studies (EPS) should be considered only after a thorough clinical and systematic noninvasive workup has been performed. EPS is most likely to be valuable in patients with syncope and organic heart disease with abnormal ventricular function and in patients with abnormal ambulatory monitoring or ECG findings. Another predictor of positive EPS results is bifascicular or bundle branch block. The presence of structural heart disease and male gender are independently associated with the finding of inducible VT in patients with syncope of undetermined origin. The diagnostic yield is low (<10%) in patients with syncope who do not have structural heart disease and who have ejection fractions >40%, normal ECG and ambulatory ECG monitoring, absence of injury during syncope, and prolonged duration of syncope (>5 minutes).

The role of SAECG has become crucial in decision making regarding EPS. In one study, an abnormal SAECG was predictive of sudden death and inducibility of VT in patients with cardiomyopathies. SAECG is useful in risk stratification post-MI, especially in those with low ejection fractions. SAECG has a very strong negative predictive value. A normal SAECG in a patient with syncope of unknown origin would indicate that the yield of performing EPS would be very low. An abnormal SAECG has a sensitivity of 73–89% and a specificity of 89–100% for prediction of inducible sustained VT in patients with syncope. SAECG has been increasingly used as a screening test for patient selection for EPS. SAECG is not very useful in evaluating sinus node dysfunction or other conduction system disease, including induced supraventricular tachycardia.

The proper interpretation of EPS findings is crucial for patient management and clinical outcomes. Prolonged corrected sinus node recovery time is suggestive of sinus node disease but the sensitivity is low. Sinus node recovery time of ≥3.0 seconds can account for syncope, especially if it is accompanied by bradyarrhythmias on prolonged ambulatory monitoring. Marked prolongation of the H-V interval of >100 msec in symptomatic patients and pacing-induced infranodal block are abnormal findings. Marked H-V prolongation is associated with subsequent complete heart block. The induction of supraventricular tachycardia, which may produce symptoms similar to syncopal episode, is regarded as a positive finding.

Sustained monomorphic VT is a presumptive finding and can identify patients who have spontaneous VT and syncope. In patients undergoing EPS, positive findings range between 18–75% (mean 60%). VT can be induced in approximately 35%, 20% have supraventricular tachycardia, while 35% may have conduction disturbances. Polymorphic VT is thought to be a nonspecific response and not helpful in defining the etiology of syncope. It can be induced by a vigorous EPS protocol in structurally normal hearts.

TREATMENT

Metabolic and Iatrogenic Syncope

Metabolic abnormalities, anemia, and hypovolemia can be effectively managed. Iatrogenic syncope is a preventable and treatable condition, especially in the elderly patients who have other coexisting chronic diseases and diminished or blunting of their cardiovascular reflexes with resulting autonomic failure. Elimination of the offending drug, changing the dosage or timing, or substitution of a patient's medication can control iatrogenic syncope. Some of the commonly offending drugs are diuretics, antihypertensive, and antiarrhythmic agents. Sustained release antihypertensive agents may be cumulative in the elderly patients with diminished renal and hepatic function. Problems in the elderly are compounded by multiple chronic diseases, polypharmacy, age-related changes in pharmacokinetics, several physicians prescribing drugs, and over-the-counter self-medication. It is extremely important to obtain a detailed drug history and worthwhile to eliminate the offending agent.

Vasovagal Syncope

Ventricular mechanoreceptor C-fibers are the primary mediators of the afferent reflex arc of vasovagal syncope. These are numerous in the left ventricle and help to modulate blood pressure, with activation taking place during pressure development and relative volume depletion. In vasovagal syncope, C-fiber mechanoreceptors are activated by catecholamines or myocardial stretch.

Avoidance or modulation of the triggers responsible for situational syncope can be effective. In some patients there are no identifiable triggers, and in such cases, patients should be advised to assume a supine position, with legs raised at the onset of warning prodromal symptoms.

In patients with carotid hypersensitivity syndrome with a predominantly cardioinhibiting response, a ventricular demand pacemaker is appropriate. If a mixed cardioinhibitory and peripheral vasodepressor response is found, an AV synchronous pacemaker is effective. In patients with a pure vasodepressor response causing hypotension, a pacemaker is not effective, but administration of fluorocortisone or aminophylline and wearing support stockings may prevent the attacks. For the treatment of glossopharyngeal syncope, carbamazepine can be effective.

Neurocardiogenic syncope, which is neurally mediated, is best treated with β-adrenergic receptor blocking agents. β-Blockers inhibit C-fiber mechanoreceptors and markedly attenuate the discharge frequency of C-fibers. This phenomenon is probably due to the negative inotropic effect of β-blockers. Disopyramide is also useful because of its negative inotropic and anticholinergic properties, and it inhibits C-fiber activation, thereby preventing hypotension and bradycardia. Hydrofluorocortisone is likewise useful, as it prevents a decrease in right ventricular preload by enhancing volume expansion. Scopolamine is another effective drug used to treat vasovagal syncope. The mechanism of action may be its effect of the modulation of autonomic outflow and be partly due to its vagolytic properties. Theophylline has also been reported to be effective in a high percentage of patients, but its mechanism of action is not clear. It may be related to adenosine receptor blockade. Fluoxetine hydrochloride (Prozac) has been reported effective in 44% of patients refractory to conventional therapy, and it is postulated that it acts by alterations in serotonin, a neurotransmitter. In refractory patients, combination therapy may be attempted in conjunction with AV sequential pacing. There are no definitive studies, however, regarding the efficacy of this treatment approach.

Syncope and Orthostatic Hypotension

Orthostatic hypotension may be treated with volume repletion and use of support stockings. Pharmacologic therapy includes low-dose fludrocortisone and β-blockade, which act by repleting volume and inhibiting vasodilation. Clonidine has been used to overcome postganglionic orthostatic hypotension. A wide variety of therapeutic approaches have been tried, with disappointing results. Patients should be taught to sleep with their bed in a head-up position, to rise slowly, to flex calf muscles on rising, and to use a lower body compression garment.

Cardiac Syncope

Significant obstruction to limit cardiac output increases with exercise can cause syncope. In critical aortic stenosis, failure of cardiac output to increase during exercise and reflex fall in peripheral resistance may cause a syncopal episode. Transient arrhythmias may induce syncope in aortic stenosis and hypertrophic cardiomyopathy. Nonexertional syncope, which is related to dynamic obstruction due to acute changes in preload, afterload, inotropic stimulation, and arrhythmias, is often observed in patients with hypertrophic cardiomyopathy.

The treatment of obstructive cardiovascular syncope can be curative in some conditions. In patients with severe aortic stenosis, aortic valve replacement may abolish symptoms and prolong survival. Hypertrophic cardiomyopathy may be treated with β- or calcium channel blockers. Recently, right ventricular pacing has been used to diminish outflow obstruction during systole by disturbing the sequence of depolarization with asynchronous septal motion. In some instances, myomectomy and mitral valve replacement may be effective.

Syncope Caused by Conduction Disturbances and Arrhythmias

Permanent pacemaker implantation is the treatment of choice when sinus node dysfunction or high-grade AV block is documented in patients with syncope. Patients with bifascicular or bundle branch block in whom EPS identifies only conduction disease appear to have a good prognosis and do not require pacemakers. Patients with syncope and bundle branch block may have inducible VT or prolonged H-V intervals. In this group of patients, the prognosis is poor and they benefit from permanent pacing and appropriate EP-guided antiarrhythmic therapy. The yield of EPS in patients with bundle branch block and syncope is good, and mortality in this group is high. However, in patients with negative EPS and bundle branch block, recurrence and subsequent mortality rates are low.

The combination of right bundle branch block with divisional or fascicular blocks of either the left anterior fascicle or left posterior fascicle constitutes bifascicular block. Block of the right bundle branch with either hemiblock and a prolonged P-R interval may be but is not always a manifestation of trifascicular block. The prolonged P-R interval may be caused by delayed conduction in the remaining fascicle or it may result from AV nodal delay. In patients with bifascicular block or trifascicular block, EPS can help define those at high risk of developing complete heart block. Patients with a resting H-V interval of 70–100 msec have up to an 8% yearly chance of progressing to complete heart block, and this risk increases to 25% when the H-V interval is greater than 100 msec. Permanent pacing is recommended in patients at high risk.

Patients with bifascicular block are at higher risk than normals for developing high-grade AV block. However, the yearly rate of progression is very low. In patients with bifascicular block and markedly prolonged H-V intervals (>100 msec), permanent pacing is recommended. In patients with trifascicular block with prolonged H-V intervals or intranodal block induced by atrial stimulation, permanent pacing is recommended. In symptomatic patients with Mobitz type II AV block or third-degree AV block, permanent pacing is required. There is no role for empiric therapy with a permanent pacemaker in patients with undetermined syncope who have a negative study or no documented bradyarrhythmias.

Electropharmacologic testing is preferred in the management of tachyarrhythmias induced by EPS. EP-guided drug selection is efficacious, and it will also assist in triaging patients who may be candidates for nonpharmacologic approaches. For recalcitrant supraventricular tachycardias, catheter-based techniques can be employed for ablation of the AV node and accessory pathways.

The other therapeutic options for ventricular tachyarrhythmias include cardiac electrosurgery, antitachycardia pacemakers, aneurysmectomy, endocardial resection, and the automatic implanted cardioverter defibrillator. Surgical techniques and catheter-based techniques, including laser and radiofrequency systems, are undergoing further refinement to manage supraventricular, ventricular, and accessory pathway mediated arrhythmias.

PROGNOSIS

Because syncope results from a wide spectrum of causes with variable outcomes, it is important to have a prognostic classification for patients with syncope. Based on several studies, patients with syncope can be categorized into high and low-risk groups. The 1-year prognosis varies between 6–33%, depending upon patient selection criteria and the cause of syncope. However, from all these studies, it is obvious that the 1-year mortality of patients with cardiac syncope is very high, ranging from 21 to 33%.

The Framingham study documented that of persons between 30–62 years followed for 26 years, 3% of men and 3.5% of women experienced syncope during their lifetime. The study showed that, in patients without apparent neurologic and cardiovascular disease, there was no increase in all-cause mortality. It should be noted that the patient population consisted of a relatively healthy group. In the Framingham cohort, the prevalence of isolated syncopal episodes increased with increasing age, being highest in men over 75 years of age. In men 35–44 years old, the prevalence of isolated syncope was 7.4 per 1000, whereas in men ≥75 years old, the prevalence was 55.9 per 1000. During the 26 years of follow-up, isolated syncope was not associated with an incidence of stroke, MI, all-cause, or cardiovascular mortality.

Syncope and sudden death are two different entities and as such should be differentiated when considering outcome and prognosis. The observed incidence of sudden death (24%) is also very high in patients with cardiac syncope, so it is extremely difficult to know whether syncope or sudden death independently contribute to prognosis. Hence, overlap is unavoidable in various diagnostic and prognostic categories. From a clinical standpoint, patients requiring cardiopulmonary resuscitation or electrical or pharmacological cardioversion should be appropriately labeled to have sudden death and not syncope. Patients resuscitated from sudden death episodes have extensive coronary artery disease and usually have ventricular fibrillation or sustained VT responsible for sudden death. Patients resuscitated from sudden death associated with ventricular fibrillation have very poor prognosis and a recurrence rate in excess of 40%. Hence, the differentiation between sudden death and cardiogenic syncope is very important, but can be very elusive.

The prognostic criteria of using high-risk, medium-risk, and low-risk categories is clinically useful, but keep in mind that syncope per se may not independently contribute to outcomes. Indeed, patients may have other associated chronic diseases. The etiology of the loss of consciousness is prognostically important. Cardiogenic syncope has high mortality, especially if it is associated with sudden death. Patients with aortic stenosis may present with exertional syncope, which is probably due to failure of cardiac output to increase with exercise and a concomitant reflex fall in peripheral vascular resistance. Transient arrhythmias can also induce syncope in severe aortic stenosis. In patients with mild aortic stenosis, one may need to evaluate for coexisting coronary artery disease as a possible cause of syncope. In patients with severe valvular aortic stenosis, the mean survival after an episode of syncope is 2–3 years without valve replacement. A long-term survival with aortic valve replacement is expected in the absence of concomitant coronary artery disease or heart failure. In patients with hypertrophic cardiomyopathy, history of syncope identifies high-risk patients, especially children and adolescents. Recurrent syncopal episodes in younger patients with hypertrophic cardiomyopathy are associated with an annual mortality rate in excess of 4%. In one study, syncope was 86% specific for subsequent sudden cardiac death. Conduction disturbance, asystole, sinus node disease, supraventricular arrhythmias, primary ventricular arrhythmias, or primary circulatory collapse are potential mechanisms for the development of syncope or sudden death in hypertrophic cardiomyopathy. Hence, a precise mechanism is rarely identified. Nonsustained VT is an excellent marker for subsequent sudden death in adult patients. Such patients can be managed with low-dose amiodarone, and with a reduction in annual mortality from 9% to less than 1%. So far, surgical therapy with septal myotomy has not decreased mortality, although syncopal episodes are decreased.

Syncope is common in patients with heart failure of various etiologies. In patients with advanced heart failure, both syncope and sudden death are very important predictors of high mortality. In a recent study, syncope predicted sudden death in patients with advanced heart failure, independent of AF, cardiac index, serum sodium, and age. In this study, the actuarial incidence of sudden cardiac death at 1 year was 45% in those with syncope, regardless of origin, compared with 12% in those without syncope (P < .0001). In one study of patients with advanced heart failure, the initial rhythm at the time of cardiac arrest was sinus bradycardia in 43% of arrests, VT degenerating to ventricular fibrillation in 38%, and second- or third-degree AV block in 10%. There are other reports in the literature that have documented both bradyarrhythmias and tachyarrhythmias as causes of syncope and sudden cardiac death in patients with heart failure. Different mechanisms play a role in precipitating syncope or sudden death in advanced heart failure. As many as 25% of these patients die suddenly within 6 months without heart transplantation. With heart transplantation, survival is significantly improved to 75% at 5 years.

Syncopal episodes are often unpredictable and sporadic. The recurrence rate is approximately 31% for patients with cardiac and 36% for those with noncardiac causes of syncope. Patients with syncope of unknown etiology have a much higher rate of recurrence, 43% at 3 years. Although recurrences do not predict sudden death or mortality, they can lead to morbidity, including fractures of skull, legs, face, and arms.

Recurrences in patients with positive EP testing and EP-guided therapy have been much lower when compared to those with negative EP findings. In one study, EP-guided therapy prevented the recurrence of syncope in 96% of patients with a follow-up of 18 months. In this study, there was one death from pump failure and no sudden deaths. However, a much higher rate of sudden death, 48% over 3 years, was reported in one study with positive EP findings. The 3-year rate of total mortality among the positive EP patients in this study was 61%, much higher than that reported in other studies. This discrepancy could possibly be related to treatment strategies or variable follow-up. Electrophysiologically guided drug therapy had a 31% cummulative rate of sudden death, and this raises the issues of patient compliance, proarrhythmia, and different or multiple arrhythmias not identified during EPS. It is hoped that the application of implantable cardioverter-defibrillator devices will alter the prognosis and outcome in patients with arrhythmogenic syncope.

SUGGESTED READING

Benditt DG, Remole S, Milstein S, et al. Syncope: causes, clinical evaluation, and current therapy. Ann Rev Med 1992;43:283–300.

Kapoor W. Evaluation and outcome of patients with syncope. Medicine 1990;69:160–175.

Kapoor WN, Karpf M, Wieand S, et al. A prospective evaluation and follow-up of patients with syncope. N Engl J Med 1983;309:197–204.

Kapoor W, Brent N. Evaluation of upright tilt testing with isoproterenol. Ann Intern Med 1992;116:358–365.

Kuchar DL, Thorburn CW, Samel NL. Signal-averaged electrocardiogram for evaluation of recurrent syncope. Am J Cardiol 1986;58:949–954.

Linzer M, Pritchett ELC, Pontinen M, et al. Incremental diagnostic yield of loop electrocardiographic recorders in unexplained syncope. Am J Cardiol 1990;66:214–216.

Sra JS, Anderson AJ, Sheikh SH, et al. Unexplained syncope evaluated by electrophysiologic studies and head-up tilt testing. Ann Intern Med 1991;114:1013–1019.

INDEX